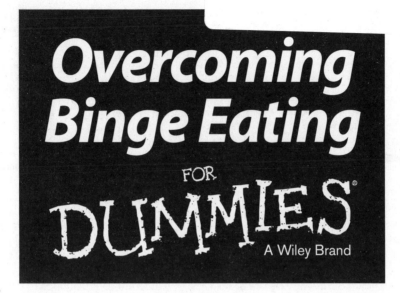

Overcoming Binge Eating

FOR DUMMIES®

A Wiley Brand

by Jennie J. Kramer and Marjorie Nolan Cohn

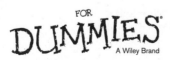

FOR DUMMIES®

A Wiley Brand

Overcoming Binge Eating For Dummies®

Published by: **John Wiley & Sons, Inc.,** 111 River Street, Hoboken, NJ 07030-5774, www.wiley.com

Copyright © 2013 by John Wiley & Sons, Inc., Hoboken, New Jersey

Contents at a Glance

Table of Contents

Introduction

•••

Do you eat when you feel stressed, sad, or angry? Do you sometimes follow strict diets only to find yourself out of control with food when you return to "normal" eating patterns? Do certain foods or situations inevitably set off an unstoppable urge to eat? Has the quantity of food you eat had a negative impact on your health? Do you feel desperate and hopeless after an eating binge? Have you ever wondered whether you have a problem with binge eating?

If you answered "yes" to any or all of these questions, you're reading the right book. Whether you're just starting to realize that there's a problem or have known it for a while, the information, ideas, and strategies we provide can help get you started on the road to healing and sustainable recovery from binge eating or any other type of overeating. This book is your road map to systematically but gently identify and change the feelings and behaviors that drive your binge eating.

If you identify yourself as a binge eater, you may be ready to take action today. But even if you don't feel that your habits completely fit with what's described as binge eating disorder, you can still benefit from these strategies as you address why you eat for reasons other than physical hunger. No matter where you are in your journey, this book can help you improve your health and well-being.

Depending on the severity of your struggles with food and eating, you may frequently recognize yourself (or someone you love) and your behaviors during the course of reading this book. Perhaps you've been formally diagnosed with binge eating disorder or self-diagnosed as an emotional eater. Left unchecked and untreated, disordered eating of any kind worsens over time, and the habits and behaviors become that much more entrenched. The sooner you seek support, the better.

Hopefully, it's heartening to know that you don't have to go it alone — we'll be with you every step of the way as you begin to understand binge eating and exactly what to do about it. We hope that this book is just what you need to finally make a difference in your physical and emotional well-being.

You may use it as a jumping-off point for seeking professional help in a more informed way. With compassion towards yourself and a deeper understanding of the fact that binge eating didn't develop overnight and will take some time to change, you can achieve sustainable results.

About This Book

Although binge eating disorder (BED) has been understood and treated by professionals for some time now, the publication of this book coincides with the first formal inclusion of the diagnosis BED in the *DSM-V* (fifth edition of the *Diagnostic and Statistical Manual of Mental Disorders*), which is used for all psychiatric diagnoses. Recognizing binge eating disorder as a diagnosable condition alongside other eating disorders such as anorexia nervosa and bulimia nervosa represents an important shift in the understanding and treatment of binge eating.

To get the most out of this book, you don't need to start at the beginning and read straight through, although reading the entire book, in whatever order you choose, will certainly benefit you in the long run. Put another way, like a good meal, take what you want and leave the rest. In fact, you often see us use food metaphors in discussing various aspects of the disorder because attitudes about food and eating extend to most other areas of life including money and relationships. That may sound strange, but as you read through, you'll undoubtedly make the connections.

Also feel free to skip sidebars and anything marked with a Technical Stuff icon. We've written them to enhance and deepen the material in each chapter, but they're not essential to understanding what you need to know.

It's useful to note that each chapter and section stand alone, so if you prefer, you can begin wherever you like, picking and choosing what's most helpful to you in learning about and reframing your long-held views and reflexive responses to food and emotions. You may even want to revisit certain sections repeatedly in order to more fully grasp new concepts, strategies, and practical ideas in a way that works for you.

Within this book, you may note that some web addresses break across two lines of text. If you're reading this book in print and want to visit one of these web pages, simply key in the web address exactly as it's noted in the text, as if the line break doesn't exist. If you're reading this as an e-book, you've got it made — just click the web address to be taken directly to the recommended web page.

Foolish Assumptions

If you picked up this book, we assume that you fit into at least one of the following categories:

- ✔ **You're a binge eater, or you suspect you may be.** Healing and recovering from an eating disorder of any kind doesn't happen overnight even if you'd like that to be the case. Whether you're at the beginning of the journey and just realizing that you may have a problem or a bit farther down the path and looking for further motivation and resources, you'll find what you need in this book.

- ✔ **You love someone who's a binge eater.** Watching someone you love struggle with binge eating in its various forms can be extremely difficult. We wrote this book not only for people struggling with binge eating, compulsive overeating, or emotional eating but also for loved ones affected by someone else's disordered eating.

- ✔ **You're a professional who treats people who suffer from disordered eating or related issues and conditions.** Perhaps you treat people with all kinds of eating disorders, related psychological conditions, and/or the physical consequences that may result. Of course you know your stuff, but this book offers a quick, practical, and layman-friendly reference guide that you and your patients can use together.

Icons Used in This Book

Throughout the book, we use icons in the margins to call special attention to certain paragraphs. Keep an eye out for the following symbols.

This book is chock full of practical information you can use now and in the future. When we use a tip icon, we're highlighting a specific idea or technique we've found particularly useful for almost everyone we've treated over the years.

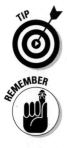

We cover a lot of ground in this book, but what we know about eating disorders and how to treat them often stems from a few key ideas and philosophies. When you see a remember icon, we're either reminding you of something we've written about before or stressing how important it is to keep one of these central ideas in mind as you read.

Eating disorders can have a long-term impact on your psychological and physical health. When we use a warning icon, we want you to take into account that your well-being is your top priority as well as ours.

Dealing with binge eating encompasses many different subjects: medicine, psychology/behavior, physiology, nutrition, cultural awareness, and more. Sometimes we delve more deeply into these areas, and we label that exploration with a technical stuff icon. You don't have to read those paragraphs to get the big picture of a section or chapter, but you certainly may want to if you're seeking more in-depth information.

Beyond the Book

In addition to the material in the print or e-book you're reading right now, this book comes with an eCheat Sheet you can access on the web anywhere, anytime at www.dummies.com/cheatsheet/overcomingbingeeating. The articles there address a range of binge-eating tips:

- Don't know where to start or need a reminder of how to eat a healthy, satisfying diet that will sustain you both mentally and physically? Check out ten ideas for eating healthfully.

- Even though it may be uncomfortable to think about, binge eating poses serious short- and long-term risks to your health. For an idea of what you need to be on the lookout for, we include a list of the most significant medical risks.

- If you're reading this book because you have a friend or loved one who suffers from binge eating, we offer tips to help you stay on the right track in your efforts to support someone else's recovery from disordered eating.

- Perhaps you're struggling with the urge to binge right now. Take this list of alternate activities with you everywhere and turn to them when you need ideas for something you can do to distract yourself that's meaningful and engaging, not just a time-filler.

Where to Go from Here

You can start wherever you like in *Overcoming Binge Eating For Dummies*; you don't have to begin with Chapter 1 and read straight through to get the information you need to understand and begin to recover from binge eating. For example, if you're interested in sampling a smorgasbord of the treatments out there, skip to Chapter 10 to get a sense of all your options. If you're looking for motivation, Chapters 7 and 9 are good starting places. If you want to dive right into nutrition, Chapter 12 has lots of tools and tips for meal planning and coping skills for dealing with food. And if you're the friend or family member of someone who binges, Chapter 21 is the first in a series of chapters about how to help someone you love get better.

Part I

Binge Eating Disorder: What It Is and What It Isn't

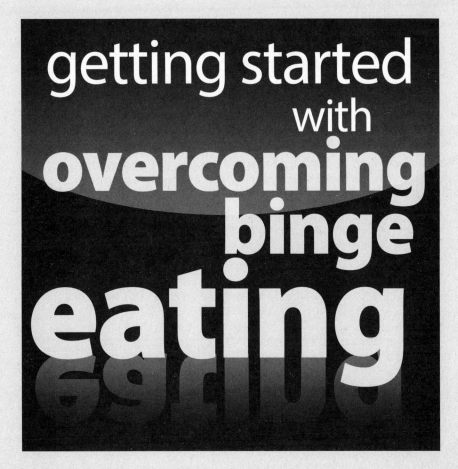

In this part . . .

✔ Identify the components of binge eating disorder (BED) and other eating disorders. Distinguish BED from compulsive overeating, emotional overeating, and the nervosas — anorexia and bulimia.

✔ Look into possible reasons for developing an eating disorder. Heredity and environment both play a role in the emergence of many eating disorders.

✔ Realize that BED is an addiction recognized by the American Psychiatric Association with a variety of effective treatment methods.

✔ Understand that BED and other disordered eating habits result in both physical and psychological ailments. In the same vein, existing physical and emotional disorders may contribute to the development of eating disorders.

Chapter 1

The World of Binge Eating Disorder

For some people, hunger is simply a physical sensation usually satisfied by a moderate amount of food. For others, physical hunger is mistaken for what we call emotional hunger, and eating food becomes a misguided attempt to soothe away the worries and upsets of life.

When you think about it, the fact that many people have eating disorders isn't really surprising. Eating and nourishment is so primal; suckling is the very first instinct you act upon after you're born. Throughout your life, eating is a fundamental part of many social, cultural, and family rituals. It therefore makes sense that many people use food as a way to get a different kind of nurturance and to self-soothe during difficult situations. Similar to drugs, alcohol, and other additive substances, food can come to be seen as a great source of temporary comfort.

But when eating becomes a primary contributor to your problems rather than a solution to them, it's a surefire sign that you need to look at your eating habits. If, for instance, you overeat to the point of physical pain or discomfort, hide your excessive eating from others, and/or feel intense shame and guilt over how much you consume, you may want to consider that you have a problem you may not be able to resolve on your own. That problem is called binge eating disorder.

In this chapter, we explore what binge eating actually means and how to determine whether you suffer from binge eating disorder (BED) or an eating disorder of any kind. We discuss a few of the many available treatments and identify who suffers from binge eating. Finally, we address those of you who may be struggling to support and help a friend or loved one who's a binge eater.

Examining Binge Eating Disorder: What it Is and What it Isn't

Binge eating disorder (BED) isn't simply having an extra piece of cake at a birthday party or overeating during the holidays or on vacation. It's a serious, progressive condition that affects both the body and mind and may drive you to eat in response to something other than physical hunger. This simple definition of binge eating, and all emotional or compulsive overeating for that matter, is a useful way to think about the whole issue. (We explain the range of eating disorders in Chapter 2.)

Simply put, *disordered eating* is eating in response to something other than physical hunger. Notice the non-judgmental simplicity with which you can start to think about disordered eating by referring to it this way.

During a binge, you lose control and can consume many thousands of calories in an attempt to numb unwanted negative emotions. Up until May 2013, clinically speaking, binge eating had been classified as EDNOS, or eating disorder not otherwise specified. As of the publication of the fifth edition of the *Diagnostic and Statistical Manual of Mental Disorders (DSM-V)*, binge eating disorder was officially recognized as a distinct and definable condition, which hopefully allows for more reimbursable treatment options as well as more research into the causes of and most effective treatments available for this complex disorder. (The EDNOS classification itself is now *other specified feeding or eating disorder*, or OSFED.)

Defining binge eating

What does it mean to binge? The criteria are clearer now than they've ever been and yet you may still have picked up this book wondering if how you eat qualifies you as someone suffering from binge eating disorder. The *DSM-V* sets out the following criteria:

- ✔ Eating a larger amount of food than normal in a short period of time
- ✔ Losing control during the binge episode
- ✔ Bingeing at least once per week for at least three months
- ✔ Not using any sort of compensatory behaviors like purging or exercising

We discuss these criteria in more depth in Chapter 2, but if this list starts you thinking about some of your own behaviors, you've come to the right place. When you're ready to embrace and tackle the issues, this book can help you not only figure out what to do but why and how to do it.

Even if you flip through these first chapters and decide that you don't technically suffer from binge eating disorder, the information you uncover about compulsive or emotional eating may still resonate strongly with you. Whatever form your disordered eating takes, you can surely benefit from the ideas and strategies in these chapters. You may even feel inspired or motivated to take a step beyond the guidance offered here and seek out professional treatment, if needed.

Dealing with the consequences of binge eating

Binge eating, compulsive overeating, and emotional eating take a toll on the mind and body. Although some binge eaters may maintain an average weight, most become overweight or obese and suffer from chronic diseases associated with excess weight. If you're a binge eater, you probably already know that you're at increased risk for heart disease, high blood pressure, high cholesterol, metabolic diseases, and diabetes among many other conditions. (Chapter 4 talks about physical and emotional health concerns.)

Perhaps you also experience some of the psychological or emotional causes and effects of binge eating. For example, depression, anxiety, attention deficit hyperactivity disorder (ADHD), obsessive compulsive disorder (OCD), and other disorders can be part of a complicated system that triggers and/or exacerbates binge eating.

In the final analysis, the whole complex of emotions, experiences, and behaviors may leave you feeling desperate, hopeless, and increasingly socially isolated, all of which can make the urge to binge even greater.

Accepting the Reality of an Eating Disorder

Many binge eaters must deal with lives that feel out of control almost all the time. Even if you try to ignore the persistent thoughts, feelings, and urges you have with regard to food, it isn't enough to overcome your drive to binge eat or overeat. However, as much as you'd like help and a way to heal yourself, it can be difficult to acknowledge that you have a problem.

If you've picked up this book, chances are you're struggling with disordered eating of some kind, and no matter what label you put on it, making changes would benefit you both physically and psychologically in the long run.

Seeing the signs

No matter the exact form your overeating takes, you may still be telling yourself that it's no big deal or that it's not a real problem (although you're reading this book, so you're at least a bit suspicious). If, in fact, you've readily acknowledged that you have a problem, you may be struggling to find some way to keep it from taking over your life. Or perhaps you're at a more advanced stage and the bingeing has already put your health and/or your relationships in jeopardy.

Whatever stage you're in, the signs that you may be in trouble from using food to soothe yourself are relatively easy to spot if you know what to look for. When you're bingeing or overeating in any way:

- ✔ **You feel out of control.** The hallmark of binge eating is a sense that you cannot stop regardless of whether you want to or your body hurts from taking in so much food.

- ✔ **You turn to food to deal with negative emotions or situations you feel you can't cope with in any other way.** At the beginning, bingeing may have helped you feel better, at least temporarily. Now, it creates as many or more problems than it resolves, but you don't know what else to do but eat.

- ✔ **You keep your eating habits a secret.** In eating as in the rest of life, if you're desperate to keep something a secret, it's probably not a good sign. You try as best you can to make sure that no one knows anything about how, what, when, where, or why you're eating, and this in and of itself suggests you may have a problem.

- ✔ **You feel utter regret when the binge is over.** You may promise yourself every time that you won't binge again, and when you do binge, you're overwhelmed by shame, guilt, grief, and desperation. What's even worse is that these negative emotions simply perpetuate the continuous cycle of feeling bad and then eating for release. Of course, it's more complicated than that, but over time, the hopelessness that descends upon you is one factor that makes the situation worse.

Deciding to make a change

If you're a binge eater, compulsive overeater, or emotional eater, you've probably already tried every diet under the sun more than once. Maybe some of them work for a while, but eventually you fall back into old routines and end up right back where you started or even worse off than where you began.

Most binge eaters mentally beat themselves up on a regular basis by telling themselves that it was just a matter of not having will power, that even trying to stop bingeing is stupid and hopeless. These conclusions are painfully and needlessly punishing and also just not so.

The reasons that diets don't work are because

- ✔ **Diets don't ever work.** Diets just create an inevitable pendulum swing of deprivation and cravings, both emotionally and physically.

- ✔ **Binge eating, as with all disordered eating, actually has nothing to do with food.** Yes, you read that right. Strange as it may sound, food is just the available weapon, if you will.

You may be scratching your head, wondering what in the world we're talking about, but as you may have already noticed, focusing only on food when it comes to tackling these issues simply isn't working. Instead, when you're ready to make a change, you have to find other reasons that will help finally flip the switch for you.

Everyone's different, and your personal motivations for slowly putting a stop to binge eating are likely quite different from the reasons that motivate other binge eaters. However, many people who've successfully put binge eating behind them have some of these strategies in common:

- ✔ **Take time to get ready.** Slowing and eventually ending binge eating or overeating of any kind is a marathon and not a sprint. Even though you may be eager to jump in and make changes immediately, if you can step back for a moment, be clear about your motives, gather any pertinent information, and make an action plan, preferably with strategic support from others, you'll set yourself up for long-term success.

- ✔ **Focus on possibility.** Whether it's imagining all you'll be able to do with your life when eating doesn't dominate your day-to-day thinking or concentrating on the small successes you have along the way, overcoming your disordered eating in large part depends on the idea that if you can see it, you can have it. If you can see it, you can be it. It's a leap of faith to imagine what until now has seemed to be unimaginable. This is an essential strategy for many areas of life.

✔ **Set realistic goals and reward yourself for meeting them.** Making major changes in the way you eat and, more importantly, the way you think about eating takes time and determination. By establishing small milestones along the way, bite-size pieces, so to speak, you give yourself time to learn new ways of being in the world and give yourself an opportunity to celebrate incremental success in ways that motivate and inspire you. In other words, portion out change rather than bingeing on it. (Caution: The food metaphors have just begun . . . many more to come!)

Chapter 7 addresses motivation in more depth.

Seeking treatment and support

Successful treatment comes in all shapes and sizes. Although some binge eaters choose to see a team of eating-disorder professionals, others may not be able or willing to tackle every issue simultaneously.

No matter how enthusiastic and ready you are to move forward, recovery can be emotionally and physically challenging, and taking an approach that makes the most sense to you and pacing yourself in a way that feels comfortable are two ways of building a foundation upon which you can evolve as you begin to heal.

In this book, we take a three-pronged approach to recovery:

✔ **Medical/Physiological:** Binge eating can take a serious toll on your health, so as you begin to think about getting better, the first stop is your doctor's office. You may already be in regular contact with your physician about ongoing health issues, or you may have been avoiding a visit for a long time. Either way, it's important to discuss the fact that you've been struggling with binge eating in addition to addressing any of the chronic conditions that may have developed as a result of overeating such as obesity, high blood pressure, heart disease, and diabetes — to name just a few.

Aside from the medical piece of healing from binge eating, there are broad physiological considerations, particularly with respect to learning how to understand your whole body. For instance, as you recover, you learn or relearn how to assess your hunger and fullness accurately and appropriately by listening to the signals your body sends you before and after meals.

You can also discover how to move your body in a way that feels healthy and positive. Over time, healthy forms of exercise and movement can help establish a better sense of self and improve your body image.

✔ **Psychological:** Healing from disordered eating of any kind, and bingeing in particular, starts with an understanding of the underlying psychological conditions, thoughts, and feelings that lead you to conclude, consciously or otherwise, that overeating is the best way to cope. Even though it may be difficult or uncomfortable at times, understanding your deepest motives and developing a willingness to address longstanding behavior and thought patterns are essential to the process of ending binge eating.

✔ **Nutritional:** A dietitian specializing in eating disorders can help you establish new strategies when it comes to food. If you're a chronic binge eater, you may have forgotten or you may never have known what it means to nourish yourself. A dietitian can give you the nutritional support you need to get started and the pointers you'll want to make changes that work for you along the way.

Chapter 10 talks about the professional and peer support system you may tap into as you head toward recovery.

Don't let yourself become overwhelmed by what lies ahead. You don't have to take it all on at once, and in fact, if you're trying to stop bingeing, it probably makes sense to tackle your recovery in bite-size pieces with the same moderate, gentle approach you're planning to take towards food, eating, and yourself now and in the future.

Taking Steps to Get Better

Recovering from binge eating or any kind of compulsive overeating isn't an overnight process. It's taken months or years to arrive at this point, and getting better takes time as well as determination. You have to be wiling to gently, but resolutely, look at yourself in the mirror and slowly change the thoughts and behaviors that aren't good for you at the same time that you learn to accept yourself for who you are. It's not a straightforward or linear affair, but with patience and hard work, you can make a healthier and happier life for yourself.

To be or not to be an addiction — that's the question

Addiction is a complicated word and one that may be overused in modern culture, but when it comes to binge eating, it can be helpful to think of it as an addictive behavior.

New research shows that the way the bodies and brains of binge eaters react to food mimics the way other addicts respond to the substances and/or behaviors of their addictions. Images of the brain, particularly PET (positron emission tomography) scans and functional MRIs (magnetic resonance images), taken during a food binge, an alcohol binge, and while using cocaine or heroin are virtually identical and show almost identical stimulation of the pleasure centers in the brain. Whether this means that binge eating is an addiction is still an uncertain, but the physiological similarities are so strong that it's certainly a useful idea to consider during recovery.

Whereas the goal for most other addictions is to achieve abstinence, this is obviously not the case with binge eating. You have to eat to survive. Coming to terms with the idea that you must establish a lifelong relationship with food is one of the complex realities of facing down binge eating, compulsive overeating, or any form of disordered eating. In fact, among Overeaters Anonymous members, one aphorism is that "when you are addicted to drugs you put the tiger in the cage to recover; when you are addicted to food you put the tiger in the cage, but take it out three times a day for a walk." To be clear, in no way are we making light of the plight of all those who take the courageous journey to beat any addiction. But those involving food are that much more complex in this way.

Continuing research into the way that eating, and certain foods in particular, activate the pleasure centers in the brains of binge eaters and into how and why binge eaters tend to gain weight more easily may ultimately result in different treatment paradigms. However, here and now, thinking of binge eating as an addiction only matters if it helps you reframe the way you think about your own relationship to food and eating and if it changes how others view your behaviors. If people in your life judge you as being lazy or having no discipline, explaining that BED is a recognized addiction may promote a more helpful attitude.

No matter how you feel about it, being flexible and curious on your journey helps you pick and choose the ideas and strategies that'll be most useful, meaningful, and motivating for you along the way.

Considering professional treatment

By its very nature, binge eating is a condition that tends to isolate its sufferers. You've probably tried your best to keep your eating habits and how you feel about yourself and food a secret from most people you know, even those closest to you. You also may have tried to get better on your own without long-lasting success. Hopefully, something in this book will help propel you into meaningful and sustainable change.

Perhaps now is the time to embrace the idea that you don't have to go it alone. It's a lot to ask of yourself to try to make significant changes in your life without the proper support and guidance from people who have more experience in this area than you do. Although you may be reluctant to reach out to professionals for a variety of reasons, asking for help from physicians, psychotherapists, dietitians, and other eating disorder specialists is truly a sign of strength and readiness. In fact, it's also a way to set yourself on the path of being kinder to yourself and more realistic about your abilities and your challenges.

The wide variety of eating disorder treatment possibilities means that there's something out there for everyone. You need to determine which makes the most sense to you and what you feel will be most effective, but whatever you decide to do, consider that you need to take care of your body, your brain, and your behavior. These are a few of the many treatment options we discuss later in the book

- **Cognitive behavioral therapy (CBT):** One of the most common and effective approaches to treating binge eating disorder, CBT begins with the premise that thoughts and perceptions lead to feelings (or avoidance of them),which then leads to desirable and undesirable behaviors. Ultimately the idea is to understand and intervene in the way you think and feel in order to affect your behaviors. A specific focus in treating binge eating and all forms of disordered eating is to learn new reflexes and new coping skills that do not hurt you in the end. Chapter 11 explains CBT methods.

- **Traditional or process-oriented psychotherapy:** Talk therapy is what you may imagine when you think of going to see a therapist. It's one thing to concentrate on changing behaviors and reactions in the here and now, but it's also critical to long-term success that you work to gently uncover the driving forces behind your disordered eating. In other words, psychotherapy is a way to uncover what the heck is so strong, so compelling, that an intelligent and successful person like you would continually take part in eating behaviors that you know will not end well. When you can step back with a different lens to view the past and realize that it does not have to predict or determine your future, there is great freedom, insight and thus an ability to steer a different course.

- **Nutritional counseling:** It's likely that you've been bingeing or eating in response to something other than physical hunger for so long that you don't remember (or perhaps you never knew) how to nourish your body in a healthy and satisfying way. Seeing an experienced dietitian can be a watershed moment for many people because it's a chance to collaborate on and help create a sustainable plan for eating in a way that supports you, has variety, is not restrictive, fits your lifestyle, and has a certain level of accountability. (Nutrition is the subject of Chapter 12.)

✔ **Family/couples therapy:** This is most often a critically important component of treatment. It's educational for those who live with and/or love you, so they can offer constructive and meaningful support, both concretely and emotionally. You all discover vital do's and don'ts that aren't so obvious and extremely helpful for the long haul. Family and/or couples therapy can be a path to enhance relationships, especially those that have suffered due to disordered eating.

✔ **Support groups:** Even if you're seeing a psychotherapist and dietitian and feel that your treatment plate is full, so to speak, a support group is a great way to find a like-minded community as you move forward. No, it's not a commiseration session. Ideally, support groups offer a relaxed, non-judgmental, safe environment where you can talk about specific recovery-related issues and get advice and ideas from others in the same situation you're in. (Chapter 10 offers advice on how to find support groups.)

This is just a tiny taste of the strategies, ideas, and techniques contained in this book. It may take some tweaking to find the perfect combination that works for you, but in time, you will.

Relapsing as a necessary part of the process

Healing from binge eating isn't a perfectly linear process, and even though it may seem uncomfortable to hear, it's likely that even if all is generally going well, you will have a relapse. Now that you know, you can stop worrying about it and consider it a part of your evolution. (Chapter 15 explains how to handle and move on after a relapse.)

But not all relapses are alike. The key to success lies in your expectations. If, for instance, you expect that things will change very quickly and that you'll get better and better and thinner and thinner, never abuse food again, be the perfect weight, and stay there and live happily ever after, you may be quite disappointed. Rather than thinking of the trajectory of your recovery as a perfectly linear process, it's probably more helpful to imagine it as a road with many with peaks and valleys. Your goal is to even out the ups and downs and make the hills and valleys less pronounced and the distance or time between them greater and greater. With a realistic attitude, you'll be better prepared for the realities of recovery and better able to keep your commitment to yourself.

A relapse is simply a sign that you need to make adjustments in your recovery plan, not a signal that it (or you) isn't working. Even though a relapse can be emotionally and physically challenging, it offers a chance to step back and reevaluate your plan. And being able to evaluate what's working well and identify what's not, both when it comes to food and when it comes to the rest of your life, is an important skill that you can use in all aspects of your life.

Many binge eaters suffer from an all-or-nothing thinking; try not to let yourself fall into this trap. If you relapse, it doesn't mean that your recovery is over, that you're a failure, that it's hopeless, useless, too late, or that it would be easier just to binge. Nothing could be further from the truth. That thinking is just one of the paths back to what is, in essence, an undesirable but comfortable set of behaviors and habits. A relapse is a setback, yes, but it's important to think about what may have triggered you to relapse, work out strategies to keep it from happening again, and move forward. Getting better is about finding a moderate, realistic path toward the future, not about being perfect.

Looking across the Population

Traditionally, anorexia nervosa and bulimia nervosa, two very common and long-recognized eating disorders, have been considered conditions that primarily strike young women (even as those statistics continue to change and become broader in scope). *Anorexia* is characterized by an extremely distorted body image and excessive dieting that leads to severe weight loss with a pathological fear of weight gain and eventually becoming fat. *Bulimia* is characterized by frequent episodes of binge eating followed by inappropriate behaviors such as self-induced vomiting, laxative abuse, or over-exercising to avoid weight gain. Most bulimics are of normal weight while those with anorexia are underweight.

However, BED is and has always been more of an equal-opportunity condition. Although the numbers aren't absolutely definitive, more than 3.5 percent of females and 2 percent of males in the United States suffer from binge eating. In Canada, the National Eating Disorder Information Centre reports binge eating disorder affects about 2 percent of all people. And the U.K. Counseling Directory states that it's thought that binge eating is more common than other eating disorders, with approximately 2 percent of adults being affected. Forty percent (and perhaps more) of sufferers are men, and binge eating affects children and adolescents, younger and older adults, and people of all races. New diagnostic criteria have certainly played a role in giving a realistic picture of who's suffering from binge eating, but it still remains to be seen why binge eating is on the rise.

Understanding that men binge too

It's tempting to separate out binge eaters by gender and describe different reasons why women and men binge. But the fact of the matter is that the underlying motivations and root causes aren't so different. Like women, men suffer from

✓ Body image insecurities and distortions

✓ Perfectionism

✔ Stress, anxiety, depression, and other psychological conditions

✔ Coexisting addictions to drugs or alcohol and/or other addictive tendencies

✔ Self-esteem issues

✔ Past history of abuse or trauma

Some specific tendencies for men who binge or compulsively overeat include

✔ **Attitude toward food:** Traditionally, men have not been conditioned to feel that certain foods are socially unacceptable or should be forbidden in a diet. Red meats, fried foods, and rich desserts are often perceived as tokens of deserved success. Consuming large quantities of food in a brief period of time is socially acceptable for men who are challenged to engage in eating contests or dared to overeat by restaurant menus and television shows. Consuming four dozen chicken wings in a half-hour may be perceived as a sign of masculinity — certainly not something to feel ashamed about. With a greater tolerance and acceptance of these behaviors, recognition of a disorder beyond one's control can be difficult.

✔ **Body image:** Although times are changing and men are beginning to feel the same sort of societal pressures that women feel to have a perfect or better body, by and large, it's still considered more acceptable for a man to be overweight or obese than it is for a woman. Unfortunately, that tolerance may ultimately backfire if a man doesn't realize that his disordered eating puts him at risk for serious health conditions.

✔ **Age:** Although most women begin bingeing in adolescence, during college, and/or as young adults, the majority of men who binge start somewhat later. The reasons vary from individual to individual but may be related to occupational stressors reflecting early socialization for men to be the primary breadwinners. Age-related hormonal shifts may also be at work as well as a change in lifestyle from typically active to much more sedentary.

✔ **Treatment**: To put it as candidly and plainly as possible, while admittedly brushing with a broad brush stroke, in general most men prefer processes that are quick and easy, concrete, and very action-oriented while women generally prefer a more measured, progressive, thorough approach. Of course there are many exceptions to this, but it is an important set of ideas to consider when designing treatment plans for both men and women.

Chapter 16 is devoted to issues faced by men who binge.

Shifting hormones in mid-life

You may think of adolescence as a time of great hormonal upheaval, but perimenopause and menopause bring about just as many changes to a woman's body and signal a new, sometimes challenging, sometimes rewarding, phase of life. It should be noted that men also experience a variety of hormonal changes at various stages that need be considered though they're often less talked about.

While in the throes of both perimenopause and menopause experiencing the predictably unpredictable estrogen surges and cascades, women suffer from mood and energy swings, anxiety and depression, hot flashes, night sweats, blood pressure and blood sugar fluctuations, muscle and skin changes, unwanted hair growth, and perhaps most frustrating, almost inevitable weight gain even though food intake and/or energy output remain unchanged. What changes is the rate of *metabolism,* the body's calorie-burning process.

It's easy to imagine that in the midst of these physical changes, which may breed feelings of being out of control, compounded by developmental, family, relationship, and professional shifts that often occur at this stage of life, someone who's vulnerable to bingeing, emotional eating, or who may have been a binge eater earlier in life may turn to overeating as a way to soothe herself, willingly or unwillingly, consciously or unconsciously.

Eventually though, menopause brings about a hormonal calm which may eventually quiet the urge to binge. Until then, treatment, both for the symptoms of menopause and for binge eating itself, can help restore balance to your life.

Bingeing and change-of-life issues are covered in Chapter 19.

Offering a Helping Hand

Few things in life are as upsetting as watching someone you love struggle with addictive behaviors she can't control. And in fact, if you're the friend or family member of someone who's a binge eater, the first step toward being able to truly help that person get better is to step back and see the situation for what it really is.

If you can see binge eating not as a lack of will or discipline, but rather as a set of addictive behaviors and habits that have developed for many different reasons, you have a good chance of being able to play a supportive, nonjudgmental role in a loved one's struggle.

It's equally important to strike the right balance between supporting another person and considering your own needs, not only for your own physical and psychological but also for that of the binge eater. Later chapters, especially those in Part V, go into much greater depth with specific strategies and suggestions to achieve these ends.

Supporting the recovery process of another

You may have found yourself thinking or saying more than once, "Why can't you just stop eating?," or "Don't you see what you're doing to yourself," or some other variation on the theme. It's perfectly normal to think something along those lines, but those sentiments belie the true complexity of the situation and undoubtedly make it harder or impossible for you to play a meaningful role in your loved one's recovery. If it were as simple as knowing what to do and doing it, the binge eater in your life would have already found a way to limit the drive to overeat and to stop the binges himself.

No matter where your loved one is along the path of changing her behavior, some general guidelines apply in most, if not all, situations.

- ✔ **Set aside blame.** There's no point in trying to figure who's at fault when it comes to disordered eating. There is no blame. Focus instead on non-judgmental listening and on efforts to get better.

- ✔ **Wait to be asked for help.** Although you can't always do this, especially if someone you love is in danger, it's better in the vast majority of cases to wait for someone who suffers from binge eating to come to you. Opening up to others is a sign that someone is ready to make real and lasting changes.

- ✔ **Encourage your loved one to seek professional help.** Like all eating disorders, binge eating disorder and its related conditions are progressive. The longer someone waits to seek treatment, the more difficult the recovery. Although it's not impossible for someone to get better on his own, it's easier to do so with carefully chosen medical, psychological, and nutritional support.

- ✔ **Accept your own limitations.** No matter how desperately you want someone to get better, you can't do it for them. Your friend or loved one has to drive this process for it to truly be effective.

- ✔ **Take care of yourself.** No matter what you do and how good your intentions, you can't make someone do something they don't want to or aren't ready to do. If someone you love is a binge eater and is resistant to change for whatever reasons, the best thing you may be able to do is to accept that for now and continue with your own life.

Understanding the role of family

Families play a unique role in the treatment of any eating disorder. A family is a system, and all families create or exist within certain physical and psychological frameworks, establishing or following patterns and behaviors that make each family system unique. Without a doubt, some of these factors are positive, but others are not, and some family environments may unwittingly contribute to (but not cause) disordered eating or other kinds of negative thoughts or behaviors.

When you're at your wit's end, the quick and easy way is to point the finger at someone else rather than doing the hard work of thinking about your own role in how a certain situation has developed. Resist the temptation to blame and focus on what you can do *now* to make things better. The past is history, and moving forward toward a healthier future is a better way to spend your energy.

Chapter 2

Defining Binge Eating Disorder

· ·

In This Chapter

▶ Understanding the clinical definition of binge eating disorder

▶ Distinguishing between binge eating, compulsive overeating, and emotional eating

▶ Exploring what it feels like before, during, and after a binge

▶ Tackling all-or-nothing thinking

▶ Taking a quiz to help determine whether you're a binge eater

· ·

*I*t's not unusual to hear the word *binge* thrown about on a regular basis in the workplace or in casual conversation. People talk all the time about bingeing not only on food but also on things like alcohol, work, television, and shopping among many other things. Ours is a society that often promotes excess rather than moderation, and the language we use day in and day out reflects that.

But the fact is that what most people describe, either knowingly or unknowingly, as a binge is more than likely an exaggeration, particularly when it comes to food. A true binge consists of far more copious amounts of food and a far more complex mix of negative emotions than most people imagine when they use the word so casually.

Until May 2013, binge eating disorder (BED) and binge eating in general had not yet been fully integrated within the spectrum of eating disorders. But with the publication of the fifth edition of the American Psychiatric Association's *Diagnostic and Statistical Manual of Mental Disorders (DSM-V)*, binge eating disorder is finally recognized as a diagnosable psychiatric condition and given a formal diagnosis code. This is an important clinical milestone for the millions of people worldwide who suffer from it, not only for the purposes of possible coverage by managed care for services related to its treatment, but also because of the effect it can have on reducing the stigmatization of binge eaters.

But for binge eaters suffering day in and day out, the DSM criteria are simply a starting point. Within the criteria themselves, there are many variations of what it means to binge or to suffer from binge eating disorder. That said, no matter how bingeing has affected your life or that of someone you love, effective treatment exists.

In this chapter, we outline the clinical definition of binge eating disorder and discuss why it's so important for patients and clinicians that BED is recognized alongside anorexia nervosa (AN) and bulimia nervosa (BN) as a defined eating disorder. We explore other forms of overeating related to but different from actual binge eating as well as dissecting what happens before, during, and after a binge. We also touch upon so-called black-and-white or all-or-nothing thinking — a primary and pervasive thought pattern that underlies and perpetuates binge behaviors.

Understanding the Clinical Definition of Binge Eating

Binge eating disorder affects millions of people around the world. At its core is the profound loss of control someone feels while eating and the distorted perception that may make it feel as if bingeing is the best way to cope with, or to delay coping with, life's difficulties. In establishing diagnostic guidelines for clinicians, the *DSM-V* recognizes both the physical and psychological components that make up BED. In doing so, the American Psychiatric Association has taken the first steps towards better promoting a clinical and societal environment in which treatment and healing can take place in a gentle, realistic, and productive way. That's not to say that treatment in its many forms has not always been available and evolving. Of course it has. But again, the formalization of criteria and a formal diagnosis make it all the more feasible.

Breaking down the DSM-V definition

Even though binge eating is a unique experience for all sufferers, the fifth edition of the American Psychiatric Association's *Diagnostic and Statistical Manual of Mental Disorders* defined, for the first time, a set of diagnostic criteria that can be used to identify binge eating disorder and diagnose those suffering from it. Prior to adding binge eating disorder as a diagnostic category, binge eating often fell into the category of EDNOS, or eating disorder not

otherwise specified, which sometimes made seeking treatment more complicated clinically and more costly financially because of the catch-all nature of
the diagnostic category.

The current diagnostic criteria for binge eating disorder as stated in the
DSM-V include:

- Recurrent episodes of binge eating. An episode is characterized by

    - Eating a larger amount of food than normal during a short period
      of time (within any two-hour period)

    - Lack of control over eating during the binge episode (for example,
      feeling that you cannot stop eating)

- Binge eating episodes are associated with three or more of the following:

    - Eating much more rapidly than normal

    - Eating until feeling uncomfortably full

    - Eating large amounts of food when not physically hungry

    - Eating alone because you are embarrassed by how much you're
      eating

    - Feeling disgusted, depressed, or guilty after overeating

- Marked distress regarding binge eating is present.

- Binge eating occurs, on average, at least once a week for three months.

- The binge eating is not associated with the regular use of inappropriate
  compensatory behavior (such as purging, excessive exercise, and so on)
  and does not occur exclusively during the course of bulimia nervosa or
  anorexia nervosa.

Many people refer to what we call *compulsive overeating* or *emotional eating*
as a binge despite the fact that by this criteria, it likely does not constitute
a binge. Regardless, it's important to note that even if your eating doesn't fit
perfectly into the clinical definition of a binge, this doesn't mean you don't
have a problem.

Recognizing BED as an eating disorder

Even though binge eating disorder hadn't been fully recognized in the medical literature prior to the publication of the *DSM-V* in May of 2013, professionals have understood and been successfully treating individuals suffering from
BED and other kinds of severe overeating for some time.

Why then, you may ask, is it so important that binge eating disorder be included in the *DSM* if good treatment is going on behind the scenes anyway? Well, consider these reasons:

- ✔ **The *DSM* provides a common language for understanding mental illness.** Clinicians, researchers, managed care companies, pharmaceutical companies, and policymakers from all over the world use the *DSM* to define, diagnose, and treat mental disorders.

- ✔ **Standardization in the DSM confers legitimacy.** Before the *DSM-V,* only anorexia nervosa, bulimia nervosa, and eating disorder not otherwise specified (EDNOS) were included as eating disorders. *Anorexia nervosa* is characterized by an extremely distorted body image and excessive dieting that leads to severe weight loss with a pathological fear of weight gain and eventually becoming fat. Most anorexics are underweight. *Bulimia nervosa* is characterized by frequent episodes of binge eating followed by inappropriate behaviors such as self-induced vomiting, laxative abuse, or over-exercising to avoid weight gain. Most bulimics are of normal weight. (In Chapter 5 we discuss the full spectrum of eating disorders and the relationship among them.)

  Incorporating binge eating disorder into that list signifies a long-overdue recognition that people who suffer from binge eating are afflicted by a true mental disorder. Hopefully, those ignorant of the disorder will now understand that the issue isn't that those with BED have no self-control, are lazy, or lack willpower and discipline. That's simply not the case.

- ✔ **Binge eaters may now be more likely to seek treatment.** If you're a binge eater, you may never have thought of yourself as someone who's deserving of specialized treatment. Now, being a formal part of a continuum of diagnosable eating disorders and knowing that you're going to be taken more seriously when you ask for help may bolster your resolve to do so.

- ✔ **Treatment will likely be more carefully considered for reimbursement by insurance providers.** The *DSM* plays a significant role in determining how insurance providers reimburse physicians, psychotherapists, dietitians, other professionals, and patients themselves for treatment. Inclusion in the *DSM* means that binge eating disorder has been recognized as an official mental disorder and that its treatment may be more fully reimbursable, thus making effective treatment available to a greater number of sufferers.

- ✔ **Hopefully there will now be greater interest in more extensive research into the root causes of and treatments for binge eating.** Although research on binge eating disorder has been ongoing, now that BED has been included in the *DSM,* clinicians and scientists may be able to get more funding for their research. In time, this could lead to breakthroughs about the origins of binge eating disorder, what makes someone vulnerable to binge eating or overeating of any kind, and which treatments are most effective.

Drawing a Line between Bingeing and Overeating

Whether you meet all the criteria for binge eating disorder, you may still have a problem with bingeing or significant overeating. Even if you haven't yet reached the clinical thresholds of BED, that doesn't mean that you won't or that you wouldn't benefit from treatment right now.

Even if you aren't bingeing according to the strict definition, you may still be using food to soothe yourself in ways that are unhealthy for your body and your mind. The line between bingeing and other forms of overeating such as compulsive overeating and emotional eating isn't always clear. However, the physiological and psychological consequences may be quite similar and just as dangerous. Because any form of disordered eating tends to be progressive, it's likely to get worse over time without treatment, and you may need or want to make changes or seek help proactively rather than waiting for things to progress.

The differences between bingeing, compulsive overeating, and emotional eating are subtle but important as you seek to understand your own relationship with food and how to address it. Try these as a start:

✔ **Compulsive overeating:** A compulsive overeater has little or no ability to recognize or respond to her own hunger and satiety cues. Many compulsive overeaters are grazers who cannot moderate portion size and may consume far more calories than their bodies need, most often without even realizing it.

As is the case with binge eating, there's undoubtedly a significant psychological/emotional component to compulsive overeating. In addition, many ongoing studies continue to explore the addictive properties of high-fat, high-sugar foods as a critical physiological driver behind overeating behaviors. Also, as you'll hear us say throughout the book, trying to undo formed habits is also a part of the picture.

In all cases though, perhaps the clearest distinction between compulsive eating and bingeing is the quantity of foods eaten at one time and the frequency of the episodes themselves.

✔ **Emotional eating:** An emotional eater is essentially a compulsive overeater whose use of food as a self-soothing mechanism occurs in direct response to an emotional event or as an attempt to avoid an emotional event. Emotional eating comes about as a way to numb or cope with perceived stressors and has nothing to do with the body and its needs.

Depending on your life and your habits, you may cycle through various forms of overeating, sometimes bingeing, sometimes overeating to a lesser degree and for various reasons that may or may not yet be apparent to you. Nevertheless, any form of overeating can be unhealthy. As you read this book, you'll discover that even if you don't meet the criteria for binge eating disorder, many of the strategies and ideas we included can help you understand and impact whatever form of disordered eating may be affecting you.

Looking at the Anatomy of a Binge

If you binge on a regular basis, your relationship with food may dominate your life in ways that prevent you from living well and healthfully and from reaching your full potential as a family member, friend, partner, spouse, parent, or employee. Although you may occasionally have short periods of time when you feel free of disordered eating, for much of the time you're either attempting to avoid a binge, in the thick of a binge, or trying to recover from one both physically and emotionally. Even though you may intellectually know all the reasons why it's not a good idea to eat so much, and even if you also know what you need to do to stop, you've probably noticed that all of your knowledge goes out the window when the binge starts and you're seemingly helpless to do anything but engage in the binge. So if you're thinking about trying to stop again, you may want to adopt some new approaches.

First, take a deep breath. Start fresh and try to suspend all self-judgment for anything that has preceded this moment. Next, consider that information can, in fact, be powerful if you can hear and process it in a new and different way so that what you know and what you do begin to look alike. Start by analyzing and learning more about how binges unfold.

Before a binge

As we say many times in this book, bingeing comes about for many different reasons: genetic vulnerabilities, psychological conditions, physiological contributors, and environmental cues to name a few. With all or many of these factors in place, if you don't have adequate and appropriate coping skills, it's possible you may turn to food and overeating instead when life becomes difficult.

At one point, bingeing or overeating was probably a valiant attempt, consciously or otherwise, to soothe yourself under some very harsh and/or unavoidable circumstances. However, over time, bingeing has probably caused more problems than it ever resolved, and you may find yourself in a damaging cycle that leads you to restrict your food intake, then binge, then gain weight over and over again. The more you binge, the more you get into the habit of turning to food when the going gets rough. Over time, bingeing can become a deeply ingrained, profoundly detrimental habit that is challenging, though definitely not impossible, to break.

Your binge eating, compulsive overeating, and emotional eating didn't develop overnight nor will it resolve overnight. In addition, you simply cannot expect to give up any set of behaviors which have been successfully in place for a long time without first understanding what drove the need to begin with and offering replacement thoughts and behaviors to help ease the loss of the old ones. This is a critical point if you're finally to be successful once and for all.

One of the concepts central to understanding what drives people to binge is the idea of triggers. A *trigger* can be an emotion, such as shame or sadness, it can be a physical feeling such as hunger, or it can simply be your reaction to or interpretation of a situation at home, work, or in another setting. The key idea is that thought leads to feeling which leads to behavior. So the trigger sets this all in motion. Certainly anyone who's a binge eater has deep-seated motives that make food and eating the weapon of choice, if you will. However, a trigger is the spark that sets a binge in motion. Sometimes, a trigger can be a one-time situation or feeling, but more often than not, binge eaters respond to the same triggers over and over again, knowingly or unknowingly.

Most often, a binge eater is usually too overwhelmed before a binge to think clearly about what may have set it off. However, having more information about common triggers before going into the next episode may at least give you some pause before bingeing. When a trigger comes, it often takes one of these four forms:

- ✔ **Physical:** A physical trigger occurs in the body and is often part of a natural biological process. Hunger, particularly the acute hunger that follows a period of restriction (like when you skip breakfast), is a common trigger for binge eaters. This is further complicated by the fact that many binge eaters confuse hunger cues with those of thirst and fatigue, thinking food will solve either of the other two.

  Endocrine abnormalities in both men and women and/or hormonal cycles in women may also play a role in triggering overeating. So the hormonal shifts of going through adolescence, perimenopause, menopause, or simply menstruation can act as a physical trigger. (We talk about the endocrine system in Chapter 18 and menopause in Chapter 19.)

✔ **Psychological:** A psychological trigger tends to be a long-standing, perhaps undiagnosed, mental condition that may ebb and flow. Examples are depression, anxiety, and ADHD (attention deficit hyperactivity disorder). Over time, these underlying conditions can manifest in many ways, including distorted body image and low self-esteem, that interfere with the activities of daily life.

Psychological triggers tend play right into the complicated emotional world of binge eating. If you don't feel equipped to recognize and dispel uncomfortable emotions, you may reflexively turn to food to quiet your mind and to relieve your sense of unease or even distress. In fact, you may not be surprised to learn that many binge eaters report that being bored is one of their primary triggers.

✔ **Situational:** If you have poor problem-solving skills, daily conflicts and/ or problems that arise may send you into something of a tailspin. That sense of fight or flight in common situations may be more than you can handle, and you may feel that if resolution feels out of reach, bingeing isn't.

And it's not just anger that may be problematic. Sadness and disappointment can also play a role in pushing you to binge. If someone says something that hurts your feelings, whether that person meant to or not, or you've been looking forward to something that just doesn't happen, you may turn to overeating to make yourself temporarily feel better.

✔ **Environmental:** One environmental risk factor is a past (or present) history of being bullied or abused in some way. Environmental triggers can also include exposure to various media which place a great emphasis on comments about weight or shape at any given time, expectations about the holidays, pressure to perform — be it at school, work, or in a competitive sport — or simply visual or olfactory cues like the food in the break room at work to the fast-food restaurants on your way home. Environmental triggers have a way of burrowing deeply into your being and can touch off thoughts and feelings that drive you to overeat whether you know it or not in the moment.

During a binge

Once a binge is set in motion, it's difficult, but not impossible, to stop. You may already know more than you'd like about the compulsion to numb your body and mind with food and eating and how powerful that impulse can be once you've begun.

The good news is that you can learn to recognize and override those impulses as part of a long-term plan to heal from disordered eating. As we repeat throughout this book, recovery is a slow and steady process that begins with gentle, incremental, manageable steps toward change. You may not be able to stop bingeing or compulsively overeating right away, but with the right therapeutic tools, time, and practice, you can slowly begin to shorten your binges and hopefully stop them altogether once you start to treat yourself with kindness and to understand what drives you to eat out of something other than physical hunger in the first place.

Eating to excess

It's natural when you begin to think about addressing and perhaps stopping your binge eating to concentrate on the amount of food you eat. Binge eating disorder does, after all, involve eating a larger amount of food than normal during a short period of time.

No matter how tempting it may be to make food the primary focus of your resolve to explore and hopefully cease binge eating, keep in mind that disordered eating isn't only about changing your relationship to food. It's about gently examining, understanding, and eventually altering the underlying thoughts, emotions, and behaviors causing you to use food in unhealthy ways.

Binge eaters eat very quickly, usually until they're uncomfortably or unbearably full, and in their haste, often do not chew their food well. They eat big portions even if they're not actually hungry, and they usually binge on foods that are high in fats, sugars, or both. Some bounce between flavors and textures such as starchy carbohydrates, creamy foods, sweets, fatty foods, or salty, crunchy snack foods. You may have heard such foods referred to as *comfort foods* or *beige foods.* These can seem comforting emotionally and physiologically for a variety of reasons, both real and imagined.

Most binge eaters don't binge on healthy foods, although some try to without much success. Sugars and fats, in obvious or hidden forms, are well-known to affect physiology and brain chemistry, which may drive the urge to continue eating long after satiation.

Don't be afraid to see a professional who specializes in treating patients with eating disorders such as a psychotherapist, physician, and/or a dietitian. Overcoming binge eating is a difficult but courageous undertaking and an initial consultation will help you get a peek at some of the insights and tools you'll need for the journey ahead, one which you need not travel alone. (See Chapter 10 for information on the professionals you may encounter.)

Other things that aren't strictly articulated as part of the clinical criteria for binge eating disorder but that often occur include

- ✔ Eating in bed or in other inappropriate places such as a bathroom
- ✔ Eating standing up in front of the refrigerator
- ✔ Eating directly out of boxes
- ✔ Eating in the car and while driving

Most importantly, those with binge eating disorder report a loss of control over what and how much they eat during a binge. Some claim they feel compulsively driven to eat — it's like an itch that must be scratched. The feelings binge eaters experience during and after overeating range all the way from intense pleasure to disgust.

Don't try to diagnose yourself. You probably know a lot about binge eating, but no matter how much you read in books, research on the Internet, or consult with other people, you're not in a good position to decide whether you suffer from binge eating or any other form of disordered eating. Although some people may be able to recover without professional help, many require support and guidance from a team of eating-disorder professionals to fully heal from short or long term binge eating.

Losing control

During the binge itself, sufferers often feel out of control or disconnected from their actions. And many describe a feeling of numbness that washes over them when bingeing. A binge may begin with the intention of just having a small or reasonable amount of a certain food. If the person then eats more than intended, it's common for binge eaters to think, "Oh well, I already messed up, so I might as well eat more," which for many turns into a full out binge episode. This is the classic all-or-nothing thinking that perpetuates and often seems to justify bingeing and overeating behaviors.

Binge eaters use food as a distraction from thoughts, feelings, or situations they find difficult to tolerate. If you're a binge eater, you've probably developed a habit of using food to distract, self-soothe, check-out, seek some relief from things that are happening in your present life, or as a way to disconnect from things that have happened in your past.

In addition to binging, you may have food thoughts to escape any or all intense feelings. For many with binge eating, the experience of planning and bingeing is a way to distract themselves. To make matters even more complicated, the guilt and shame after a binge also work as a distraction and keep a distance between the binger and experiencing life in a more fulfilling way.

After a binge

Even when a binge ends, it's not really over. The physical and psychological effects of chronic disordered eating are pervasive, and bingeing can slowly take over your life. Over time, bingeing and dealing with the consequences of bingeing can feel more urgent and become more important than other activities such as your professional life, your family life, time with friends, or pursuing hobbies and interests.

Feeling shame and guilt

The remorse that comes on after a binge can be intense. The chasm between what binge eaters know versus what they do can be deep and wide (our working definition of addiction), no more so than in the minutes and hours immediately after a binge when it feels as if there may not ever be a way to build a bridge between the two.

Shame and guilt are two hallmark emotions for binge eaters. Those who suffer from binge eating, compulsive overeating, and/or emotional eating often feel embarrassed and humiliated after an episode of bingeing. Most also experience anger, frustration, disgust, helplessness, and most often self-castigation for being unable to control their own eating. Ironically, these are some of the very feelings you may be trying to avoid by the very act of bingeing, so a binge eater's despair and self-loathing from the binge itself may drive him to turn yet again to food for comfort. The result is a vicious cycle that eventually leads to both physical and psychological problems including a significant level of depression. It often takes outside help from a treatment provider or team to overcome the negative self-talk and emotions that binge eating brings on.

Keeping a secret

Most people with binge eating disorder need treatment, but many people who have an eating disorder try to keep it a secret or deny that they have a problem. Bingeing is most often a solitary act; therefore, many binge eaters are able to keep it a secret. There are many reasons why someone with binge eating disorder eats in secret. The two most common are a sense of relief and calm that bingeing brings on for the binger and an overwhelming fear of being judged negatively for binging.

Secret eating involves someone intentionally separating or isolating from the world. By severing or markedly decreasing communication and emotional connections with friends and family, those with BED end up disconnecting from important parts of themselves because they feel so ashamed of their binges and their weight. For those suffering in silence, confiding in someone may feel like too much of a risk to take even with the most kind, compassionate, and nonjudgmental friends and family. The resulting shame and secrecy compounds the fear of being discovered and consequently rejected and abandoned.

Although many people suffer in silence and are never found out, keeping a secret over a long period of time ultimately undermines important relationships. Strong relationships are built on a bedrock of trust, and without it, it may be difficult to develop lasting intimacy and companionship, romantic or otherwise. Instead, a binge eater may spend a great deal of time covering up her behavior and ultimately eroding relationships from the inside out.

Feeling physical discomfort

Bingeing almost always leaves someone with physical discomfort and gastrointestinal distress. The human body is not equipped to rapidly digest a high volume of food and becomes easily overwhelmed. Generally, lethargy and fatigue sets in, and chronic bingeing can intensify feelings of depression, anger, sadness, and loneliness — all of which contribute to physical discomfort and disease development.

Perhaps the most critical consequence of binge eating is unwanted weight gain. Although some binge eaters maintain a normal weight, most who routinely binge eat become overweight or obese, which results in medical complications and conditions such as heart disease, high blood pressure, high cholesterol and triglycerides, diabetes, and back and joint pain. If a binge eater routinely consumes high-fat foods, he may also be at risk for gout, gall bladder and liver diseases, and certain types of cancers.

Purging for relief

Purging is brought about by the need to compensate for overeating by attempting to reduce the effects by vomiting, using laxatives, or over-exercising. It's also an attempt to decrease or eliminate the negative feelings associated with the overeating. Most binge eaters do not purge, and bingeing and purging are behaviors attributed to bulimia rather than binge eating disorder.

All or Nothing: Bingeing as a Way of Life

All-or-nothing thinking is one of the primary factors that can drive you to binge in the first place and may be perpetuating the dieting-bingeing-gaining weight cycle that's become so damaging to you. Seeing the world in black-and-white is something that's common to most people with eating disorders, and it's one of the principle targets you can consider focusing on if you want to make a change.

The distorted thinking that makes all-or-nothing thinking seem so reasonable to you is the same mindset that can drive the extremes of your eating and behaviors and may underlie some of the negative thoughts and feelings you have toward yourself and your body.

Some clues that you may be an all-or-nothing thinker:

- ✔ You often use the words *always, never,* or *every* to describe situations or people.
- ✔ You jump to conclusions with little or no supporting evidence from your life or your experience.
- ✔ You think habitually negative thoughts about yourself and others.
- ✔ You see a single negative event as a never-ending pattern of defeat.
- ✔ You anticipate that things will turn out badly.
- ✔ You feel a need to blame yourself or others as if everything must have a cause or culprit.
- ✔ You view yourself and others as good/bad or superior/inferior rather than simply accepting certain characteristics of being a human being or just being curious about them.

Just as you're thinking about changing your eating habits, you may also need to consider changing some of the more self-destructive ways you think about yourself, who you are, and what you can accomplish. As you read this book, we dedicate many sections to working in gentle, but productive ways to change negative thought patterns and establish new ones.

Deciding whether You Have Binge Eating Disorder — A Quiz

You've arrived at the moment of truth, but this quiz is just a starting point when it comes to identifying and changing the feelings and behaviors that may lead you to binge or compulsively overeat. No matter what your results, it's important to be gentle with yourself as you embark on this journey and acknowledge that admitting you have a problem is an important step toward a healthier, more stable life. So when you're ready, get pen and paper or open a note-taking app to record your answers to the following questions:

1. When I feel stressed or depressed, I eat large amounts of food without thinking about it.

   A. Most of the time

   B. Sometimes

   C. Rarely

2. When I overeat, I always promise myself I will never do it again.

   A. Most of the time

   B. Sometimes

   C. Rarely

3. When I start eating, I feel out of control and find it hard to stop eating.

   A. Most of the time

   B. Sometimes

   C. Rarely

4. I tend to keep food hidden, so others won't find out how much I eat.

   A. Most of the time

   B. Sometimes

   C. Rarely

5. I feel embarrassed about the amount of food I eat.

   A. Most of the time

   B. Sometimes

   C. Rarely

6. When I feel urges to eat excessive amounts of food I don't make healthy decisions about my food.

   A. Most of the time

   B. Sometimes

   C. Rarely

7. I prefer to eat alone.

   A. Most of the time

   B. Sometimes

   C. Rarely

8. When I'm upset or stressed, I want to eat even when I'm not hungry.

   A. Most of the time

   B. Sometimes

   C. Rarely

9. When I binge I stop feeling negative emotions, I feel numb.

   A. Most of the time

   B. Sometimes

   C. Rarely

10. I think about food even when I'm not hungry.

    A. Most of the time

    B. Sometimes

    C. Rarely

Tally up your score, giving yourself 1 point for every A answer, 2 points for every B, and 3 points for every C.

If your total is between

   10–14 points: You struggle with binge eating.

   15–23 points: You have binge-eating tendencies.

   24–30 points: You're not a binge eater.

If you scored between 10 and 14 points, you can benefit from this book. You may also wish to seek the advice and counsel of a trained eating disorder psychotherapist, medical doctor, psychiatrist and/or dietitian. This book alone can help you get started for sure but may not be enough to stop your binge eating.

If you scored between 15 and 23 points, this book can help you. You may want to consider meeting with a professional, but you can also try to gain an understanding of what drives your disordered eating and try to successfully change patterns on your own with our suggested tips and strategies.

If you scored between 24 and 30 points, you probably don't need this book for your own purposes, but even so, there are excellent strategies for just a tune-up in terms of your relationship to food and body image as well as helpful tips and routines for daily life. Also, if you know someone who struggles with binge eating, this book can be a highly valuable resource for supporting and helping that person move forward in her recovery from binge eating.

Chapter 3

Who Binges and Why

In This Chapter

▶ Considering the relationship between nature and nurture

▶ Looking at reasons the number of people who binge is growing

▶ Understanding physical and psychological triggers

▶ Answering the classic chicken-or-egg question about bingeing and psychological factors

There's no simple answer to the question of who binges and why. Unlike other eating disorders, the statistics for binge eating and other overeating disorders are not quite as clear cut as those for anorexia nervosa and bulimia (which we describe in Chapter 2).

Some research indicates the numbers are roughly split 60/40 between women and men and among races. And interestingly enough, although the bulk of binge eaters are middle aged, the rest of the population that suffers from binge eating disorder and/or compulsive overeating is divided fairly evenly among adolescents and older adults. A study by the U. S. National Institute of Mental Health reports that 3.5 percent of women and 2 percent of men will have BED in their lifetime.

As we state during the course of this chapter and this book, it takes a complex mix of genetic vulnerabilities, socioeconomic and environmental factors, emotional and psychological influences, and physical/medical conditions for binge eating or compulsive overeating to take hold of someone's life. In each and every case, the underlying causes and how they come together to trigger disordered eating are unique for each person.

Taking time to discover what triggers binge eating in general and then exploring what underlies your own specific binge behaviors is a critical step towards regaining balance in your own life and restoring your sense of well-being. You may already have a sense of what drives your eating behaviors or you may never have taken the time to consider what underlies your behavior. But in order to heal, learning about yourself and how you deal with stress, sadness, loneliness, anger, and other emotions and feelings can help you figure out how to replace binge eating as a coping mechanism and to move forward with your life.

In this chapter, we explore some of the factors that drive binge eating as well as the complex questions about whether nature, nurture, or both are at work in promoting binge-eating behaviors. We also examine the two primary types of trigger: physical and psychological.

Debating Nature versus Nurture

As the understanding of the human genome has expanded in the past several decades, so has the race to discover links between genes and disease. Never have scientists known so much about the role of heredity in determining mental and physical health. What people may have suspected for a long time about genetics and their relationship to medical and/or psychological conditions is being proven in ongoing studies, some of which show that obesity, eating disorders, and mental illness tend to run in families.

However, genetics is not destiny. Let us say that again — genetics is *not* destiny. Just because your mother or father suffered from depression or an addiction or even an eating disorder doesn't mean that you will. A family history of a disorder merely means that you have a greater likelihood of suffering from that condition or a similar one. You can't catch the disorder from someone or give it to anyone — it's not communicable so far as we know! Can you contribute inadvertently? Sure. Are you fated to suffer? No, but it's important to be realistic about the likelihood given certain circumstances. This is an important point to consider if you suffer from disordered eating and/or if you're the parent or loved one of someone who suffers. Forewarned is forearmed.

If you're feeling frustrated, angry, and hopeless about yourself and your relationship to food, it may be tempting to try to figure out who to blame for why you started bingeing or overeating. Whether binge eating occurs because of nature or nurture no one quite knows, and you may spend a lot of time and energy trying to answer an unanswerable question about whose fault it is. If you can set aside a need to blame someone, including yourself, you can focus on positive changes and a new start.

If you're thinking about making a change and putting a stop to binge eating, after you examine your family history and patterns, you may discover that some of them were set in motion when you were quite young. You may even discover family norms that were in place before you were born.

But as with all heritable tendencies, the family customs you grew up with may not serve you very well. The good news is that you don't have to live with them for your whole life. You may fear that old, ingrained habits and ways of thinking are holding you back from overcoming your eating disorder, but you can, in fact, change them and adopt new, healthier ways of living. It's not easy but it is simple. Making major changes can sometimes be painful or challenging, but with support, guidance, and concrete strategies and techniques, you can find ways to take charge of things and live a life you love in a healthy way.

Comparing Bingeing and Associated Disorders

The underlying emotions, triggers, and drives that define the four major eating disorders — anorexia nervosa, bulimia nervosa, other specified feeding or eating disorder (OSFED), and binge eating disorder — are far more similar than you may think. We explore the full range of the eating disorder spectrum in Chapter 5, but in the following sections, we outline the similarities and differences among the four.

Finding common ground

If you're suffering from disordered eating, it's likely that your behaviors and thinking may not always fall neatly into one diagnosis or the other. Instead, over time, you may travel along the eating disorder continuum from restricting your food intake to bingeing to purging to bingeing to gaining weight and cycle back again to restricting. What each of these points along the continuum have in common is an obsession with food and a distorted sense of your own body image, size, and appearance, and their overall importance in the scheme of life. In each phase, you have a need to feel a greater sense of control and a desire to find ways to numb yourself or self-soothe. These issues come to dominate your life in unhealthy ways.

For example, there's an overlap between people who suffer from bulimia and those who binge. In fact, bulimics are frequently binge eaters who attempt to rid their bodies of the food they've eaten through laxatives, vomiting, or the use of other compensatory behaviors. Both bulimia and binge eating disorder come about as attempts to cope, albeit unhealthy ones, and both do significant damage to both the mind and the body in the short and the long run.

Developing more than one disorder

Many people with an eating disorder experience more than one disorder due to the fact that there are some common and predictable shifts for long term sufferers. For example, more than one-third of people with anorexia nervosa go on to have bulimia nervosa. And if you're diagnosed with bulimia, you may have suffered from binge eating disorder in the past or may be more susceptible to it in the future. Moving along the continuum is one way for someone with an eating disorder to attempt to control behaviors, symptoms, or weight. The shifting between disorders can occur any time and for many different reasons.

Another possibility, although less common, is for binge eaters to diet and become anorexics after some weight loss and the experience of successfully controlling their minds and bodies. The sensation of control can be a first for binge or compulsive overeaters, and they may go too far. Unfortunately, this is sometimes the case after various forms of bariatric surgery and largely driven by fear. It's important to note that anorexia is not only defined within the context of total body weight as it pertains to weight loss, but also how much weight is lost over a certain period of time, total food intake, perception of oneself, and the tenacious need to be thin.

Binge eating to anorexia and back again

Sarah has struggled with binge eating her whole life. Now 31, she's obese and has been on more diets than she can count. After the death of her father, she lost her appetite, which was a new experience for her. Up until then, she had always been able to eat her way through her feelings, but something was different, and for the first time ever, she didn't cope with her sadness that way. Within the first month, she lost a significant amount of weight and began getting compliments about how great she looked. Even though she had longed to hear that kind of thing all her life, she felt ashamed and guilty for feeling good about the way she looked as a result of her father's death. Nevertheless, she joined a gym, started to see a personal trainer, and changed her eating habits even more.

Over time, her exercise increased to two-to-three hours a day, and she was eating very little. About eight months after her father died, Sarah had lost so much weight that she was in the normal range for her height. However, she stopped menstruating and was significantly malnourished. Although she wasn't anorexic according to height-to-weight ratio criteria, her doctor considered her dramatic weight loss and the associated thoughts and feelings to be anorexic-like and watched her cautiously.

Now, a year and a half after her father died, Sarah has started bingeing again. Within four months, she had gained back all the weight she lost and was bingeing most days. The reasons are many and varied no doubt, not the least of which is that she had spent so much time focusing on achieving a new body, she most likely never took the time to grieve the loss of her father. In addition, it's likely that her body and her emotions felt so restrictively deprived that the pendulum made its inevitable big swing.

Diagnosing a Rising — and Varied — Tide

With the change to the diagnostic criteria in the fifth edition of *Diagnostic and Statistical Manual of Mental Disorders (DSM-V),* binge eating disorder has finally been distinguished as its own diagnosis with its own specific criteria. As a result, the number of binge eaters is on the rise statistically as they are now being properly diagnosed and categorized. Not only have the diagnostic changes shifted statistics, but because binge eating disorder (BED) is now a recognized condition, more people are coming out of the shadows and seeking treatment.

Bingeing across genders

Much has been written about the ways in which young women are vulnerable to disordered eating due to factors such as hormonal changes that occur in adolescence, perceived high expectations for women and girls to be perfect and thin, messages conveyed in the media, and more. When these influences as well as inherited tendencies, psychology, and other circumstances collide, some young women turn to food or the avoidance thereof to ease the discomfort and angst of growing up and what it means physically and emotionally to leave girlhood behind and become a woman. The same is now also true in growing numbers for boys and men but not yet at the same rates as for females.

It's no secret that if you look at the numbers across the eating disorder continuum, more women suffer from anorexia, bulimia, binge eating disorder, and other specified feeding or eating disorder (OSFED) than men. However, unlike the other eating disorder diagnoses, binge eating disorder tends to be somewhat more evenly divided between the sexes for a multitude of reasons that support the idea that the underlying triggers may be extremely similar. Like women, men who suffer from binge eating disorder can also be overachievers and perfectionists or suffer from psychological conditions such as anxiety disorder, OCD (obsessive compulsive disorder), depression, substance abuse issues, or ADHD (attention deficit hyperactivity disorder).

Recognizing men who binge

Although men comprise an estimated 5 percent to 15 percent of people with anorexia or bulimia, current statistics suggest an estimated 40 percent of those with BED are male. Further, recent studies show that the overall incidence and prevalence of all forms of eating disorders are increasing among men.

It's hard to know if men have always suffered from disordered eating at these rates or if the number of men affected by disordered eating is rising simply because more men are coming forward and seeking treatment. Whatever the reasons, binge eating in men isn't that different from binge eating in women even though there's a tendency to try to separate out the sexes when researching and studying any sort of psychological condition.

The reality is that men and women are often exposed to both similar and uniquely different triggers, and men may suffer from the same psychological conditions that contribute to women's need to binge or compulsively over-eat. However, overeating of any kind may be more socially acceptable for men than for women in certain cultures and circumstances. This can be dangerous for men who have a problem because social convention may mask the fact that they need to seek treatment.

If you're interested in learning more about men and binge eating, Chapter 16 is dedicated to that topic. However, the strategies and techniques in the entire book apply equally to men and women, and both can be helped by the ideas in every chapter.

Focusing on older women

Just as hormonal shifts affect girls and young women during adolescence, a similarly dramatic change in hormone levels occurs as women experience perimenopause and menopause.

Fluctuating levels of estrogen, which occur during pregnancy, menstruation, and during menopause, can make a woman more vulnerable to having obsessive thoughts, anxiety, depression, fatigue, cramps, headaches, and hot flashes — to name a few. Every single one of these normal side effects a woman experiences as part of the hormonal changes during the course of her life is also a trigger for bingeing.

If you're a woman, be aware of your menstrual cycle and note the moods and feelings you have at different points throughout the month. These changes in your cycle can greatly affect bingeing symptoms.

Furthermore, the lives of women in their 40s, 50s, 60s, and beyond tend to be complicated by life challenges such as simultaneously caring for parents and children, working longer hours to pay for their children's education and/or to try to save for an ever more elusive retirement, and accepting the realities (and also privileges!) of aging in a society that places a great deal of emphasis on youth and beauty. (Cynthia M. Bulik explores these issues in *Midlife Eating Disorders: Your Journey to Recovery* published by Walker & Company.)

Knowing the numbers

Finding accurate statistics for eating disorders is difficult for many reasons. First, a large percentage of people who suffer with an eating disorder are secretive about it. Their family members and even close friends may be unaware of the problem. In addition, because eating disorders such as anorexia and bulimia were linked to relatively wealthy, well-educated young women between the ages of 14 and 25, when they were first identified, the general assumption was that if you didn't fall into this demographic, you were unlikely to be a sufferer.

Research proves that these generalizations are incorrect, but the numbers still largely depend on people coming forward and seeking treatment — something that continues to be difficult due to shame and stigma.

In our rapidly and ever-changing modern society, most people must reinvent themselves again and again during the course of a long life. For an older woman in particular, that can be challenging not only as she moves through different stages of her personal, family, and professional identities, but also because, statistically speaking, women tend to live longer than men. A woman with a male partner faces significant social, financial, logistical, and emotional changes if he passes away before she does.

Because binge eating is often a response to stress, depression, anxiety, and/ or isolation — all of which occur as people age — it's not a surprise that more older women (and men) turn to (or return to in some cases) disordered eating or other addictive behaviors as a way to cope. In addition physical factors such as thyroid problems or other undiagnosed medical conditions that come with age may be at work.

Growing numbers

Binge eating disorder may very well be the most common eating disorder, and diagnoses of the disorder are increasing. Although people of any age can suffer from varying degrees of binge eating disorder, it is in fact more common in adults. It's somewhat more common in women than in men. Statistics indicate that BED affects blacks as often as whites, but researchers don't yet know how often it affects people in other ethnic groups. The overall incidence, however, is on the rise across cultures.

The majority of those who suffer from binge eating, compulsive overeating, or emotional eating usually become overweight or obese. However, by no means are all those with BED overweight; some sufferers maintain what's considered a normal weight, but they can and do have the disorder.

Understanding Physical Triggers

Often, seemingly unrelated behaviors or biological processes can lead to bingeing for a varied set of reasons. Bingeing behaviors then develop in response to distorted perceptions of these events as well as myriad other contributing factors that can affect certain individuals in negative or troubling ways. Over time, the interplay between physical and psychological forces becomes stronger, and the tendency for patterns to repeat themselves and become habit can be very compelling.

No single trigger — the physical ones we talk about here, or the psychological and environmental triggers we discuss in upcoming sections — is enough to cause binge eating on its own, but when several come together, they can bring about a powerful compulsion to binge as a way to self-soothe and/or numb negative feelings. In many cases, you can't control what triggers may be present in your own life, but you can be aware of the forces driving you to eat out of something other than physical hunger. Just observing your feelings and behaviors is the start of being able to change them over time.

Wash, rinse, spin, repeat: The cycle of bingeing, obesity, and dieting

Do a survey of people on the street, and you're likely to discover that fully half or more are on a diet. Most adults and even many children have dieted repeatedly and will probably do so again. In a desperate attempt to avoid and/or live with the effects of prevalent high-fat, high-calorie processed foods that dominate the typical U.S. diet, and are becoming ever more available around the world, extreme and severe dieting trends and methods abound. Although such diets are inevitably futile and expensive, for those physically or psychologically susceptible to binge eating, dieting can be the primary gateway behavior that leads to further disordered eating and obsessive and unhealthy thinking about food, body, and self.

For this group, dieting can set off a pendulum swing between restricting food intake and bingeing that can become ingrained and result in a relentless cycle of dieting, bingeing, gaining weight, and then dieting again. The cycle often looks like this: in a desperate attempt to lose weight you refrain from eating all the foods you love and often not enough of the foods that would be beneficial. Eventually, desires and cravings become too difficult to override, which usually leads to binges on high quantities of unhealthy, refined, fatty, and/or sugary foods (often called *binge* or *comfort foods*). The temporary aftereffect of a binge often *feels like* a sense of relief. This is rather short-lived and in the long run, hardly worth the high as the subsequent feelings of shame, guilt, and embarrassment lead you right back into a binge.

Drinking alcohol and bingeing

If you're a binge eater, you may already know that alcohol is a trigger for bingeing on food (as well as on more alcohol). Alcohol reduces inhibitions and stimulates appetite. Alcohol is also a depressant, although most people don't think of it that way. It can grossly alter your mood, and, as you may know, strong negative feelings are one of the primary triggers for bingeing or compulsive overeating.

If becoming tipsy or even drunk doesn't trigger you to binge, the hangover the next day may. Often a hangover incudes fatigue, head/body aches, dehydration, inability to concentrate, and many other overall negative feelings, any of which may lead to a post-alcohol consumption binge.

Feeling hungry

Think about normal, healthy hunger. It happens to you every single day, probably several times a day. This natural reaction is a healthy and constant reminder of your body's need for nourishment. However, for binge eaters, hunger signals are hard to recognize and often get confused with feeling starved.

During the course of treatment for BED or related eating disorder, one of the primary nutritional goals is to eat at regular intervals so as not to experience extreme levels of hunger. Even if you don't seek professional nutritional counseling, consider eating regular meals and snacks so that by modulating normal hunger, you can also successfully modulate binges. This, of course, also requires that you eat your regular meal in a mindful and moderately paced way.

Sensing Psychological Triggers

Binge eating or any kind of compulsive overeating isn't something that materializes overnight. The seeds of the psychological, environmental, biological, and genetic factors that drive you to eat out of something other than physical hunger may have been present as early as birth, may have developed in childhood, or may have only taken root as you grew and changed during adolescence, young adulthood, and beyond.

Understanding your unique psychological triggers is important as you consider moving forward and leaving binge eating or compulsive overeating behind. If you can begin to recognize the situations, feelings, and circumstances that make bingeing feel as if it's the only option, then you can begin the process of learning how to anticipate and counteract those impulses while developing new habits along the way.

That's not to say it will be easy, but with a gradual and gentle approach to managing and eventually replacing your negative thoughts and behaviors toward food, eating, and your body, you can recover and live a healthier, more peaceful life.

As you discover more about yourself and understand more about why you use eating as a way to soothe yourself, try to resist the urge to place blame on any one individual (including yourself), situation, or feeling. By cultivating a gentle, loving curiosity about who you are, you lay the groundwork for a life in which you don't have to live with overwhelming shame, guilt, anger, and seemingly uncontrollable urges.

Seeing the body for what it isn't

When you look in the mirror, what do you see? For many binge eaters, it's difficult if not impossible to align their own negative perceptions of their bodies with reality. Depending on the underlying reasons you binge, you may feel a deep sense of shame or disgust about your physical being. Bingeing may seem like a way to suppress those feelings, but ultimately, overeating in any form only serves to reinforce those perceptions.

Comparing yourself to others

You know that comparing yourself to others in any arena is ultimately a no-win situation. What may seem to be a source of healthy motivation and competition is more often than not a source of debilitating envy and discouragement. People who perpetually measure themselves against others are rarely able to find the true sources of their own self-worth and often are unable to acknowledge their own attributes or accomplishments.

Measuring yourself against others becomes particularly problematic when it comes to body image and weight. In most of the English-speaking world, being thin is prized, and that ideal is enforced in the media, in various social circles, and most pervasively in your own mind. Of course, the paradox is that health and beauty are uniquely individual to each person. To coin a cliché, beauty truly does lie in the eye of the beholder.

Unfortunately, people who suffer from disordered eating of any kind tend to see only their deficiencies, finding it much more natural and productive to criticize all that is wrong with themselves (and others) rather than to acknowledge and be grateful for all that is positive and possible. As you can imagine, this despair and hypercriticism perpetuates the binge behaviors the sufferer reviles, and the negative self-image may in fact be a primary source of a binge-eater's problems. Such a lack of self-worth also makes even more elusive any sense of hope or possibility that life may someday be better.

Feeling blue

Depression is one of the known triggers for binge eating, and it comes in many forms. *Situational depression* can appear as the result of a specific or traumatic event; *chronic depression,* with its many causes and contributing factors, can be part of your life for years. Either way, some people use food in an attempt to ease feelings of despair, emptiness, and hopelessness.

Unfortunately, binge eating or compulsive overeating of any kind tends to make depression worse, not better. Really take that in for a minute. Perhaps intellectually this makes perfect sense. But emotionally, it's hard to remember that the very thing you thought would ease your sadness actually makes it worse. In the long run, the shame, guilt, and hopelessness that bingeing tends to bring on can make your depression significantly worse. Which causes which? It's a chicken-versus-egg question to which the answer is both. Yes, both depression and binge eating, (and anxiety for that matter), feed each other. It's impossible to find the starting point when looking at the infinite number of points that comprise a circle.

In the past, talking about depression was taboo, but many physicians routinely screen their patients for mental illness during physicals, so if you've seen a doctor recently, you may have already discussed the possibility of a link between disordered eating and depression. Whether you've been diagnosed with depression or have never considered it as a possible reason to overeat, as you continue your journey, you may need or want to tackle this problem as part of your plan to stop bingeing.

Fighting the big B — Boredom

Ask any binge or compulsive eater what's her biggest trigger and almost all say, "Boredom." But boredom is a perception and nothing more. Boredom is really just an inability to or discomfort with being with yourself and your thoughts. It's also an inability to just be — to simply relax and enjoy the moment. It's funny that if, heaven forbid, you were told that you had a short time to live, you would likely savor time. Yet when time feels endless, boredom results from the fear of having too much of it.

At the beginning, overeating may simply be a way to pass the time, but over time, you may come to depend on bingeing as a way to avoid any uncomfortable sensation. When bingeing becomes a habit, it's usually difficult to stop.

Losing track of routine

Life inevitably includes some routines, deadlines, and milestones. As a child, adolescent, and young adult, you probably lived with the structure of school and the demands of homework, but as you get older and your familiar routines change or are disrupted, you can find yourself vulnerable to binge eating.

This disruption is most pronounced when someone goes away to college and no longer has the predictable structure of home and family life but instead must forge new paths and relationships. A similar set of challenges often occurs when you enter the work force for the first time and face creating new schedules and routines. Further along the developmental timeline, empty nesters may find themselves at loose ends when their children go to college or when they retire and no longer have the same perceived sense of purpose, identity, and routine.

Whether these major shifts lead to feelings of depression, sadness, boredom, or a sense of being lost in the world, they can also prompt you to turn to food to make yourself feel better, to fill a void, or to create order in what feels like a chaotic storm. This common reaction is one you may have the inner resources to resolve on your own, but it can also be effectively addressed and worked through in a therapeutic setting.

Experiencing Environmental Triggers

Environmental triggers vary from person to person, day-to-day, and hour-to-hour. An *environmental trigger* describes an external situation, event, or location that causes a negative reaction that leads to the need to use unhealthy but automatic soothing behaviors. For example, seeing a billboard for a burger and fries may be a trigger that awakens the urge to binge for one person; another person has the binge urge along with a sense of panic and anxiety when he gets a call to go to the boss' office. Or perhaps it's simply getting some bad news that seems too hard to wrap your mind around. Maybe you could handle any one of these situations on its own, but seeing the billboard after being reprimanded by your boss or getting bad news and having to deal with your boss on the same day is too much to handle.

Knowing what factors in your environment may trigger an urge to binge can help you plan how to handle those situations.

Chapter 4

Physical and Psychological Effects

*D*isordered eating has far-reaching effects on the body and mind. As we say over and over again in this book, eating disorders aren't only about food, eating, and the body; they're an expression of deeper, unresolved psychological issues. You try to manage or avoid these issues though the use and abuse of food and your body. So it's not enough to look only at how binge eating breaks down your physical being. You also need to consider how disordered eating and its consequences have impacted the way your mind and your emotions affect your perceptions of yourself and the world around you.

On the physical side of things, it's pretty straightforward to understand how binge eating, compulsive overeating, and emotional eating take a toll. Although some binge eaters maintain a normal weight, most become over-weight or obese. Excess weight gain leads to myriad health problems, many of them chronic, such as high cholesterol, type 2 diabetes, and heart disease, but carrying extra weight can also impair the activities of daily life, making it difficult and sometimes painful to move around.

Not being able to participate fully in activities with family and friends and feeling limited by your own body exacts its own emotional price. And that's one of the primary reasons that understanding the psychological compo-nent of binge eating isn't quite as simple as looking at the physical effects. Although binge eating and disordered overeating often go together with depression, anxiety, and other psychological conditions, it's difficult to say that one is the definitive cause of the other. Instead, the two create a vicious cycle in which you eat to soothe negative emotions but in the process create other unwanted feelings such as shame and regret due to the actual binge behaviors that were meant to soothe.

In this chapter, we explore the physical effects of binge eating, focusing primarily on conditions associated with obesity and overeating in general. We also talk about binge eating's effects on the mind, on emotional states, and on relationships.

Harming the Body

Over time, the effects of binge eating can impact every system in your body including your cardiovascular, endocrine, digestive, and musculoskeletal systems to name a few. Whether these effects are temporary or permanent largely depends on the length of time you binge and how frequently the episodes occur. However, eating disorders are progressive, and without treatment or intervention, they usually get worse over time as the thinking that drives them becomes more entrenched and the behaviors become more habitual.

Stretching the stomach

One of the hallmarks of binge eating is the uncomfortable, even painful, feeling in your stomach during and after a binge. In fact, if you're a chronic binge eater, severe discomfort may be the only thing that makes you realize that you must stop eating and brings you back from the feeling of being numb, out of control, and powerless over food and the emotions that may have led you to eat out of something other than physical hunger in the first place.

Even mild to moderate overeating can stretch the stomach up to three times its normal size, but compulsive overeating, emotional eating, and particularly binge eating can have serious side effects. Over time, a stretched stomach can hold more and more food, thus requiring more calories and greater volume to feel full. A gradual increase in stomach size or capacity can lead directly to weight gain, which may eventually cause overweight if not obesity.

Binge eaters are also susceptible to other conditions that may damage the digestive system including

✔ **Acid reflux and heartburn:** *Acid reflux* is a condition in which the muscles between the stomach and esophagus, also known as the *esophageal sphincter,* do not function properly and allow food, liquid, and stomach acid to flow back into the esophagus. In the case of a binge eater, acid reflux usually occurs due to overstuffing, which leads the muscle to become blocked so that it cannot perform its usual function.

One of the most common side effects of acid reflux is *heartburn,* an inflammation of the esophagus that causes a painful burning sensation. Often severe heartburn is mistaken for a heart attack. Long-term or repeated instances of heartburn may also damage the delicate tissue that lines your esophagus, leading to ulcers, heightened sensitivity to food and eating, and even esophageal cancer.

✔ **Gas, bloating, constipation, diarrhea:** The human body isn't equipped to digest a great deal of food all at one time. Bingeing can be extremely taxing to the digestive system, resulting in inefficient function, slow digestion, malabsorption, and unpleasant side effects that may persist for hours or up to several days.

✔ **Nausea:** A common side effect from any kind of overeating, nausea is one of the first signs that the stomach is overly full. Depending on how long you've been bingeing and the severity of your disordered eating, you may or may not developed the habit of ignoring the sensation of nausea, which tells you that you've eaten more than your stomach can handle.

✔ **Pain:** Although stomach size varies from person to person, human stomachs generally have a volume of about one liter, which is a little bit more than one quart. Binge eating may cause intense stomach pain due to pressure on the stomach walls if you eat more than this. Many bingers become familiar with the pain and discomfort caused by their binge episodes and eat through them or take short breaks to allow the stomach to empty a bit so that they can eat more.

✔ **Stomach rupture:** You may have wondered to yourself during a binge if it's possible for your stomach to explode. Many bingers have asked themselves this question at least once. Although it's an extremely rare scenario, a severe incident of binge eating occasionally leads to esophageal or stomach tearing or rupture, which is a medical emergency and may result in death due to infection when the stomach's contents seep into the abdominal cavity.

Without a doubt, bingeing takes a toll on the entire digestive system, but the good news is that even a dramatically stretched stomach can return to normal size over time. It may take a couple of days or a couple of weeks of not bingeing and eating normal-size meals to feel a difference. However, it's much easier on your body to eat smaller, more frequent meals while you heal, get used to new eating habits, and while the stomach returns to a more normal size. With time and improved nutrition, you will once again be able to respond to your body's biological signs of both hunger and feeling satisfied.

Eating to obesity and all of its risk factors

Although some binge eaters maintain a normal weight, the vast majority suffer from overweight and obesity. In addition to the multitude of medical risks associated with this condition. For many obese people, overall quality of life is affected as well.

Throughout this book and specifically in Chapter 20, we explore the relationship between obesity and bingeing and outline some of the strategies you may want to try if you're struggling with both weight and binge-eating issues.

Lowering your quality of life

No matter how you slice it, being obese can make day-to-day life difficult, and that's particularly true if your weight is a result of binge eating or another form of overeating. Dealing with both physical discomfort and the emotional conditions that triggered you to binge can make it feel as if you're carrying the weight of the world, not only on your shoulders, but also in your mind, heart, and body.

Some weight-related issues that may affect your overall quality of life include

- ✔ Physical disabilities
- ✔ Physical discomfort when moving around
- ✔ Sexual functioning or resistance to intimacy
- ✔ Sleep disturbances
- ✔ Social isolation

Most obese people are not able to do the things they enjoyed when they were at a normal weight. In general, life is harder both physically and emotionally for someone who is obese. If you've become obese during the months and years you've been bingeing, you may have trouble participating in family activities or socializing with friends. You may avoid public places. You may even encounter discrimination. In addition, you may be affected by low self-esteem and suffer from other more serious mental health problems such as depression and anxiety among others.

To make matters worse, bias against overweight and particularly against obese people may be one of the last acceptable forms of prejudice, particularly in Western societies but also around the world. Whether consciously or subconsciously, many assume that obese people are to blame for their own condition and take for granted that obesity is a sign of a lack of will power, overindulgence, or laziness.

Finally, obese people tend to have fewer social plans and romantic relationships compared to others due to social isolation, shame, and other factors
that negatively impact participation in their families and communities. One
insidious component of both discrimination and isolation is that career
and earning potential are often negatively affected by obesity and for obese
women in particular.

Impacting your health

The effects of obesity on physical health are well-known, well-studied, and a
frequent source of public conversation and debate in countries all over the
world, due in large part to the rising rates of both obesity and the accompanying medical conditions that result.

The World Health Organization (WHO) reports that 65 percent of the world's
population live in countries where overweight and obesity kills more people
than underweight. In 2010, the Stanford Hospital reported that obesity causes
up to 300,000 premature deaths a year in the United States alone. The poor
eating habits that typically plague people who struggle with binge eating,
compulsive overeating, and emotional eating can lead to serious long-term
health conditions. Most are the result of obesity and include but are not limited to

- ✔ Arthritis/Osteoarthritis
- ✔ Certain types of cancer including cancer of the uterus, cervix, ovaries,
  breast, colon, rectum, and prostate
- ✔ Decreased mobility, joint pain/swelling
- ✔ Fatigue
- ✔ Fatty liver
- ✔ Gallbladder disease or gallstones
- ✔ Gastro esophageal reflux disease (GERD)
- ✔ Gout
- ✔ Heart disease
- ✔ Herniated discs
- ✔ Hiatal hernia
- ✔ High blood pressure
- ✔ High cholesterol
- ✔ Menstrual problems and fertility problems
- ✔ Poor wound healing

- ✔ Shortness of breath
- ✔ Sleep apnea
- ✔ Stroke
- ✔ Type 2 diabetes

Depending on how long and how frequently you've been bingeing, you may have already either experienced some of these conditions, received warnings from your physician about them, or done your own research about the risks to your physical health.

As we say many times in this book, putting a stop to binge eating isn't just about gathering more information and knowing more. You probably know plenty right now. Making a change is about bridging the elusive gap between what you know and what you do.

Educating you about the potential risks of obesity and bingeing is part of our responsibility as eating disorder professionals, but we know that it's rarely an effective strategy to scare someone who binge eats with the threat of disease. Besides, we're willing to bet that you've heard it all before from your doctor or perhaps from well-meaning friends or relatives.

Instead, our plan for you and for this book is to lay out the information you need to know but more importantly, to provide practical, real life strategies to help you cope with stress, anxiety, and all of life's difficulties without turning to food.

Going up, up, up: The rising incidence of chronic conditions

Obesity doesn't affect just the individual; it also affects society, healthcare costs, and the social fabric of our communities. At the same time, obesity has deep roots in demographic differences, societal and familial expectations, and socio-economic factors. Although it may be tempting to focus only on the ways obesity has affected rising healthcare costs (certainly it has played an often-discussed and well-studied role), an obesity epidemic has also come about due to a complex set of forces that has been growing and developing over time and seems to have exploded during the past few decades.

As you probably know, obesity has direct effects on overall health and disability and markedly impacts the increasing rates of chronic diseases such as diabetes and heart disease. The World Health Organization (WHO) states that "obesity and overweight pose a major risk for chronic diseases, including type 2 diabetes, cardiovascular disease, hypertension and stroke, and certain forms of cancer," that reduce quality of life and cause sizeable healthcare costs. In short, obesity itself is the primary and most substantial risk factor for many other chronic diseases.

The socio-economic contributors to obesity are complicated at best. Many studies have attempted to explain the development of an *obesogenic environment*, which simply means that the combination of industrialization and rapid economic growth has resulted in more sedentary work and leisure activities as well as less activity overall for most people. The reduction in physical activity coupled with dietary changes during the past half century, such as the consumption of higher calorie foods with more fat and sugars, are all part and parcel of a culture that promotes obesity.

Dem bones, dem bones: Facing structural damage from chronic overweight

Just as overweight and obesity can strain other systems in the body, they also tax the musculoskeletal system by accelerating wear and tear on the bones, joints, and spine.

Osteoarthritis of the knees is particularly common among individuals suffering from excessive weight gain, and obese people have difficulty with many issues related to mobility. Squatting, a motion required for sitting down and standing up from a chair or car, is particularly troublesome as are walking, running, and climbing stairs.

Biomechanically, the knees bear the brunt of the pressure on the body because when you walk, the force between the kneecap and the rest of the knee is about three times your body weight. When someone with knee problems performs even more strenuous activities, the force on the knees can reach six to ten times their body weight. For example, the force on a 200-pound (90.7 kilograms) person's knees while walking is 600 pounds (272 kilograms), and when climbing, running, or squatting, the force can be up to 2,000 pounds (907.2 kilograms). Multiply those numbers by the number of years a person has been overweight, and you get excessive wear, pain, swelling, and eventually arthritis.

In addition to knee problems, obesity also affects the spine. Abdominal obesity, in particular, causes compression of the spinal column, which leads to back pain and disc bulging. Over time, carrying around excess weight in your abdomen is like constantly wearing a 50-pound (22.6 kilogram) backpack backwards for years at a time. The spine hasn't evolved to support that kind of weight, and eventually it becomes compressed, causing herniated discs.

Although losing weight can't reverse all the damage to joints and bones that can be caused by overweight and obesity, research shows that even moderate weight loss can have a dramatic effect on the relief of joint pain.

Confusing your metabolism

If you're in the throes of a struggle with binge eating or any kind of overeating, you've probably wondered if you've somehow damaged your metabolism. You're not alone. One of the primary fears of most people with an eating disorder is that by using eating as a way to cope with emotional difficulties, you've done irreparable damage to your metabolic system. You may have even fallen into the pattern of thinking, "Oh well, my metabolism is already slow anyway. I might as well go on eating." If you recognize this kind of all-or-nothing thinking, read on.

The good news is that it's pretty much impossible for you to permanently damage your body's ability to regulate its metabolic rate. Certainly, when you're bingeing or overeating, your metabolism likely isn't working as well as it could be, but it's not accurate to think of it as permanently broken. In reality, your metabolism is ready and waiting to be activated again, but it needs some TLC to get going.

Extreme patterns of eating work against your metabolism for a period of time but not forever. Consistent healthy eating patterns help your body readjust itself.

Think of your metabolism as a wood-burning stove or fireplace. If you've ever used a fireplace to keep warm on a cold winter's night, you probably lit it with a small amount of kindling, then kept it burning bright and hot for hours by throwing small logs on it at regular intervals. And you probably know that if you were to throw a huge log on the fire, it would smoke, fizzle out, and not burn very well. That's exactly how your metabolism reacts when you binge. It's not that your body has lost the potential to burn energy forever, but rather that it can't burn evenly when you're feeding it too much — or not enough.

Once you reduce and eventually stop bingeing altogether, your metabolic rate returns to a normal range. Of course, many factors can affect your metabolism: hormone-based conditions such as hypothyroidism, polycystic ovary syndrome (PCOS), and others as discussed in Chapter 18. If you've been diagnosed with one of these endocrinological conditions or any medical problem, you can work with your doctor to develop a plan specific to your situation.

Even if you're not suffering from any particular medical condition, rebalancing your physical being and restoring your metabolism requires patience, understanding, and loving kindness toward your body and the natural process it's undergoing. Of course, you're hoping for instant results, but your body needs time to heal. Realizing and accepting the gradual nature of this process is an important part of the new approach you're taking.

Working with a registered dietitian (RD) who has experience with eating disorders can help you feel calm and confident during this time of transition. An RD can collaborate with you about what and how to eat to recover your metabolic rate and how to slowly add moderate physical activity to your life. You may need to make adjustments to your meal plan over time, but with support and persistence, change is possible.

In order to reenergize your metabolic rate, start by observing these three key practices:

✔ **Discover how to recognize your true hunger signals.** This seems simple, but it's actually one of the most difficult challenges you face if you've spent years unable or unwilling to respond to your body's hunger cues. Many binge eaters find they can't tell the difference between physical hunger and emotional hunger, and so they eat without knowing or understanding what they need to sustain themselves. Many also confuse hunger, fatigue, and thirst cues, so it's important to mindfully check in with yourself about which is really the primary need.

With practice, you can begin to recognize when your body truly needs sustenance and when you want to eat out of something other than physical hunger. Over time, your awareness will grow, and you can learn for the first time or relearn what physical signs appear when you really need to eat for health and energy.

✔ **Eat well-balanced meals throughout the day.** If you've been bingeing for some time, it may feel scary or even counterintuitive to eat throughout the day. You may be thinking, "What? Eat throughout the day instead of saving my calories for my night eating? Then, I'll truly become as big as a house!" In fact, the reverse is true. Eating regularly can very effectively disrupt the pendulum swing between restricting and bingeing that's been dominating your life, your eating, and your behavior.

Although your ultimate goal may be eating three meals and two snacks every day, you need not master this immediately to have success in the long run. In fact, making radical changes from one day to the next can ultimately undermine your objectives if you feel the changes you're making aren't manageable or realistic.

Instead, break your day down into segments — dare we say bite-size portions? — and make changes you feel you can stick to. For example, rather than trying to eat three meals right away, you can start by eating breakfast within 30 minutes of waking every day for two weeks. Once you feel that you've integrated that habit into your life, then you can broaden the scope of your plan.

We discuss these issues in depth throughout this book, but if you're interested in finding out more about getting started with a recovery plan and nutrition, you can refer to Chapters 7 and 12, respectively.

✔ **Eat nutritious foods.** If you're in the habit of eating high-calorie, high-fat foods both when you binge and as a part of your daily life, you may want to rethink your habits and slowly introduce more nutritious alternatives.

First and foremost, you need to stock your fridge with healthy, high-fiber, nutrient-dense foods, and then you may need to work on actually getting into the habit of eating them. If you've spent years craving and eating junk food, you may need to retrain your body and brain to enjoy different tastes, smells, and textures. Not every healthy food will appeal to you, but keep in mind that being flexible and curious is an important part of putting a stop to your binge eating.

Clouding the Mind

When it comes to binge eating's relationship to psychological conditions, it's ill-advised to make neat assumptions about cause and effect. At the beginning, binge eating may have worked as a strategy to soothe yourself and calm feelings such as sadness, loneliness, anger, or stress. There may also have been influences and conclusions you drew that you weren't consciously aware of in the moment. It's only over time that binge eating becomes less and less effective as a way to temporarily resolve your emotional issues. In fact, it may become a problem in and of itself rather than something that helped you cope.

Without taking time to address the underlying psychological and emotional issues that caused you to binge in the first place, you may feel permanently stuck in the cycle of negative emotions that trigger binges and compulsive overeating. It's only when you break that cycle that you may begin to understand and reimagine yourself, your body, and your place in the world.

Although it's possible to slowly work through issues on your own, you may want to consider seeing a psychotherapist who specializes in eating disorders if you can. We discuss how to research eating disorder professionals in Chapter 10 and offer ideas for other kinds of treatment and support throughout this book.

Shifting personality and mood

By now, you know that many factors contribute to what we loosely call *cravings*. It's the old chicken-and-egg story (although neither chicken nor eggs are common food triggers as far as we know!). In other words, are you overeating because you're sad, anxious, or avoiding/experiencing so many other emotions and eating makes you feel tired and unmotivated, and so on. Or are inherent physiological issues such as unstable blood sugar, hormonal abnormalities, digestive abnormalities, and the like that contribute to your propensity to overeat? Even though it feels as if it would be easier to point to one or the other, the truth is that your triggers and the binges themselves are more likely a cyclical combination of all of the above. Everything feeds off of everything else, both physically and emotionally.

As we explore in later chapters in this book, research shows that binge eaters often suffer from other psychological disorders that compound the difficulties inherent in their disordered eating. To name just some of the more common ones

- ✔ ADHD (attention deficit hyperactivity disorder)
- ✔ Anxiety in its many forms
- ✔ Bipolar disorder (across the spectrum)
- ✔ Depression in its many forms
- ✔ OCD (obsessive-compulsive disorder)
- ✔ PTSD (post-traumatic stress disorder)

Just because you have unresolved psychological issues doesn't mean that you'll turn to food to cope with them. However, if food does happen to be your weapon of choice, so to speak, addressing and treating any psychological vulnerabilities can have a significant and beneficial effect on the feelings that drive you to binge or overeat.

Impacting relationships

One of the struggles you may face is the sense of shame and secrecy you experience about your eating behaviors. As your bingeing became more frequent and perhaps more severe, you may have retreated from the world as a way to protect yourself from the criticism and scrutiny not only from friends and family but also from complete strangers and the world at large.

At times, everyone gets tired and wants to stay home and hibernate, but if you've ever cancelled an outing with friends because you have nothing to wear that fits properly or ignored the phone because you're in a post-binge haze, you may already know that you're isolating yourself for different reasons.

As with any psychological conditions that accompany and exacerbate binge eating or any disordered eating, isolation tends to build on itself over time. Unfortunately, spending more and more time alone tends to reinforce negative or hypercritical feelings about yourself and your perceptions about how you think other people see you.

Isolation affects both personal and professional relationships. You may have experienced some of these common scenarios:

- ✔ **In your personal life:** Because binge eating profoundly affects your self-image, if you feel terrible about yourself and your body, you may have withdrawn from your partner. You may be protecting yourself, but you may also have come to feel that you're not worthy of love and affection — two ideas that, in addition to not being true, may rob you of the emotional support you need.

- ✔ **In your family life:** Binge eating reaches into all aspects of family life, whether that be in the family you've created for yourself or in your family of origin. You may avoid family get-togethers for fear of criticism, or you may be worried that you're passing on a predisposition for disordered eating to your own children. Whatever your concerns, you take on more than your fair share of blame, which tends to make you feel even worse.

- ✔ **In your professional life:** Whether your self-esteem was low before you started binge eating or it plunged after you turned to overeating as a coping mechanism, feeling bad about yourself keeps you from asserting yourself in professional situations. You may be so preoccupied with eating and with what others may think of you that you can't do your best work. And not doing your best work may prevent you from getting ahead at your job. Unfortunately discrimination may also be a factor.

Be assured that, no matter where you are in this process, you're not alone and there are ways to put binge eating behind you and live a fuller, healthier, and happier life.

Chapter 5

Distinguishing Binge Eating Disorder from Other Eating Disorders

*I*f you live in the Western world, you live in a culture obsessed with thinness and dieting, and many men and women across the United States and around the world fall into the trap of equating their self-worth with how slim they are. For many people, it doesn't go any further than that; they go on with their lives, and although they do think about their bodies and their weight at times, worrying about food and body image doesn't necessarily get in the way of living well and enjoying all that life has to offer.

Unfortunately, many individuals become entangled in the complicated and dangerous web of disordered eating. Although anorexia nervosa (AN), bulimia nervosa (BN), other specified feeding or eating disorder (OSFED), and binge eating disorder (BED) all express themselves differently, they have much in common. They can be triggered by many different factors, but oftentimes, it's the combination of biology, hereditary or genetic likelihoods or vulnerabilities, life circumstances, and underlying psychological conditions that creates the fertile ground in which eating disorders can put down roots and grow.

Why some people are more susceptible than others is still a complex question. Certainly after an eating disorder has been diagnosed, it's possible to go back and figure out what may have led someone to use an unhealthy relationship to food and body to cope with difficulties in her life. However, it's impossible to pinpoint just one reason — that lightning bolt moment or magic answer — that draws a person to disordered eating and its accompanying thoughts and behaviors as a way to self-soothe.

We focus primarily on binge eating disorder, emotional eating, and compulsive overeating throughout this book, but in this chapter we discuss the other three most common eating disorders — anorexia nervosa (AN), bulimia nervosa (BN), and what's called other specified feeding or eating disorder (OSFED) — to provide the backdrop for the continuum of disordered eating on which binge eating lies. For each diagnosis, we review the signs and symptoms, the associated behaviors, and some of the psychological and medical consequences. We give careful attention to what they have in common and also show you more about what makes the disorders and the individuals who suffer from them different from one another.

Traveling Along the Eating Disorder Continuum

Although each of the three eating disorders is undoubtedly different from the others, anorexia, bulimia, and binge eating disorder lie on a continuum along which many sufferers travel during the months and years that they may use restricting food intake, overeating, and/or purging as a way to cope with psychological conditions such as anxiety, obsessive-compulsive disorder (OCD), distorted body image, depression, and ADHD among many others.

As we've said before and we'll say many times again, eating disorders aren't really about food, eating, or weight. They're actually an expression of psychological and emotional distress in which the sufferer uses food as a way to cope with difficult situations — food, or fear of food, is just the weapon of choice, if you will.

Although we don't know exactly why someone gravitates toward one eating disorder or another, many working theories suggest that a combination of factors such as personality, temperament, genetic and/or biological factors, family culture, learned behaviors, and other psychological conditions can play a part in the underlying drive to use one's relationship to or perceptions of food and body as a way to express emotional or psychological pain.

Although explicit diagnostic criteria exist for each disorder, there can be overlap in the thoughts and behaviors of all eating disorder sufferers. In the next sections, we talk about the specifics of each of these illnesses and help you understand how all four are related.

We use definitions and criteria from the fifth edition of the *Diagnostic and Statistical Manual of Mental Disorders (DSM-V)* as a jumping-off point for our discussion. Published by the American Psychiatric Association, the *DSM's* classifications are reviewed and updated periodically, most recently in May 2013 with the publication of the *DSM-V*. The *DSM* is important because it provides common language and diagnostic criteria for medical and psychological professionals in the United States and around the world. Along with several other revisions and additions, the most recent edition included binge eating disorder as an official diagnosis for the very first time. This matters not only because it is an acknowledgment of the experience of millions of sufferers but also because the diagnosis opens up the possibility of more favorable insurance reimbursement for treatment.

Exploring Anorexia Nervosa

If you're a binge eater, emotional eater, or compulsive overeater, you may be asking yourself what anorexia could possibly have to do with you. From the outside, it may seem that you can't have anything in common with someone who starves himself, but the fact of the matter is that you've much more in common than you think.

If you've ever participated in the dieting-bingeing-gaining weight cycle, and chances are that you have, then you know what it means to restrict or limit your calories in an effort either to lose weight or to compensate if you think you've overeaten. Perhaps the period of time in which you've controlled your eating may have been briefer than that of someone who suffers from anorexia, but the emotional experience is probably very similar.

What's more remarkable and more important is understanding what's going on at the root of things. Eating disorder sufferers are often plagued by emotions and impulses that dominate their lives. On the outside, an anorexic and a binge eater may seem very different; on the inside, they both suffer from all-or-nothing thinking and understand themselves and their self-worth only through the hypercritical lens of how much they weigh, eat, don't eat, or how they think others see them.

Understanding what it means to be anorexic

Anorexia nervosa is a complex emotional disorder that affects both mind and body. Over time, anorexics become obsessed with a need to lose weight at all costs.

As stated in the *DSM-V,* anorexia can be diagnosed if the following criteria are present:

- ✔ **A restriction of energy intake (also known as calories):** Intense restriction of deprivation of calories can lead to a significantly low body weight. Significantly low weight is defined as a weight that is less than minimally normal or, for children and adolescents, less than that minimally expected.

- ✔ **Intense fear of gaining weight or becoming fat:** This phobia manifests itself even though the sufferer may be normal weight, underweight, or severely malnourished.

- ✔ **A distortion in the way the sufferer sees her body:** A disturbance in the way the anorexic person sees her body weight or shape, placing too much emphasis on body weight or shape when evaluating herself, and/or denying how serious the problem has become.

Furthermore, the DSM-V defines two types of anorexia nervosa:

- ✔ **Restricting type:** If you're suffering from this form of anorexia, you control your weight only by cutting calories, restricting your food intake, and over exercising.

- ✔ **Bingeing/purging type:** In this form of anorexia, you cannot tolerate eating food in any amount even though you try to do so. You then attempt to purge what you eat, through vomiting or the use of laxatives, diuretics, or enemas.

Recognizing the signs and symptoms

Without a doubt, when most people think of eating disorders, they think of anorexia. With the publication of several groundbreaking books and the death of beloved celebrities including singer Karen Carpenter from heart failure as the result of anorexia nervosa, anorexia burst into public consciousness in the 1970s and 80s and defined what the general population knew about eating disorders and the toll they can take on the body and mind.

For many people, the malnutrition associated with anorexia makes it the most feared of the three eating disorders (that is, feared by loved ones and those in the health field but often wrongly envied or revered by those who wish they were thinner). In fact, it does have the highest rate of death of the three and of *every* other psychiatric diagnosis — including schizophrenia and severe depression. However, it may still be difficult for loved ones of an anorexic to see the symptoms of the disease or to recognize how serious the illness has become.

In addition to the official diagnostic criteria, you may be able to recognize a friend, loved one, or even a stranger suffering from anorexia. A person with anorexia

- ✔ Can never be thin enough.
- ✔ Is obsessed with food even though he does not eat.

✔ Develops complicated and precise rituals regarding food.

✔ Has a distorted body image and believes she's fat — even if she is obviously very thin.

✔ Exercises excessively even when injured or exhausted.

✔ Suffers from fatigue, insomnia, dizziness, and/or fainting.

✔ May have a bluish discoloration of the fingers.

✔ Has hair that's thinning, breaks, or is falling out.

✔ May grow *lanugo,* a layer of soft, downy body hair , due to low body temperature.

These are just some of the most obvious symptoms that may signal that something quite serious is going on. As with all eating disorders, anorexia is a progressive disease, meaning that without treatment it gets worse over time. There are also less obvious medical consequences from anorexia and anorexic-like thinking and behaviors. These are best detected through medical examination, lab work, etc.

While an anorexic's inability to eat may seem minor, inconsequential, or even just like everyone else at first, over time, it may spiral into a full-blown health crisis. Very often anorexics deny that there's a problem and may be proud of how thin they've become, seeing it as a sign of power and control. Nevertheless, if you know someone who you think may be in danger from anorexia, it's important to intervene when appropriate even if it's difficult to bring up the topic.

Facing the consequences of anorexia (and yes, this pertains to binge eaters)

Anorexia is, in all its variations, starvation, which has devastating effects on both the body and mind. Some of the consequences include

✔ Damage to the heart muscle, including a risk of heart failure

✔ Low blood pressure

✔ Severe dehydration that may lead to kidney damage or failure

✔ Organ failure in severe cases

✔ Disruption in menstruation and/or fertility

✔ Osteoporosis

Unfortunately, existing data show that even with treatment, not all anorexics recover, and many have only a partial recovery, meaning they may be able to work and maintain some relationships but remain overly focused on food and weight. They may continue to abuse laxatives, diet pills, or to over-exercise and remain underweight. Those who do not recover may remain dangerously underweight and often develop severe medical conditions related to the disease.

Eating disorders have the highest mortality rate of any mental illness. A study by the National Association of Anorexia Nervosa and Associated Disorders (ANAD) reported the following statistics:

- ✔ Five to ten percent of anorexics die within ten years after contracting the disease and 18 to 20 percent of anorexics are dead after 20 years.

- ✔ Anorexia nervosa has the highest death rate of any psychiatric illness (including major depression).

- ✔ The mortality rate associated with anorexia nervosa is 12 times higher than the death rate of *all* causes of death for females 15 to 24 years old.

Understanding Bulimia Nervosa

Like anorexia, bulimia is generally well-known. As a binge eater, it may be easier to understand what you have in common with bulimics. After all, bulimics binge, and the feeling of being out of control around food is something that's easy for you to relate to.

The main difference is that bulimics purge what they've eaten while binge eaters don't. Purges come in many forms — vomiting, using laxatives and diuretics, and abusing exercise are all ways that bulimics seek to compensate for the effects of their binges. Although you may have never purged, you probably understand the sense of despair and self-loathing that descends upon you after a binge.

You probably also intuitively understand the shame and secrecy that lead a bulimic to hide her behaviors. In that way, bulimia and binge eating are very different from anorexia in which sufferers don't seem to mind if others know that they're starving themselves even though anorexics certainly endure their own shame because of their perceptions of their bodies and how they think others will see them.

However, if you binge by yourself, as most do, so that no one will discover what you're doing, then you know the isolation and loneliness of all eating disorders. Like anorexics and binge eaters, bulimics also equate their weight with a sense of self-worth and may live in a world that's black-and-white with no middle ground that might help lead them towards healthier thinking and a sense of balance.

Understanding what it means to be bulimic

Like anorexia and binge eating disorder, bulimia has formal diagnostic criteria that have been defined for health care professionals by the *DSM-V*. For the lay person, the most recognizable symptom of bulimia is the cycle of bingeing and purging; however, because a bulimic may conduct these activities in private, it can sometimes be difficult to be sure that someone you know suffers from bulimia.

The *DSM-V* criteria define bulimia as

- Recurrent episodes of binge eating characterized by

  - Eating, in a discrete period of time (for example within a two-hour period), an amount of food that's definitely larger than most people would eat during a similar period of time and under similar circumstances

  - A sense of lack of control over eating during the episode, defined by a feeling that you cannot stop eating or control what or how much you're eating

- Recurrent inappropriate compensatory behavior to prevent weight gain

  - Self-induced vomiting

  - Misuse of laxatives, diuretics, enemas, or other medications

  - Fasting

  - Excessive exercise

- The binge eating and inappropriate compensatory behavior both occur, on average, once a week for a period of at least three months

- Self-evaluation is unduly influenced by body shape and weight

As with anorexia, there are two types of bulimia:

- **Purging type:** During the current episode of bulimia nervosa, the person regularly engages in self-induced vomiting or the misuse of laxatives, diuretics, or enemas.

- **Non-purging type:** During the current episode of bulimia nervosa, the person uses inappropriate compensatory behavior such as abuse of exercise but has not regularly engaged in self-induced vomiting or misused laxatives, diuretics, or enemas.

Recognizing the signs and symptoms of bulimia

Unlike anorexics and binge eaters, who may wear their disorders on their sleeves, many bulimics succeed in hiding their eating disorder, however severe it may become, due to the fact that many maintain a normal weight and keep their disordered eating and its associated behaviors secret.

However, some exterior signs and symptoms can lead you to suspect that someone is a bulimic. A bulimic

- Engages in binge eating.
- Is secretive about his eating in general. A bulimic may not eat in front of other people or may hide food.
- May gain or lose large amount of weight in a short period of time.
- Often goes to the bathroom immediately after a meal.
- May have a swollen jaw, salivary glands, or cheeks as a result of purging.
- Has teeth marks or other signs of injury on his or her hands due to self-induced vomiting.
- Often suffers from co-occurring illnesses such as depression or anxiety.
- Abuses alcohol, drugs, or other substances and often engages in self-harming behaviors.

Facing the long-term consequences of bulimia

As with all other eating disorders, bulimia starts slowly and builds over time. Because bulimia can be associated with other psychological disorders such as depression or anxiety, treatment is a critical part of a successful long-term recovery. The effects of bulimia can be quite damaging and include

- Damage to the heart, primarily due to unstable blood pressure and electrolyte imbalance which may lead to an irregular heartbeat and heart failure.
- Kidney damage.
- Acid reflux as a result of damage to the esophagus due to self-induced vomiting.

✔ Digestive problems including IBS (irritable bowel syndrome), the inability to digest foods (lazy bowel syndrome), and/or laxative dependence, which may cause bloating, constipation, or diarrhea.

✔ Anxiety or depression — although these may be part of what caused someone's bulimia, they can also be exacerbated by it.

Including the Other Specified Feeding or Eating Disorder (OSFED) Category

Although eating disorder professionals have recognized for a number of years that binge eating disorder is an illness on par with anorexia and bulimia, it's only in the fifth and most recent edition of the *DSM* that the American Psychiatric Association officially included it as a diagnosable disorder. *DSM-V* also eliminates the diagnosis of eating disorder not otherwise specified, or EDNOS, and replaces it with other specified feeding or eating disorder (OSFED).

Until now, binge eating disorder has been considered part of a catch-all diagnosis that eating disorder professionals called eating disorder not otherwise specified, or EDNOS. EDNOS has been used to describe disordered eating and other behaviors that don't exactly meet the criteria of anorexia nervosa, bulimia nervosa, and/or other eating disorders. However, the *DSM-V* has now designated these diagnostic categories as other specified feeding or eating disorder, or (OSFED).

Getting a diagnosis of OSFED doesn't mean that your disorder isn't serious or that it doesn't require treatment and/or medical attention. It just means that your symptoms don't fall neatly into a single category or meet the exact criteria of one of the other eating disorders.

Happily, it's worth noting that some of the criteria for anorexia and bulimia also changed in the new *Diagnostic and Statistical Manual of Mental Disorders* and render the use of the new catch-all diagnosis of OSFED much less frequent.

One of the complications of OSFED is that treatment for it isn't as well-covered by insurance providers in comparison to the AN or BN diagnoses even though those aren't always reimbursed at optimal levels either as it takes time for the practical applications of diagnostic criteria to be properly taught and discussed with the managed care representatives who determine coverage for these cases.

Understanding what it means to be diagnosed with OSFED

Practically speaking, until the introduction of the newest diagnostic criteria of the *DSM-V,* EDNOS — the old catch-all diagnosis — was the most commonly diagnosed eating disorder and accounted for up to 40 percent of patients suffering from diagnosed eating disorders. Now that BED is a separate category, those numbers will go down, but the new OSFED diagnosis will likely still be used in less clear-cut cases of disordered eating.

For all practical purposes, an OSFED diagnosis simply means

✔ Although symptoms fall into the category of anorexia, bulimia, or BED, the symptoms themselves have not yet become acute.

✔ Symptoms and behaviors may not be extremely serious but likely closely resemble those of anorexia, bulimia, and/or BED.

Furthermore, the *DSM-V* defines OSFED as

✔ All of the criteria for anorexia nervosa are met except that, despite significant weight loss, the patient's current weight is in the normal range.

✔ All of the criteria for bulimia nervosa are met except that the binge eating and inappropriate compensatory mechanisms occur less than once a week or for less than three months.

✔ All of the criteria for binge eating disorder are met, except that the binge eating occurs, on average, less than once a week and/or for less than three months.

✔ The patient has normal body weight and regularly uses inappropriate compensatory behavior after eating small amounts of food (for example, self-inducing vomiting after consuming two cookies).

✔ The patient has recurring episodes of night eating, also known as night eating syndrome, that occur after awakening from sleep or after the evening meal.

Linking the Various Disorders

If you're reading this book in order to determine whether or not you have binge eating disorder and to figure out what to do about it if you do, you may be still be wondering what anorexia, bulimia, and/or OSFED have to do with you even if you've recognized some of your own behaviors and thinking in the descriptions in this chapter. As you many know from your own experience, many people who suffer from disordered eating shift from eating disorder to eating disorder or pass through phases in which they exhibit symptoms of one or more disorder.

In fact, many binge eaters, compulsive overeaters, and emotional eaters report that at one time in their lives they were anorexic or bulimic, or at the very least tried to restrict and/or purge. If you notice some anorexic or bulimic tendencies in your own behavior, you're not alone. Most people with an eating disorder have symptoms that do not fit solely into one of the three main eating disorders. More often symptoms travel along the eating disorder continuum, ebbing and flowing over time.

Most people know that at some point for a binge eater restrictive dieting leads to bingeing. The binge-diet cycle, illustrated in Figure 5-1, is, in some ways, an example of how different eating disorders are co-conspirators. While the dieting, or restrictive part, of this cycle may not be profuse enough to be considered actual anorexic behavior, it's nonetheless a symptom and contributes to BED as a whole.

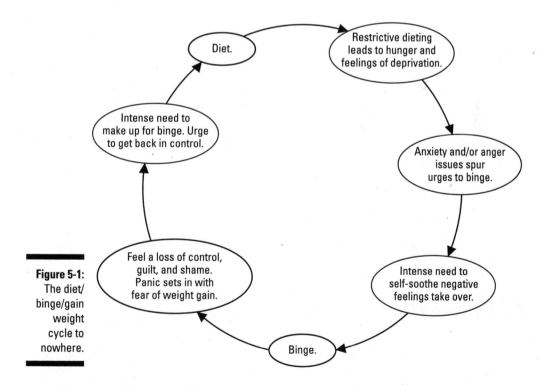

Figure 5-1: The diet/ binge/gain weight cycle to nowhere.

Bingeing to bulimia and back again

Erin is 42 years old and has struggled with eating her entire life. She often describes herself as a failed bulimic. Erin's first memory of bingeing was when she was eight years old. She would sneak food into her bedroom after dinner and eat it all after the house had quieted down. As a result, she began to gain weight, and during the course of pre-pubescence and her early teen years, she became significantly overweight.

By the time she was 14, her bingeing was what she described as out-of-control. At that time, Erin went on a diet that persisted on and off for several years. Although the diet began with making healthy changes to her eating habits that resulted in weight loss, after about six months, she began to restrict her food intake more severely. She also started exercising for up to three hours per day every day.

By the time she was 17, Erin wound up weighing less than 100 pounds and was admitted to an inpatient eating disorder facility for what was to have been a long-term stay. Regrettably, she only got to stay a relatively short time, in part because of her insurance plan and in part because she had become restless and wanted to get back to real life. Although she had received intensive treatment psychologically, nutritionally, and educationally; had gained sufficient weight to be discharged; and was able to maintain a reasonable weight for her height and age for some time, she continued to be restrictive with her food, counted calories, and exercised every single day. (Note: many reading this might be thinking, "So what? I know lots of people who count calories, are careful about what they eat, and exercise regularly." Context, history, and motivations are key considerations to keep in mind as you read on).

In college, Erin excelled, but she experienced an unusually high level of anxiety, stress, homesickness, and academic pressure that sent her spiraling back into the familiar safety of her eating disorder. The difference was that this time Erin went back to bingeing the way she had when she was eight years old. For fear of weight gain, over time Erin started to use laxatives as a failed attempt to compensate for overeating. She also began exercising again for up to three hours per day as a compensatory mechanism and as a perceived sense of penance, restricted her eating for days at a time, and also sometimes attempted to purge — all of these in order to try and maintain what she perceived as a normal weight.

When she began working after graduate school, Erin no longer had time to keep up with her cycles of bingeing, restricting, exercising, and fasting, so her symptoms slowly narrowed to bingeing only. She continued to gain weight until she finally went back for treatment — this time with an even longer history of symptomatic behaviors under her belt, a new sense of determination, and an understanding that this cycle was likely to continue for the rest of her life if she did not finally give it the time and attention it required.

So it's easy to see that over the course of Erin's eating disorder history, she's migrated from bingeing as a young child to anorexia as a teen to bulimia as a young adult to bingeing. But it's also plain to see that these are not hopeless situations. There is help available but it does, in fact, take becoming sick and tired of being sick and tired for treatment to take hold. It's also important to start treatment as early as is humanly possible since it's the best way to unearth some of the root causes and the behaviors before they become even further and chronically entrenched.

Part II
Do You Have Binge Eating Disorder?

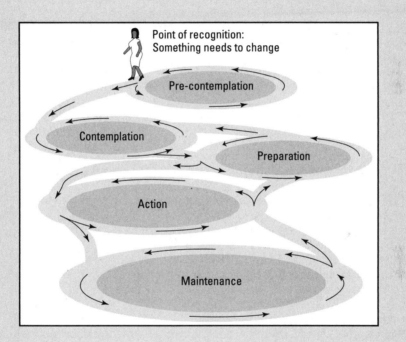

Debunk myths about binge eating disorder at www.dummies.com/extras/overcomingbingeeating.

In this part . . .

✔ Recognize the symptoms of binge eating disorder (BED) and find ways to treat them.

✔ Find motivation to change unhealthy behaviors. Tap into an assortment of effective tools and resources that get you on the path to recovery and help you through its twists and turns.

✔ Accept that obesity is often a result of binge eating disorder. Find out how to counter the effects of the range of physical and emotional health issues that attend obesity.

✔ Realize that not every BED sufferer is overweight. Some BED sufferers have developed habits that keep them at a normal weight despite bingeing. Find tools that can help this type of BED sufferer.

Chapter 6

Understanding the Symptoms of Binge Eating

In This Chapter

▶ Breaking down the behaviors associated with binge eating

▶ Bingers at every size: moderate weight, overweight, and obese

▶ Examining the relationship between bingeing and obesity

▶ Getting started on ending the overeating

*M*any tried-and-true techniques exist to help you slow and eventually stop binge eating or any form of compulsive overeating. However, successful improvement over time, whether with a professional treatment team, through strategies you find in books, on websites, or in support groups, often depends on tailoring a plan to your individual needs and continuously evaluating the most sustainable course of action for you.

Whether you identify yourself as a binge eater, recognizing and understanding your triggers to overeating is one of the first steps towards finding solutions. You may have flipped through the first chapters of this book looking for clues to help you determine if you suffer from binge eating disorder or other forms of disordered eating. Perhaps you've found some evidence that suggests that you do, or maybe you know simply from your own intuition that you use food as a coping mechanism. For some people, being able to put a name to their problem is a significant step in beginning to come to terms with it and finding long-term ways to solve it.

If, on the other hand, you're still not sure whether you suffer from binge eating or where you fall on the eating disorder spectrum, keep in mind that even though great similarities exist among binge eaters and compulsive overeaters in general, you don't have to suffer from every symptom to benefit from the ideas in this book or from treatment, should you so choose to seek it out.

In this chapter, we delve into the behaviors and emotions associated with binge eating and offer several opportunities for self-assessment. We also discuss the underlying similarities of moderate weight, overweight, and obese bingers. Finally, we'll offer a number of practical suggestions for creating greater awareness of your bingeing behaviors and beginning to curb them as you decide how to move forward with your life.

Listing Common Signs of Binge Eating

No matter how bingeing or compulsive overeating has affected your physical health, emotional wellbeing, or appearance, most sufferers seem to have some symptoms in common:

- **Feeling out of control and/or unable to stop eating:** No matter what you put into your mouth, you can't stop eating even though you'd like to. You know that bingeing isn't good for you, and you wonder why what you know doesn't seem to have an impact on your actions. You eat until you can't eat anymore, and it feels terrible.

- **Eating quickly and/or continuing to eat even when you're already full:** If you're eating as a way to cope with uncomfortable or painful feelings, it probably seems as if you can't eat quickly enough to make them go away or to numb yourself out, whether you're conscious of what you're doing or not. It doesn't matter if you're starving or full, you can eat no matter what your body is telling you (if you're even aware of the signals it sends before being so full you can't go on).

- **Using eating as a coping mechanism when you feel stressed, angry, sad, or simply unable to tolerate any variety of emotions:** When you feel bad, you eat. Though you may not have connected the dots yet as to exactly which emotions trigger a binge, it's hard not to notice that during or after a bad day, you turn to food to try to soothe yourself. Unfortunately, over time bingeing doesn't free you from negative emotions; it only brings about other uncomfortable feelings that may, in turn, generate even more bingeing.

- **Hiding food and keeping your eating habits secret:** You feel ashamed, guilty, sad, angry — you name it — about your eating habits, and you can't let anyone know, so you sneak food and hide it somewhere you can eat it later where no one will see you or question you about your actions. If you're left with empty food wrappers, maybe you bury them under other trash or make sure to take out the trash before anyone sees how much you've eaten. If someone discovers what you're doing, you may pretend you don't know what that person's talking about.

✔ **Feeling guilt, regret, disgust, or other negative emotions after bingeing:** The most common emotional experience binge eaters describe is feeling regret, guilt, and/or even disgust after a binge. Regardless of what and how much you're eating, if you experience these types of feelings after what you think may be a binge, if you don't get help, you may end up dealing with bigger and more devastating binges at some point.

Realizing that if it feels like bingeing, it's a binge

Whether or not you've ever used the word *binge* to describe your eating habits, people who binge eat generally know what a binge feels like for them. In spite of the clinical description, which includes calories consumed and the amount of time in which that occurs, binges are still a very subjective, personal experience, and what's a binge for one person may not be for another.

The technical definition of a *binge* is eating an amount that's significantly larger than most people would eat in a discrete period of time. Together with the food consumption itself, most binge eaters describe feeling an extreme loss of control during the episode.

The feelings associated with the episodes can be very similar from person to person. The guilt, distress, embarrassment, hopelessness, isolation, and other negative feelings that occur after a binge are quite typical and are the key focus of the disorder rather than the specific quantities of food ingested. The sooner you can target what eating behaviors cause the most trouble for you, the sooner you can begin to figure out how to change them.

Identifying a binge regardless of what you eat

Everyone overeats every once in a while, and many people know the feeling of having one too many helpings during the holidays or eating dessert on your birthday even though you're already full.

But binge eating is a whole different ball game, and although it may be tempting to normalize your overeating and pretend that everyone's doing what you're doing because eating to excess is sometimes part of modern life, if you're honest with yourself, you eventually have to rethink that assessment of things.

The shame and secrecy associated with binge eating or any kind of disordered eating can keep you from acknowledging — even to yourself — that you have a problem. However, denying the seriousness of binge eating's consequences on your emotional and physical health isn't good for you in the short or long term.

It's enormously brave to admit that you have a problem you can't solve on your own. Read that sentence again. Acknowledging an eating disorder isn't for sissies, so it's important to recognize what a huge step it is to even just explore the possibility of change and to be curious about what a life without bingeing might look like. Although it may feel like a cliché, owning your own behavior and beginning to break it down into manageable components (or bite-size pieces seems fitting here; sorry — we warned you about a lot of food metaphors!) may make the problem feel less overwhelming and can inspire you to continue on your journey towards wellness even if it's sometimes uncomfortable.

If you're reluctant to think of yourself as a binge eater, perhaps one way to understand what you're doing is to examine one episode and think about the feelings and behaviors that accompanied it:

- ✔ Did the episode start with a negative feeling that was coupled with the urge to fill yourself up or, more likely, did that occur to you only in the aftermath of the binge state?
- ✔ Did you continue to eat more and more when you knew you weren't hungry?
- ✔ Did you eat in secret or hide the evidence afterward?
- ✔ Did the episode feel out of control?
- ✔ Does this happen often and at predictable times such as at night or whenever you're alone?

If you answered yes to one or more of these questions, you may be binge eating, compulsively overeating, or experiencing binge-like episodes. Regardless of the amount of food or the number of calories you consume, unchecked overeating can harm your physical and emotional health. If you recognize your own eating patterns in these questions, you may want to start thinking about how to curb and ultimately put a stop to these behaviors. Easier said than done for sure but very, very possible.

Recognizing your eating patterns

Over time, most binge eaters develop certain patterns of behavior. It may be the place and/or time of day in which the eating takes place, the order in which you eat whatever foods you consume during the binge, and/or just the rituals you develop around everything to do with the binge.

Understanding the finer details of your binges is an important step in making positive changes and eventually regaining control of these eating behaviors. Once you have an awareness of what your tendencies are during binge episodes, you may be able to address them one at a time.

Keep in mind that you can make real, measurable progress long before you're able to stop binge eating completely. Most people don't go from bingeing regularly to never bingeing again, and if you're trying it at this early stage, the immensity of that goal could be daunting and overwhelming. Instead, success can first be a matter of bingeing fewer times during the week, bingeing for less time each time, or consuming fewer calories during each binge. Slow and steady wins the race.

Your journey towards slowing and eventually stopping binge eating or overeating of any sort most likely won't be a perfectly linear process with constant improvement and no setbacks. Long-term success at recovering from any eating disorder means celebrating small steps along the way, anticipating slips, gently getting back on track without being too hard on yourself, and being flexible and realistic about making adjustments to your plan as you go.

Keeping a food and emotions journal as we discuss in Chapter 12 is one way to begin to identify and keep track of your eating habits even if you don't want to or can't make any changes right away.

Don't worry about the food and emotions journal being perfect. You can use the template we suggest in the appendix of this book, but if you don't have access to a computer or a way of making a grid, it's still a great start to jot down notes on what you're eating, the time of day when you eat it, and how you felt before, during, and after you ate. It's important that you do this in real time rather than from memory at the end of the day. It's unlikely that you'll remember exactly what you ate, and more to the point, you probably won't remember what you were thinking and feeling.

Documenting your eating habits is an important method for starting to understand patterns in your eating behaviors. When you know exactly how much you're eating and when you're eating it, you may be able to develop a different perspective on your binge episodes. Although in the moment it may feel like an out-of-control binge, when you see your eating as part of the larger picture, you can move forward instead of feeling stuck.

Calling all overeating episodes binges discourages a change in perspective. Being realistic about exactly what a binge is for you helps you move out of the cycle. For many binge eaters, if triggering emotions are present eating even a typical amount of food can feel like a binge. Knowing the difference between a binge-like episode, and an actual binge is important for your success. It boils down to calories consumed but also, and perhaps more importantly, context. Is the eating in response to physical or emotional hunger? During the eating, is it at a pace that allows you to identify being satisfied or full versus feeling stuffed? These are the types of questions to ponder.

Looking at Moderate-Weight Bingers and the Binge/Diet Cycle

Although many binge eaters eventually become obese, not all binge eaters end up obese or even overweight. If you've decided you can't possibly have a problem with bingeing because you've stayed more or less the same size over years of binge behavior, think again. Overweight and obesity are likely side effects of bingeing, but they're not an absolute certainty.

If you binge on the weekends and make up for it by dieting or otherwise restricting your intake during the week, you may be able to maintain a normal weight. This doesn't mean that you're not a binge eater, compulsive overeater, or emotional eater.

It's also important to note that the physical consequences of binge eating, even when they don't cause obesity, can be uncomfortable or even severe. Many binge eaters who maintain a moderate weight have just as many physical discomforts and medical consequences as obese bingers including acid reflux, digestive problems, high cholesterol, diabetes, and high blood pressure to name a few.

Dieting as a trigger

It probably isn't difficult to identify any number of contributing factors, both physical and emotional, that may trigger a binge. Some triggers are extremely specific and personal, but one common trigger for anyone who binges or compulsively overeats can be unacknowledged or exaggerated hunger. *Unacknowledged hunger* is exactly what it sounds like — you're hungry and know you're hungry, but you avoid eating in an effort to lose weight. *Exaggerated hunger* is similar in that it starts off as unacknowledged hunger that becomes extreme because you wait too long to eat and become so hungry you simply can't stop yourself from bingeing.

Even though it may seem counterintuitive, dieting, especially restrictive and extreme dieting, is almost always a trigger for those with a tendency to binge. Just think of a pendulum and how naturally it swings from one extreme to the other simply by gravity. If you've ever declared any food off limits, not eaten it for a certain time period, and then found yourself overeating or bingeing on it, you know what we're talking about.

Restricting calorie intake, as in extreme diets, tricks your body into thinking it's starving. Even though you know that's not the case, on a cellular level, your body is hormonally similar to someone who's malnourished. The absence of energy-producing food causes the brain to go into food-seeking overdrive — which almost always results in uncontrollable or ravenous eating.

If you've ever experienced this cycle, you may be able to look back and identify how long you normally last on your diet before you succumb to a binge. Is it a day? A week? The ever magical two-week norm? Do you start the day doing "good" and end it being "bad"? No matter what your routine, restrictive dieting is a particularly potent trigger.

Swinging from binge to diet and back again

If you're a long-term, normal-weight binger, you've probably figured out a bingeing formula that keeps your weight in check and your eating behaviors secret. For most people, these strategies include extreme and often unhealthy dieting of some sort to offset the effects of bingeing or overeating.

If the "dieting, bingeing, gaining weight, dieting again" cycle is familiar to you, now is your time to get off the merry-go-round. Many bingers fear that if they stop dieting after a binge they will continue to binge and gain more and more weight. Although this fear is normal, the bingeing-dieting cycle can never work for the long term. Without breaking the cycle, you may easily find yourself trapped and unable to stop swinging back and forth between starving yourself and overeating.

Use these practical tips to gently start to put the brakes on your behaviors and slowly disturb and eventually stop the cycle.

> ✔ **Eat by the clock until you're ready for intuitive eating.** Although it may seem counterintuitive, eating more often and at regular intervals can be one of the first and most important ways to regulate your hunger levels and ultimately your urge to binge. Make a schedule for yourself so that you eat at the same times and the same intervals every day. For example,

have breakfast at 8 a.m., eat a light snack at 10:30, lunch at 1:30, plan for another snack at 4, and then sit down to dinner at 7 p.m.

You may be thinking, "Are you kidding? If I eat all of that and then binge later, I'll blow up like a house." Actually, it's not true. Eating more predictably is your ticket to being *much* less likely to binge in the first place. By having a regular eating schedule, your blood sugar stays stable, you won't feel as deprived physically or nutritionally, and you'll simply feel more regulated in every way.

Your eventual goal is to successfully read your own hunger and satiety cues, which takes time to master, but until then, eating by the clock is a great way to get started.

✔ **Seek out positive stress-management techniques that work for you.** Unfortunately, dealing with stress is part of life. In order to function, most people develop coping mechanisms that help them relieve the anxiety and fear they feel in stressful situations and get themselves and their lives back to normal. If you turn to food and eating to help soothe yourself during life's ups and downs, perhaps this is an opportunity to consider different ways to face stress and its consequences. In Chapter 10, we discuss alternate coping skills and give some ideas for other ways to handle the pressures that sometimes make life hard.

✔ **Give up dieting for good.** If you've been dieting for most of your life, it may seem normal to bounce between restricting your food intake and bingeing, but by now, you know that traditional diets don't work and that making small, realistic, incremental changes to your eating habits improves your chances of maintaining these new, healthier habits during the course of your entire life. The all-or-nothing mentality that may have led to your binges in the first place is the same way of thinking that can sabotage your attempts at recovery. Even though it can be difficult at first, it's important to think about food in a more reasonable, realistic way.

✔ **Don't beat yourself up.** Feelings of guilt and hopelessness and negative judgments about your eating behaviors can wear you down and perpetuate your unregulated eating in a powerful way. At some point during the cycle, it's important to give yourself a break and try to slowly let go of the guilt. Again, we know this is easier said than done, but your way has simply not been working. It may be time to dismiss the judge and jury that's always taking up space in your head with a running commentary and just start fresh.

✔ **Make plans with others during your vulnerable times.** Overcoming bingeing is difficult to do alone. Set yourself up for success by scheduling your time in a way that limits bingeing opportunities. Remember, you don't necessarily have to announce to others that your express intention is to hang out as a way to prevent a binge. Instead, focus on doing something positive and fun, this way you're better able to take your mind off the urges you experience.

Bingeing on activities is not going to be the long-term solution to not bingeing on food. Eventually, your goal is to be able to be with yourself and all of your thoughts and feelings without having to numb out. After all, as the title of Jon Kabat-Zinn's famous book says, "Wherever you go, there you are." Hopefully, this will soon become a lovely thought rather than a dreaded one.

Considering Overweight and Obese Bingers

There's no doubt that for many, if not most people, binge eating or any kind of overeating eventually leads to overweight or obesity. In fact, obesity is the most obvious side effect associated with binge eating disorder even though obesity may also come about for other reasons. The effects of bingeing are certainly more visible for those who become obese, and with this comes an even deeper level of shame, denial, isolation, and thus, a perpetuation of the behaviors to soothe some of those uncomfortable thoughts and feelings.

Seeing through the illusion of control

If you're obese, you may feel even more vulnerable to bingeing, which can suck you into a deeper cycle of weight gain, negative feelings, and then bingeing to temporarily relieve those feelings. Unfortunately the long-term consequences of uncontrolled overeating can put you at greater risk, not only for depression and anxiety, but also for heart disease, diabetes, high cholesterol, and high blood pressure — and a combination of these ailments can be quite serious. You probably already know this.

The big question becomes how to have what you know match up with what you do. We make many suggestions throughout this book, but frankly, for meaningful change to happen, some switch has to flip in your own brain and your own heart. You have to find your own motivation, be it fear of medical consequences, concern about your relationship with food being mimicked by your children, feeling as if you are somehow being passed over for promotions or other professional opportunities, feeling socially isolated, noticing the toll these addictive behaviors are taking on other important relationships in your life, or just simply being sick and tired of being sick and tired.

When you decide you're ready to make changes for the long haul is when the real therapeutic work begins to take hold. Sure, you still have to address behavioral aspects, which is why an intelligently regulated meal plan and sleep schedule are so very helpful. You also need to explore a host of alternate coping skills in an effort to reprogram your automatic food responses. That's also why focusing on eating without distractions by television, computer, telephone, and the like during meals and snacks is also an important behavioral change. Over time, new behaviors will replace old, less productive ones.

We cannot reiterate enough that at some point in your life, whether you knew you were doing so or not, you chose to use food for comfort because it seemed like a good idea at the time. Perhaps you thought it would offer some sense of control in a sea of otherwise chaotic thoughts or life situations. It must have felt necessary for whatever the reasons, and so it is important to sort through whatever the influences or situations were at the time, or still are, that led to all of this. It's not enough just to decide . . . . If only. That's the stuff Monday morning diets are made of. Notice those usually end by 4 o'clock or so.

Dealing with the issues that led you to binge eating or compulsory overeating is where the support and skills of a psychotherapist skilled in eating disorders and/or a therapeutic support group can be key. These people can help you move your emotional mountains, although at your own pace. It need not happen over the course of years and years on the couch. The results can be surprisingly rewarding and forward-moving even in the short term with the use of techniques such as art therapy, psychodrama, talk therapy, lots of homework/exercises that engage your interest, and more.

Keep in mind that the binge or overeating behaviors didn't appear overnight, and they won't go away overnight. Be gentle with yourself and with the process and don't expect quick fixes, and you will be very much more likely to experience sustainable change at a very deep and meaningful level.

Dealing with extended binges: What are you really hungry for?

Although many binges have a discrete beginning and end, a binge can be prolonged, extending for days or even weeks. An extended binge typically consists of constant grazing including large, high-calorie, high-fat meals coupled with constant snacking in-between. An extended binge can go on for so long because the binger never feels she has completely filled up, so within a short period of time, there is more grazing. The excessive snacking is also a way for bingers to hide their behaviors in public or social situations since it seems a lot less obvious that there may be a problem when someone overeats by grazing rather than by eating a very large amount at one time.

A key question to stop and ask yourself when you become aware of the grazing and constant eating is, "What am I hungry for?" Although you may be tempted to say that you're hungry for whatever your favorite binge foods are, food isn't the answer. Some other hunger isn't being addressed, so it feels impossible to ever be full until you satiate that hunger.

Are you hungry for love? Companionship? Peace of mind? Acknowledgement? Affection? A change in your professional identity? Further education? An expanded view of life through travel? The list can be endless. And in fact, you may only be able to figure out what void you may be trying to fill by making such a list. You may be surprised at what you hunger for, and it's okay to allow yourself to want these things without thinking that you're insatiable or selfish. One thing is for sure, no food on the planet is sufficient substitute for what you really hunger for. Perhaps after you write your list, you will be less likely to seek emotional sustenance through food. Then you can seek out support to help put some of the things on that list into action.

Getting Back to Normal

For someone who binges, getting back to normal may sound totally unattainable at first. Chances are a binger may not even know what is normal, much less how to get there. Of course, talking with a therapist and working with a dietitian can help a binger work towards a less conflicted emotional life, improved coping skills, and a healthier day-to-day routine.

Even if you aren't currently in treatment or are undecided about what your plans are for seeking help, you can take a number of steps to try to slow and eventually stop your bingeing behaviors:

- ✔ **Don't skip meals.** Skipping meals and/or snacks almost always causes you to overeat at the next meal. Eating just one (or two) big meals per day causes your blood sugar to be unstable which hinders weight loss. Aim for three meals per day plus one or two snacks.

- ✔ **Make sure to eat breakfast within one hour of waking.** Breakfast literally makes or breaks your day. You must eat within an hour of waking up to set your endocrine system up to have healthy, balanced blood sugar throughout the entire day.

- ✔ **Practice distinguishing between hunger and cravings**. Cravings are generally for something specific (or a specific category of foods such as sweets). However, if you're truly hungry, you'll be satisfied by other foods including raw veggies dipped in hummus or a turkey sandwich.

The lines between hunger and cravings blur for binge eaters, especially when they're faced with an abundance of food options. Listen to your body and learn to distinguish between cravings and hunger.

✔ **Be mindful while eating.** Be aware of what you're eating and how much. Focus on your food and minimize any other distractions:

- Avoid eating in front of the television or computer.

- Clear off the kitchen table.

- Don't read, study, write, or talk on the phone while you eat.

Eating mindfully allows you to taste your food, enjoy your meals, notice fullness faster, and experience a higher level of flavor and satisfaction, and feel less of a desire to overeat.

✔ **Keep a food and emotion journal.** We can't emphasize enough how important it is to collect data on your own eating habits, so you can analyze them and make simple, lasting changes that work for you. Knowledge is power, and by documenting what you're eating together with when you're eating it and why, you'll begin to understand yourself and the pattern of your eating behaviors in a new and important way. You may be able to make some changes yourself, but you may also need a psychotherapist and/or a dietitian to help you strategize about techniques that will work to help you curb binge eating. (We talk about journaling in Chapter 12.)

Chapter 7

Becoming Motivated for Change

● ●

In This Chapter

▶ Discovering what flips your switch and lights the way to recovery

▶ Preparing yourself for change and setting SMART goals

▶ Feeling better inside and out

▶ Staying on track over time

● ●

*M*aking significant changes to your lifestyle takes time, patience, and a positive, flexible attitude. If you recognize yourself as a binge eater or a compulsive overeater and know that you've been abusing your body with food, you may be wondering, "What's next?"

Perhaps you've already hit your breaking point, and you're ready to begin a new journey. Or you may just be contemplating or considering what you can do to stop the abuse of food and your body without having fully committed to the process of change yet. Maybe you just don't want to deal with what feels like the overwhelming task of understanding and putting an end to your disordered eating. If this last one resonates with you, keep reading anyway. You never know what will finally flip that switch.

Whatever your stage of readiness, you're probably looking for motivation and a reason to stop bingeing that will sustain you as you embark upon a process that takes time, honesty, energy, financial resources, and courage.

As you probably already know instinctively, there's no one-size-fits-all answer. For each and every person who eventually discovers or rediscovers how to cope with life's ups and downs in ways that don't involve the abuse of food and body, there's a unique set of motivations, some external and some internal. Your individual motivations and reasons are all driven by you and what you want for your life.

In this chapter, we explore some of the most common reasons people want to stop binge eating. You may not think you'd need to see such a list, that you know these reasons already. But it can be quite reassuring to know that you share similar thoughts, doubts, goals, and obstacles with others who struggle with disordered eating. We also offer several practical steps to help you target exactly which incentives or motivations may be most meaningful to you personally if you're thinking about trying to end your dependence on bingeing. Lastly, we discuss easing into gradual but significant change and offer ways to set realistic and attainable goals that help you build your confidence and sustain you for the long haul.

Finding Your Personal Reasons for Change

If the desire to stop bingeing were enough, this would all be pretty easy. However, by now you know that using food as a coping mechanism is harder to give up than you'd imagine. Perhaps you've tried to stop bingeing before and maybe you've had some temporary successes, but if you've picked up this book because you've fallen back into bingeing or compulsive overeating, you may need to take a step back and figure out what will motivate and really sustain your new commitment to yourself.

No matter whether you've been bingeing for months, years, or decades, you probably already know what overeating is doing and will continue to do to your physical health. Binge eating or compulsive overeating can also negatively impact your relationships, your professional life, and/or how you feel about yourself every minute of the day.

For the most part, binge eaters understand, at least intellectually, that overeating isn't a good idea, and that although they may not know why they overeat, most realize that their relationship to food is not a healthy one. Obviously, the challenge arises when it's time to compare what you know with what you do. If you take a moment to consider the gap between the two, and the inability to match up them up even though you may desperately want to, you'll have a practical, working definition of *addiction*. If you can understand your situation in this way, then it's much easier to approach finding solutions in a gentle and loving way rather than with self-blaming or hopeless cynicism.

Getting ready

One of the biggest mistakes people make when they want to change longstanding habits or ways of thinking is to think that they must change everything at once in a black-and-white, all-or-nothing way. If you've ever binged and awakened the next morning thinking, "That's absolutely the last time. From now on, I won't binge anymore," then you know what we're talking about. The dilemma comes later in the day or later that week when your resolve weakens and suddenly the radical change you so desperately wanted to make doesn't seem to be such a good idea anymore. If this is a familiar scenario, you probably haven't clearly defined the reasons why you want to make changes nor do you have any real strategies or supports to fall back on. That's why getting ready is so important.

Even if you feel that you've hit your breaking point and you want to stop bingeing right this minute, your long-term chances for success improve greatly if you take some time to act not out of desperation but rather out of a gentle resolve to heal yourself in a nurturing and healthy way.

Figure 7-1 illustrates some of the stages along the road to recovery.

REMEMBER

As you begin to reach out to and discover a variety of professional resources to help you on this journey, keep in mind that your emotional eating did not develop overnight nor will it go away overnight.

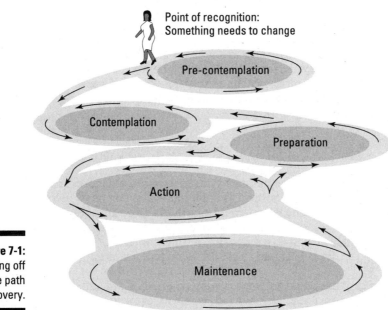

Point of recognition:
Something needs to change

Pre-contemplation

Contemplation

Preparation

Action

Maintenance

Figure 7-1:
Setting off
on the path
to recovery.

Some ideas for getting ready include

✔ **Identifying the reasons that you want to make a change.** In the next pages of this chapter, we offer several exercises to help you come up with motivators uniquely meaningful to you. You can also find other worksheets on the Internet, in a therapy or support group, or you can create your own from books or any other source you find. The most important thing is to be honest with yourself.

One person may want to lower her blood pressure because her sister just had a stroke, another may be motivated by wanting to be able to buy only one plane ticket instead of two to his daughter's destination wedding. Your reasons to stop bingeing will change over time, and success, however you define it, depends on having multiple, specific motivators that fit with you and your goals.

Try not to assume that any one motivator is more important than another. The bottom line is that the only motivator that matters is the one that speaks to you in that moment. Some days you'll just want to fit into a smaller pair of pants, some days it will be being able to get up and down from your sofa more easily, and on others, you may dream of playing catch with your kids without panting breathlessly. Just find the one that's meaningful to you right now.

✔ **Keeping a food journal before you attempt to stop bingeing.** In Chapter 12, we discuss the benefits of keeping a food and feelings journal during the course of slowing and eventually stopping the binges, but it's also a tool you can use even before you get started. If you numb out while you binge and can't remember exactly how much you ate and when, documenting every food, thought, and feeling, however onerous that might seem initially, is one of the keys to a greater understanding of what and why binges take place.

✔ **Deciding on a plan.** Successful, long-term change often depends on making incremental adjustments. Your first impulse may be to change everything all at once, but that kind of all-or-nothing thinking is part of the mentality that may underlie your disordered eating. Instead, consider making seemingly minor changes, one at a time, in a way that's manageable and realistic.

If you're unable to put your finger on two or three small changes you can make on your own or if you feel overwhelmed and unable to narrow down your goals, it may be time to ask for help from a professional.

✔ **Making an appointment with a psychotherapist.** Even before you've done anything at all, congratulate yourself for engaging in the initial stage of trying to examine and adjust entrenched eating behaviors, thoughts, and feelings. For many people, constructing a professional team consisting of an psychotherapist, a physician, a dietitian, and/or other professionals who work with patients who suffer from disordered eating is an important part of the process. (We talk about the types of professionals you may encounter in Chapter 10.)

If you've been considering making an appointment with a therapist but haven't yet done so yet, perhaps today is the day to make the call. And if you don't yet have referrals, perhaps your goal for this week and next is to find a couple either through some of the online resources we suggest in this book or from other trusted professionals.

Even if you aren't able to work with a professional eating disorder team for financial, geographic, or other reasons, you can in part mimic the support you would receive from these professionals on your own, if need be. You can set emotional and nutritional goals for yourself, and if you feel comfortable with your physician, you can include her in the health objectives you want to achieve.

Rating your reasons

It would be nice if slowing and eventually ending your binge eating or compulsive overeating was a matter of simply deciding to stop. However, always remember that the emotional and psychological forces at work which perpetuate your disordered eating defy logic, intellect, and good intentions. It takes something other than pure desire to shake up some of those habitual, automatic responses.

In Table 7-1 we suggest some of the most likely reasons you may want to stop overeating, but we left space at the bottom for you to write your own reasons. In the second column, rate each reason from one to ten with one signifying the reason doesn't matter to you at all and ten indicating that it's a very important reason.

Table 7-1 Pinpointing Your Reasons to Stop Bingeing	
Reasons for Wanting to Stop Bingeing	*How Much Does It Matter to Me?*
I will improve my overall physical health.	
I will be able to do more activities with my friends and loved ones.	
I hope to live longer.	
I will make a difference in the lives of my children by setting a better example of how to cope with life's ups and downs and also how to be kind to oneself.	
I will strengthen my relationship and will enhance intimacy with my partner or spouse.	
I will feel better about myself in so many ways by silencing my inner critic.	
I won't be afraid to go food shopping or attend social events at which I may be exposed to a lot of food.	
I won't have to listen to negative comments about my size or health from my friends, family, or strangers.	

(continued)

Table 7-1 *(continued)*

Reasons for Wanting to Stop Bingeing	How Much Does It Matter to Me?
I will enjoy shopping for clothes and won't have to wear only those things that drape and cape.	
I will be able to reduce or stop taking certain medications that became necessary to better manage my ill health due to obesity.	
I will be able to dine out with family and friends without feeling uncomfortable.	
I will be able to look in a mirror that shows more than just my head and chest.	

Take a moment to write out several copies of the five most important reasons on note cards that you can carry in your wallet or purse, leave in your desk drawer at work, and put any place you can use them to remind yourself of your goals when you find yourself wavering.

Setting SMART goals

Many binge eaters and people with disordered eating habits describe an all-or-nothing mindset that feeds the destructive eating habits they use to soothe themselves and numb pain, anxiety, shame, and/or other negative emotions. If you're an all-or-nothing thinker, you may feel as if you will never know what it is to eat specific portions or what it is to know when you're hungry or full; that you must either eat everything in sight or simply never eat again. If this description fits you, it probably seems like there's never a middle ground where you can slowly work up to your goals.

One way to work your way out of all-or-nothing thinking is by learning to set SMART goals, a technique that can help you get and stay motivated to change. SMART is an acronym for

  ✔ **Specific:** It's easier and more satisfying to meet a specific goal rather than a general one. A specific goals lays out exactly what you hope to achieve and why. For example, rather than saying, "I'm going to stop bingeing today," you can reframe your objective and decide, "I will eat regular meals and snacks this weekend."

✔ **Measurable:** Can you keep track of how you're doing on your goal? If your goal is to eat regular meals and snacks this weekend, you can document your progress in a food and emotions journal so that you know exactly what's going well and what you might need to pay attention to.

It's easy to fall into the trap of weight changes as the measureable goal here. Although losing weight may in fact be part of your health plan, it's a mistake to focus on it exclusively.

✔ **Attainable:** It can be overwhelming and indeed sabotaging to try to make huge changes overnight. That's why setting attainable goals is so important. Goals that are too small or too big become meaningless and may cause you to lose motivation. On the other hand, achieving a goal that's well-matched with where you are in your journey can help boost your confidence and sharpen the skills you'll need to continue.

✔ **Relevant:** Take time to determine what goals are important to you. Think about what goals make the most sense in your life right now, and set aside for later those that may be more important in the future. If, for instance, your long-term goal is to stop bingeing, developing a regular schedule of meals and snacks that you eat every day is an important new habit that you'll work on over time. Therefore, working on eating meals and snacks at the same time for a few days matters in terms of finding out how you'll feel as you practice this new habit and begin to adjust some of the ways you interact with food.

✔ **Time-bound:** Attaching a timeframe to a goal allows you to start and achieve objectives in discrete chunks or should we say "bite-size pieces?" If you set goals that must be achieved by a certain date, you not only give yourself an appropriate sense of urgency, you also have the opportunity to reassess and refine the goal and to set it again with slightly different parameters depending on what worked and what didn't. This also allows for your inevitable humanity and allows for slips without beating yourself up. Instead, you just reboot.

Setting SMART goals takes practice, so you'll learn as you go even if you have to make adjustments to the goals you set out for yourself. Your SMART goals format isn't meant to be a separate journal from the food and emotions journal, but merely a guide. You can record some of the successes and challenges you face as you begin to establish a new framework for your life. You can look back over time at how these goals change, how they influence your food selections, and how you feel about eating and yourself. Often taking a positive steps to achieve any goal helps you with all your other goals.

Just because you're trying to stop bingeing doesn't mean that all your goals must be related only to bingeing — or to food, for that matter. In fact, for true success, emotional goals are also necessary. Any and every goal has the potential to make you feel better. And feeling better, directly or indirectly, helps further your recovery.

Using multiple motivators for success

Just as most people who binge have a long list of reasons for turning to food for comfort, most also have several significant reasons why it makes sense to stop. Depending on what's going on in the rest of your life, these reasons may shift in priority. That's why it's important to identify several key motivators that can keep you going in the short and long term.

Try this exercise to begin to narrow down what will be meaningful to you as you move toward putting an end to binge eating in your life.

1. **Write down ten reasons to stop bingeing. (Write more if you can).**

   These can be anything from pants size, to medical health, to simply being able to get in and out of your car more easily or going out with friends more.

2. **Circle or highlight at least three reasons you find most compelling.**

   It's important to be honest with yourself here. Don't feel bad if something important like a serious health condition such as pre-diabetes, doesn't particularly move you to change your behaviors. Everyone is different so it's critical to zero in on what matters to you.

3. **Rank your motivators from Step 2 in order of importance.**

   Doing this sets the framework for what motivations you will use and when.

4. **Write a few sentences about each of your motivators, including why, how, and when each one is meaningful for you.**

   Ask yourself:

   - Why is this a motivator?

   - How does it motivate me?

   - When do I feel most motivated by it?

 Your answers provide you with a solid framework you can use to motivate yourself on a daily basis. Knowing what motivators to focus on is incredibly helpful when you're in the throes of an urge to binge. With practice, you can put your key motivators to use when you're struggling.

Feeling Better About Yourself

One of the simplest ways to feel better about yourself is to follow through on a goal. Maybe it's a food-related goal such as planning a healthy lunch and sticking with the menus you came up with. Or maybe you made use of the coping skills you've been practicing from Chapter 10. Or it could be cleaning out that closet you've been meaning to clean for the past six months. Whatever it is, big or small, following through on a goal you created for yourself is an esteem builder that can make you feel better about yourself.

Emphasizing the positive

As you begin to dig deeper into the reasons to seek help in ending binge eating, you may be thinking quite a bit about what you're giving up rather than what you may receive or gain in the long run. It's normal for your focus in this initial stage of change to be on the behaviors and thoughts that must come to an end rather than on welcoming the new habits, new joys, new pleasures, and new ways of thinking that will eventually take their place.

In addition, over time you may have gotten into the habit of berating yourself for many reasons. Binge eaters typically report shame, sadness, anger, and disgust with themselves before, during, and after they binge, and the accompanying negative self-talk that leads to compulsively overeating may be one part of what holds you back when you're trying to achieve any sort of goal, not just one that relates to disordered eating.

One strategy for reinforcing the positive and retraining yourself to think more about where you're going than where you've been is to plan for what you *will* do rather than what you *won't* do.

You may want to develop affirmations you can use to support your reasons for stopping bingeing. An *affirmation* is a short, positive statement that reminds you of your objectives and your ability to achieve them. If you've taken time to pinpoint your reasons for wanting to stop bingeing by using the exercise in Table 7-1 in the "Rating your reasons" section earlier in this chapter, then you're on your way to making positive changes that will improve your life in ways you can't yet fully understand. Using the primary reasons you decided on for ending the binges and your specific goals, you can develop affirmations that reinforce the small, manageable steps you're taking to end your binge eating.

These general guidelines for developing affirmations can help you get started:

- ✔ **State the affirmation in the present tense.** Begin with "I am" or "I can" to emphasize that the change you are seeking to make is happening now and not in the future.

- ✔ **Make the affirmation short and sweet.** You probably have many goals for yourself, but an affirmation is meant to reinforce a finite truth rather than to encompass everything you wish to change. The tighter the focus of the affirmation, the more likely it is to be effective.

✔ **Keep the words and the tone positive.** Though it may seem obvious, an affirmation is a positive statement. For example, if your goal is to take a five-minute walk around the block every time you feel the urge to binge, instead of telling yourself, "I won't binge, I won't binge, I won't binge" during the walk, a positive affirmation might be, "I enjoy walking" or "I feel healthy and strong."

✔ **Write the affirmation to reflect the way you speak.** No need to get fancy and poetic if that's not the way you talk. You may very well be a part of the swirling universe, but the affirmation should feel natural enough to you that it's easy to say and/or write repeatedly and makes you feel that you are able to achieve your goals.

✔ **Never suggest the possibility of failure.** No matter how much self-doubt you may be struggling with, an affirmation is an opportunity and a first step toward being all that you can be. Stay away from phrases like "I'll try" or "Maybe I'll . . . ."

If you've never worked with affirmations before, you may feel a tiny bit silly when you get started, especially if you've gotten used to negative self-talk that has reinforced some of the bad feelings you have about yourself. It takes time and patience to reverse and overcome the habit of beating yourself up, so do your best to be open to new ways of thinking and doing and give affirmations a try.

You can change and adjust the following affirmations to fit your thinking and your situation:

✔ I am strong and healthy.

✔ I am my own coach, not my own inner critic.

✔ I am eating healthy foods because they make me feel better.

✔ I am choosing my health and vitality over food.

✔ I am taking care of my body.

✔ I am enough.

✔ I choose moderation instead of regret.

✔ I can decide bite by bite if I want more.

✔ I can start over right now.

Finding ways to reward yourself

Now that you're thinking about finding meaningful motives and setting SMART goals, you may also want to plan for new ways to reward yourself when you reach those goals. If you typically celebrate your successes by eating or overeating, now's the time to consider other ways to celebrate meeting your objectives.

Although it may seem obvious, if your ultimate goal is to reimagine your relationship with food and to discover how to nourish yourself in healthier ways, you'll want to come up with pleasurable ways to honor your successes in life, not just those related to your recovery from binge eating, but also the other moments when something wonderful happens.

REMEMBER

That doesn't mean that you shouldn't ever have a piece of cake on your birthday or at a wedding, it just means that hopefully the cake won't be the most important part of the celebration to you.

In theory, your improved well-being should be reward enough, but let's face it, we're all human, and sometimes we need a little push. Over time, you'll come to know and appreciate the intrinsic or internal rewards of slowly and steadily bingeing less and less often, but sometimes extrinsic or external rewards can help motivate someone when the going gets rough.

No doubt you have ideas of your own, but we include a few of our favorite ways of rewarding yourself without food:

- Send yourself flowers. Sign them "from a secret admirer." (This one's our favorite, hokey as it is. Try it!)
- Enjoy a manicure and a pedicure — whether you're male *or* female!
- Take a long, relaxing bath.
- Buy yourself tickets to the theater, a sporting event, or some other big event you've been waiting to see.
- Go to the movies with a good friend or family member.
- Buy yourself some new music by a favorite artist, group, or composer.

No matter what it is, rewarding yourself is an opportunity to build on your success and slowly retrain yourself to live your life in a different way.

Improving Your Physical Health

There's no doubt that improving your physical health can be one of the most important and most meaningful reasons to make changes in your life. Your health may have declined over time as your cholesterol, blood pressure, and weight slowly crept up, but it may take a crisis or a diagnosis of a serious medical condition before you really decide that you needed to stop bingeing or compulsively overeating once and for all.

You probably already know that by improving your physical heath you'll live longer and live better with fewer medical conditions and less discomfort. And without a doubt, the benefits you realize from taking care of your body also spill over into other aspects of your life. If you spend time now identifying not only the physical improvements you'll experience when you take care of your body but also the psychological and emotional ones, the more motivation you'll have during the times when you are susceptible to your urges.

Psychological and emotional benefits, at times, are even more important than the physical benefits. Physical improvements such as weight loss, improved blood pressure, or a reduction in other health conditions such as sleep apnea, need time to occur whereas psychological and/or emotional benefits can be immediate. For example, noticeable weight loss may take weeks or even months, but feeling more upbeat because you're not bingeing or communicating more effectively with your spouse can happen right away. Focusing on this can help you get through those first few weeks or months until you do have noticeable physical improvements.

 Make a list of all the benefits you'll experience if you stop bingeing. Start with the physical improvements but also include the psychological and emotional pluses as well. Chances are, the list is endless when you stop to think about it. The most important part of this exercise is to prioritize the improvements that speak to you and are meaningful in your life.

Removing the Stigma from Binge Eating Disorder

While much progress has been made for other groups in society, if you're an overweight or obese binge eater, you probably already know that bias against people who are overweight is one of the last socially acceptable forms of discrimination.

Finding motivation in the next generation

Edna has type 2 diabetes, and when she binges, it can take two or three days to get her blood sugar back to an acceptable range. Even though she visits her doctor regularly and understands the risks to her health and how much better she'd feel if she gave up bingeing, she still can't stop. Recently she tripped in her garden and slashed her leg against a rock. One of the side effects of diabetes is slow wound healing, and it took a long time for her leg to heal and for her to be up and around again. Her kidney function has also slowed considerably, and sometimes she goes for several months without bingeing after she sees the nephrologist because she's so fearful of what might happen if she doesn't stop. Unfortunately, these periods never last.

Edna's daughter has pleaded with her to stop overeating and emphasizes that Edna is doing terrible damage to her health and to her body. Even though Edna agrees, when she's in the throes of a binge, her concerns about her health go right out the window, and she forgets all about her blood sugar.

The only thing that seems to keep her from bingeing is the desire to see her grandkids grow up and to participate in their lives. Even though she's tried for years to stop bingeing, now that her grandson is playing t-ball, something clicked for her, and she's determined not to binge so that she feels well enough to attend his t-ball games on Sunday afternoons. Edna knows that if she has a binge on Saturday night, she'll feel too sick on Sunday to attend. In the moments when Edna really wants to binge anyway, she focuses on her grandson and imagines him and his teammates in their uniforms.

Even though controlling her blood sugar and managing the effects of diabetes was a motivator for her, it wasn't quite enough. Instead, by focusing on her grandson instead of on her personal health, she can work though the urges without bingeing, attend the games, and lower her blood sugar.

For many years, people assume that if someone is overweight or obese, that means that person is lazy, undisciplined, or unmotivated to lose weight. If you've ever heard anyone use those words or other kinds of disparaging language toward you or someone else struggling with disordered eating and/or weight issues, you know how hurtful comments like this can be — especially because they're not true.

With the inclusion of binge eating disorder in the most recent *Diagnostic and Statistical Manual of Mental Disorders (DSM-V),* hopefully there will be greater opportunities for research that may offer a window into the minds and bodies of people who are vulnerable to binge eating or compulsive overeating disorders.

In the meantime, you can find ways to protect yourself and ensure that your civil liberties remain intact no matter what your size or shape. Apart from limiting relationships with people who make you feel bad about yourself, you can also be aware of bias in the following situations:

- ✔ **Medical care:** Studies show that in spite of their training, doctors suffer from the same degree of anti-fat bias as the rest of the population. The results can be devastating for your health and well-being if you're obese and seeing a biased physician. In addition to not getting the care you need for conditions that may be the direct result of obesity, if you feel judged by your physician, you may skip preventative care and routine screenings for diseases such as cancer.

  What can you do? No matter how long you've been seeing the same doctor, you may need to make a change. Get recommendations and research potential physicians online, then interview them and get a sense of how they might approach you and your medical needs.

- ✔ **The workplace:** Discrimination in the workplace for any reason is unacceptable. Many overweight or obese individuals have experienced difficulties at work due to their weight no matter the quality of the work they do. A study published in the *International Journal of Obesity* showed that women are 16 times more likely to report weight discrimination than men and that starting salaries and leadership potential are negatively impacted for obese people.

  If you think you are a victim of workplace discrimination, the first place to check in is with your human resource contact. Review the workplace discrimination materials to find out exactly what your rights are.

- ✔ **Travel**: Many airlines charge double if you don't fit in a seat with an extension belt or with the armrest down. Some airlines require you to purchase two seats.

Motivational Tools to Start the Process of Change

As you begin and hopefully continue the process toward making sustainable progress, your goals will inevitably change as you slowly and reasonably implement new eating habits and new ways of thinking about food and your body. Several months and years from now when you look back on the exercises and journals you're working on right now, you may be surprised to find that what motivates you then may be much, much different than what motivates you today.

Part of the journey towards ending the binges is understanding that nothing — not even your strategies toward disordered eating — stays the same. Over time, as you hopefully come to terms with the way you use food to cope with stressful situations, your mindset may shift and you may need to come up with new, more compelling reasons to keep going.

Some strategies to keep your motivation strong and current include

- ✔ **Reading, reading, reading:** You can find countless books about disordered eating and individual paths towards recovery. Not every story will speak to you, but many may have some kernel of knowledge or truth that strikes a chord as far as your own struggle and your own progress. Even if you don't know exactly why something seems meaningful to you, you can keep a reading journal where you jot down quotes from and impressions of the books you read. If you feel stuck some time in the future, looking back at the journal may give you renewed energy and perspective.

- ✔ **Going online:** The Internet offers myriad opportunities to connect with other people and find inspiration and ideas. Many of the most prominent and respected eating disorder organizations offer chat rooms and online support groups geared toward binge eaters. In addition, you can find articles, blogs, and essays about personal transformation of all kinds.

- ✔ **Acknowledging your accomplishments regularly:** Self-reflection is a powerful tool for continued motivation. Self-reflection is an opportunity to examine the past, but it's also a way to keep you grounded in how far you have come. Taking time to remember and acknowledge your success and all the lessons you've learned may very well be the thing that keeps you motivated in those moments you're feeling more susceptible to your urges to binge. Keep a running list that you update every few months as a way to see the large-scale changes you've made.

- ✔ **Using technology:** If you have a smartphone or tablet, you already know that thousands of apps exist for fun, work, shopping, games, and almost anything else you can think of. If you haven't taken time to explore the many apps for personal health, you may be missing out on great tools to support your efforts to end binge eating. You can keep your food and emotions journal on your phone, learn mindfulness techniques, practice alternate coping skills, download a meditation timer, or explore many other apps designed to help you set and meet your goals.

  As you're exploring apps, avoid downloading and using calorie counters. They're not productive and may lead to feelings of deprivation.

- ✔ **Watching inspiring movies:** Sometimes checking out and tuning into a heartfelt positive and inspiring movie can help reset your mind frame during those times that you are not feeling particularly motivated.

If you find that reading stories about others with eating disorders fails to inspire you over time, remember that struggling with and overcoming a challenge isn't something that's unique to binge eaters or people struggling with disordered eating. Inspiration can come from all sorts of stories, so don't forget to look beyond books and websites about food and eating.

Chapter 8

Deciding to Seek Treatment

· ·

In This Chapter

▶ Figuring out the initial steps

▶ First things first: who ya gonna call?

▶ Adopting a new slow and steady attitude about food and body

▶ Thinking about a more comprehensive approach

· ·

*W*hen you decide that enough is simply enough, and you're really ready to stop bingeing or compulsively overeating, you may still be conflicted, confused, and overwhelmed about who to contact first and how to move forward. You may also be equally afraid of both success and of failure. That may sound strange, but read on.

If you're reading this book, you've probably been on more diets than you can remember, and you've more than likely tried and been unsuccessful at eating in a way that better serves you for the long haul. What's happened before doesn't matter now. Let's say that again in another way: The past need not predict the future and, in fact, will likely only get in your way if you're punishing yourself rather than just being curious about what can be different from here on out. What counts most is that today you remain committed to doing what you need to do to follow a new path. No matter how determined you are, that may still take regular reminders and pushing the restart button each and every day.

The way you approach your recovery can be a blueprint for how you begin to think about your relationship to food (and stressors) for the rest of your life. First and foremost, before you begin, it's important to take a step back, learn about your treatment options, make reasonable, well thought-out decisions about how to proceed, and then follow through on the plan — one bite-size piece at a time.

Believe it or not, if you jump in too fast, it's possible to "binge" on treatment! That's not to discourage you in any way from moving forward with enthusiasm, energy, and optimism. However, how you approach treatment can be a metaphor for everything else in your life. If you're trying to make a fresh start, consider that the process is a marathon — not a sprint — and that your long-term interests are best served by a moderate approach.

In this chapter, we discuss first steps and introduce you to the different types of professionals you may wish to see along the way. We discuss the benefits of medical monitoring, targeted psychotherapy, group support, and/or nutritional counseling as well as touching on other modalities that may help you. Finally we talk about the last resort — the very last resort — of bariatric surgery, its pros and cons, and a new non-surgical alternative, Virtual Gastric Band (VGB) or Gastric Band Hypnosis (GBH).

Taking the First Step

Research shows that eating disorders across the spectrum often go undiagnosed and/or untreated. That's particularly true for the more than eight million people in the United States alone who suffer from binge eating disorder. As you may know from your own life or from the lives of those you care about, binge eaters can go for years without ever being formally diagnosed or treated for what's really taking a toll on their health.

Taking the first step is easier than you think. Whether it's been a few days or a few years since you've seen your primary care physician, your first stop should be a visit to your doctor for a comprehensive medical exam that can be a benchmark as you begin to make changes. Figure 8-1 shows treatment paths and possibilities.

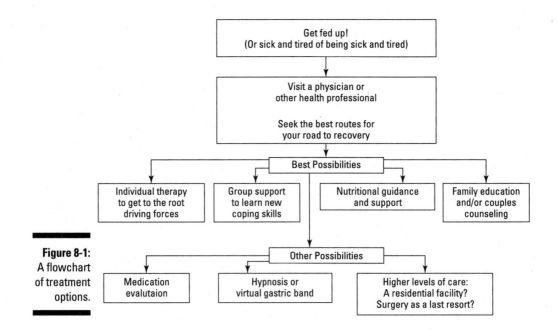

Figure 8-1:
A flowchart
of treatment
options.

As you get into the rhythm of recovery and find new patterns and ways of being, hopefully it will get easier and easier to incorporate self-care into your life.

Seeing your doctor

Having support from your physician is important as you attempt to stop binge eating.

Over the years, you may have been treated for conditions you suffer as a result of overeating, and perhaps you've already been candid with your physician about your disordered eating. If that's the case, then bravo to you — being open and honest with at least one person even before you attempt to make a change is a huge step and one that you can be proud of. Now that you want to move forward and stop bingeing, you should plan to meet with your doctor again to develop a plan for the physical and/or medical part of your journey.

And if you're just now realizing that you have a problem or if you've been keeping the truth from your doctor, now is the time to be upfront with her. Knowing more about the extent of your disordered eating and associated conditions such as depression or anxiety that may be exacerbating the situation is a crucial component of the strategies you and your physician develop together.

Although doctors are well-trained and very well-intentioned, if you find that any discussions with your doctor seem inadvertently punitive or scolding, see if you can have a frank conversation about dealing with each other in a more encouraging, respectful way. If an honest, forthright talk doesn't do the trick, you may want to consider seeing someone who can be both kind and firm. It may sound like mattress-testing, but having a supportive doctor is important to your success.

Although it may seem foreign to you at the beginning of this process, learning to respect and care for your body is one of the key pieces to the puzzle. Over time, and in a thoughtful way, you can slowly nurture and heal yourself from the effects of binge eating and/or compulsively overeating. But as we say throughout this book, there's no need to take everything on at once, and you shouldn't feel that you must resolve each and every issue simultaneously. If you've been bingeing for years, it will take time to slowly and steadily discover new coping mechanisms and more effective ways to approach eating and being in the world.

You'll obviously have goals specific to your situation, but if you're looking for a jumping off point, keep these objectives in mind:

 ✔ **Take a good look in the clinical mirror.** First things first, you need to know what your weight trends have been (gains/losses and over what period of time). If it's too triggering to know your actual weight, your clinician can track it blindly as long as someone is tracking consistently. It's also vital (no pun intended) to know your blood pressure and cholesterol levels and whether your bingeing has put you at risk or has caused the beginnings of heart disease, diabetes, or any number of other conditions that accompany being overweight and/or obese.

Making that first appointment may seem daunting, but it's important to have this information both because it's one way to mark the beginning of your journey and also because it can be a way to motivate yourself as you see these markers change.

✔ **Find ways to track and monitor your progress.** Develop a plan with your doctor to do regular blood work and have regular checkups. Although your weight may not change immediately, easing out of the binges can have immediate, beneficial effects on your blood sugar, cholesterol, digestion, and other physical indicators. Having accurate records of your progress is one way to keep yourself motivated.

Even though you may be eager to lose weight, it's important to remember that your weight may not change immediately when you stop bingeing. Although it may be a new way of approaching your health and your body, stay focused on your overall physical well-being and be aware of your energy level, digestive or bowel habits, breathlessness when it occurs, and the cholesterol and blood sugar. Try not to pay much attention to the scale.

✔ **Keep up with your regular screenings.** If your energy is refocused on your new commitment to your health, you may feel as if you don't have time for extra doctor's appointments for seemingly unrelated and less important screenings such as gynecological and urological exams, mammograms, skin checks, and other preventative health care. Think again. Your total healthcare picture can determine your success.

Scheduling time with specialists

Depending on what's been bothering you most, your physician may refer you to specialists to address some of the effects of binge eating and compulsive overeating. Hopefully most of these appointments aren't urgent or life threatening, but that doesn't mean that they're not important. Some of the basics to check on include:

✔ **Balancing your hormones:** Often binge eating can negatively affect your endocrine system, leaving your hormones and your body out of balance. Your physician may refer you to an endocrinologist to monitor and treat these conditions.

✔ **Taking care of your teeth:** Bingeing can take a toll on your dental hygiene, and even if you've never had a discussion with your dentist about bingeing, he may have long suspected that you suffer from disordered eating based on certain findings. Whether you choose to tell your dentist directly that you suffer from binge eating disorder or another form of compulsive overeating, if you've avoided regular dental appointments until now, consider seeing your dentist more regularly.

✔ **Seeing things more clearly:** As you may already know, unregulated blood sugar from binge eating can cause changes in your eyesight, making your eyes cloudy and your night vision poor. If you've stopped bingeing recently, you may have noticed that your vision has improved, and you'll want to visit your ophthalmologist or optometrist for a checkup and possibly a revised prescription.

✔ **Moving beyond the conscious mind:** As researchers learn more about binge eating and other eating disorders, many physicians and psychotherapists have enlisted hypnotists to work with their patients. If you have an eating disorder, you may have rationalized your behavior for so long that it seems right and reasonable to you, and you may easily be able to explain your logic to anyone who asks. Hypnosis seeks to engage the subconscious mind as part of the process of retraining you to think and behave differently. It's worth asking about and/or considering if a member of your treatment team suggests it for you.

Seeking Psychological Support

Finding psychological and emotional support is one of the most critical parts of changing your relationship to food. If you've tried and failed to stop bingeing before, you probably already know that disordered eating has little to do with food itself. Food is just the weapon you're using against yourself and the feelings that make you most uncomfortable.

Although the specifics are different from person to person, bingeing, compulsive overeating, and emotional eating often arise as unhealthy coping mechanisms when life gets difficult. The central principle underlying your own healing is to become aware of this, to uncover more about your own triggers, and to come up with new ways of dealing with negative or troublesome emotions.

Psychological support comes in many forms. Many people with disordered eating seek out one-on-one counseling with a psychotherapist who has specific training and experience with eating disorders. Others go to therapy groups or support groups, and others find Overeaters Anonymous, other 12-step meetings, and/or Weight Watchers meetings for the encouragement and support they seek. Over time, you may experiment with one or all of these as you put together a plan that works best for you and your life.

Figuring out where to start

After you see your doctor, the next step is to put together the other parts of your treatment team. Experience counts when it comes to treating disordered eating, so as best you can, try to find specialists who frequently work with these and related issues. If you're unable to locate anyone with this expertise in your geographical area, you can search for professionals who work with addictions or at the very least have experience treating anxiety, depression, and/or mood disorders.

In addition to considering psychotherapy, if your doctor has access to excellent dietitians, then you can also start there. If she refers you to a support group at a local hospital, that's another great jumping-off point. You may have your own contacts, and you can feel good about reaching out to someone recommended to you by a friend or who you heard about through the grapevine.

Physicians, psychotherapists, psychiatrists, nutritionists, and other practitioners have informal or established professional networks, so no matter where you begin, you can tap into a group of experts who can help you on your way when you're ready. It may be that you see only one specialist at a time or you may find that you need the support of a full team — whether under the same roof or several roofs. Whatever works for you and your life is the right kind of treatment, so you can be confident that taking definitive action will lead you in the right direction with time and persistence.

Understanding why psychotherapy matters

If you're ambivalent about psychotherapy of any kind, you may want to reconsider your point of view, especially if the way you've been living and the ways you use food to soothe yourself no longer are viable and are, in fact, ruining your life and your health.

As we say, eating disorders are not about food; they're about using food as a way to cope with what's difficult in life. In fact, research consistently shows that in addition to the isolation, stigma, and physiological changes that occur when someone suffers from disordered eating, sufferers also experience higher rates of other mental disorders including anxiety, depression, and alcohol or other substance abuse.

Being nervous about or even afraid of seeing a psychotherapist or participating in a support group is normal, especially if you've spent years hiding or self-soothing uncomfortable behaviors and/or feelings. Although it may take time to understand why you've been bingeing and to develop other coping strategies, you may still experience an extraordinary sense of relief almost immediately when you have an opportunity to talk about yourself and find that you are not alone.

Recovering with the help of a therapist

You may or may not feel that psychological counseling should form the basis of your recovery or you may need time before you're ready to explore the reasons behind your thoughts and behaviors regarding food and body issues.

Therapists work in many different ways, and whatever your ideas about psychotherapy — positive or negative — we suggest developing openness and flexibility with respect to this kind of treatment. First and foremost, a psychotherapist can determine whether your disordered eating is putting your life or your health at serious risk. If that's the case and you haven't yet worked with your doctor, a psychotherapist can help you get the medical monitoring you deserve.

Therapeutic approaches can be varied and carefully targeted. You may work together using cognitive behavioral therapy (see Chapter 11), focusing on keeping track of your behaviors and your triggers in order to understand and eventually alter them. Or depending on your situation, you may need to dive right in to the underlying psychological issues that drive your binge eating or other forms of overeating, what we call a more psychodynamic approach. Treatment will more than likely include a combination of these and other techniques. That's why working with a therapist who knows and understands disordered eating is so important.

Over time, therapy may uncover other conditions that exacerbate or trigger your binges. For example, understanding that undiagnosed attention deficit hyperactivity disorder (ADHD), depression, anxiety, and/or other psychological issues can be a watershed moment in recovery since these conditions can be treated and managed with therapy and sometimes with medication if necessary.

"What?" you say. "No medication for me. I don't want to be drugged or doped up!" We couldn't agree more. The idea of being evaluated psychopharmacologically when recommended, is merely to identify and address any inherent or acquired neurobiological abnormalities that may be directly affecting your moods and behaviors. It's not for everyone by any means but may need be considered in any no-stones-unturned approach.

Enlisting Nutritional Support

Alongside psychotherapy, beginning to understand your eating behaviors and creating strategies to make changes is crucial in the effort to put binge eating behind you. Depending on what's readily accessible to you geographically or if you're psychotherapy-resistant, you may prefer to start by seeing a registered dietitian. If that feels right to you and addresses your immediate needs, then nutrition counseling may be the best entry point for your treatment process. A good dietitian can help you get started and refer you to other specialists over time if he or she feels you need additional support.

If you've been binge eating for some time now, seeing a dietitian, collaborating on structured, but manageable, meal plans, and reporting back on your progress and challenges can really help change the way you think about food. You may be thinking, "Yeah, but if I could just follow a plan, I wouldn't have a problem to begin with. Isn't that the same as all my failed diets?" Actually, no, because a big part of this process is relearning and then practicing when, how, what, and where to eat. You may find that regular visits to a dietitian help you understand and implement everyday practical skills you can use for a lifetime.

Dietitians trained in dealing with eating disorders can offer

✔ **Accountability:** Regular appointments with a dietitian encourage you to be accountable for helping develop and follow your eating plan and readily acknowledging what may be challenging for you as you move forward. If you've never kept a food diary before, reviewing it regularly with a dietitian in a compassionate, non-judgmental, and constructive way will make a big difference in your success. Over time, you'll learn to nourish your body in a more consistent and thoughtful way and to become responsible to yourself rather than to another person.

At the start, you may need to be in touch with your dietitian every day, and new, easily accessible apps and technologies allow a clinician to check up on you between appointments if you need it. In addition to in-person visits, either due to schedules or geography, you may also be able to work with someone by video chat or phone on a regular basis, which may more readily ensure consistent sessions.

✔ **Personalization:** Because there's no one-size-fits-all strategy, by tailoring a plan to suit you and your specific life situation, whether you're following a meal plan or learning how to master intuitive eating, an experienced nutrition professional can suggest and apply the methods that work best for you.

- ✔ **Motivation:** At the beginning, you may find yourself extremely motivated to change, but over time, motivation can fade for even the most dedicated person. The goal is to keep you engaged and enthusiastic for the changes you're making even when you get discouraged or frustrated. Sometimes all you need is the perspective and wisdom of someone who's seen others work through the same situations and feelings that you're experiencing.

- ✔ **Safety:** If you're eager for immediate results, it can be tempting to go on a radical or fad diet even if you know that starving yourself is nothing more than a one-way ticket to bingeing. A dietitian's role is to step in and teach you how to eat regular and moderate meals and snacks rather than engaging in eating practices that may be dangerous and ultimately self-defeating.

Working with Your Insurance Provider

If you've done research into the cost of treatment, you may feel a bit overwhelmed. There's no doubt that treatment for binge eating or any disordered eating can be costly, and you may need to take on treatment in stages so that you can afford to get what you need over a period of time.

Most, if not all, practitioners understand these concerns and can help you in various ways. Some have *sliding scale payment plans,* which allow you to pay what you can afford rather than the regular fee. Others can help you navigate the world of managed care so that your treatment is either covered by, or at least fairly well reimbursed by, your insurance carrier.

One of the first calls to make is to your insurance provider. Now that binge eating disorder has been recognized as a diagnosed eating disorder alongside anorexia and bulimia, change is coming to the way that insurance providers cover treatment. Even so, every insurer is different, and you need to find out the specific rules for your coverage so that you know whether psychotherapy, nutrition counseling, and/or other therapies are a part of your plan.

Ultimately, if you're serious about making a change, you may need to come to terms with dedicating some financial resources to your own health and well-being even if you must work on your budget to find the money you need for yourself and your treatment. It may be that if you're bingeing less, your food costs diminish and you can find resources there. Or you could decide to spend less in other areas to make up the shortfall. Whatever it is, if you can, please make yourself and your health a priority. Interestingly, most people report that they discover that their attitudes and practices about money and food often parallel each other. Just food for thought.

Finding Free Resources

As you embark upon your journey of recovery, keep in mind that you may be able to find therapeutic and nutritional support groups or meetings at little or no cost to you. Whether these meetings or groups become your primary forms of therapy due to financial constraints or whether they become simply additions to your overall plan, they can be extremely helpful and provide a good opportunity to get ideas from others:

- ✔ **Joining an online group or chat room:** Some of the many online support groups and/or chat rooms allow you to drop in as needed while others are closed and have set times every week when you meet online with the other members and maybe a group leader. You may need to do some research and try various groups until you find the right one. We discuss online groups in Chapters 10 and 14.

- ✔ **Visiting an Overeaters Anonymous (OA) or other 12-step meeting in your area:** OA is a nationwide support group for people who suffer from binge eating, compulsive overeating, and emotional eating among other forms of overeating. You can find a local, in-person meeting online at www.oa.org, or you may want to consider joining a telephone or online meeting if it fits better into your schedule. Other helpful 12-step groups may include Co-Dependents Anonymous or CoDA (www.coda.org), Al-anon (www.al-anon.alateen.org), and Eating Disorders Anonymous or EDA (www.eatingdisordersanonymous.org).

- ✔ **Making use of free nutrition or food diary programs online:** You can log your food intake on websites including www.myfitnesspal.com and www.recoveryrecord.com. Some sites display calories, and some don't. Not every program will be right for you, so take time to try out a few different ones to see if there's one way of logging your food that feels best.

Most of these sites include forums on topics such as emotional eating or binge eating. If you don't like online food logging, consider signing up for the forum only. This way you can get some support for free in an anonymous program without having to use the food diary part of the program.

Investigating Other Treatments

Hopefully, once you begin this process, you'll be comfortable with the idea of reasonable, measured progress. However, at times, you may also feel desperate and wish for a solution that can solve your problem in one fell swoop. Many people feel this way, but in practice, these solutions are few and far between, and rarely, if ever, work without the steady commitment we discuss here.

Although the therapies we talk about in the next sections may be warranted in extreme cases, keep in mind that although they provide what seems like a quick fix, in the long run, they won't keep you from having to do the work of exploring and learning to adjust your tendency to eat in response to emotional triggers. You still need to find your own way to eat in response to physical hunger instead of emotional need. That's not to say that these treatments may not be right for some; however, you need to make your decision in conjunction with experienced professionals who can help you examine all the pros and cons.

Investigating bariatric surgery

Bariatric surgery is an option you may have considered if the challenge of dealing with your intense binge eating feels insurmountable. Surgery may seem like an easy way to solve your eating and weight problems quickly with minimal effort on your part; however, weight loss surgery is risky and very much a last resort. Although it's appropriate for some people, bariatric surgery is probably not for most people no matter how extreme your bingeing may have become.

The three most common surgeries include

- ✔ **Gastric bypass:** Gastric bypass is a surgery performed to limit both the amount of food you can take in and the way the food is absorbed. The stomach is generally divided into one large and one small pouch and the small intestine is reattached to both, with the smaller stomach being the primary controller of how much food you can take in.

- ✔ **Laparoscopic gastric banding (lap band surgery):** Lap band surgery works by making the stomach physically smaller, which then limits the amount the stomach can hold. During the surgery, an inflatable band is placed around the top portion of the stomach. The surgery is minimally invasive and reversible.

- ✔ **Vertical sleeve gastrectomy:** This surgery involves removing the left side of the stomach, leaving a much smaller stomach about the size and shape of a banana.

Although many patients report good short-term results after bariatric surgery, because surgery patients don't necessarily develop new nutritional strategies or address the underlying reasons that drive their abnormal eating, a large percentage of patients usually regain a portion of the weight within the first three years of surgery, especially in the case of lap band surgery.

You must evaluate for yourself whether those odds are worth the risks and costs of surgery. It's also worth noting that in a large number of cases, other addictions surface subsequent to the surgery. There are a number of theories about why, but you can understand that in order for real, sustainable change to occur, it's vitally important to keep getting support to get at the heart of what drives you to eat other than out of physical hunger. Other potential long-term complications can include

- Ulcers
- Gallstones
- Malabsorption of nutrients, protein, vitamins, and minerals in food including vitamin B12 and iron, which cause anemia and muscle wasting
- Hernias and bowel obstructions
- Leaks at one of the staple lines in the stomach or between the stomach and the small intestine that can cause intractable and repeated infections

Considering another alternative: Gastric band hypnosis or virtual gastric band

Hypnosis for weight loss is a very effective and innovative technique to treat compulsive overeating or binge eating. Treatment called GBH (gastric band hypnosis) or VGB (virtual gastric band) involves using hypnosis as a viable alternative to invasive surgical procedures.

A significant trial is being conducted under the auspices of The National Health Service of Great Britain. Long-term effectiveness of GBH and VHB seem to far surpass long-term results of actual surgeries, although the study results weren't published as this book goes to print.

Elements involved in the procedure include

- Undergoing careful psychological pre-screening.
- Four consecutive weekly one-hour sessions performed by a certified hypnotist who suggests that the surgery has taken place. The patient is completely awake and aware but in a highly relaxed state, and the hypnotherapist can speak to the patient's receptive preconscious mind.
- Listening to a short CD once or twice a day for 28 days.
- Willingness to follow nutritional and body movement guidelines and practices specific to the methodology.

Make no mistake: Although GBH/VGH is much less costly and does not carry any of the risks as actual surgery, it too will fail over time if other supports are not put in place as part of a responsible and sustainable program such as the treatment modalities we discuss throughout the book. These may include support groups, targeted psychotherapy, body movement, and/or nutritional counseling and education.

Considering a residential or inpatient setting

If other options have been exhausted and/or have not produced the desired results, or if your health is beginning to fail because of the effects of the binge or overeating and accompanying overweight, or if you feel you've hit rock bottom either physically or emotionally, you may want to consider inpatient or residential treatment in which you attend a specialized facility for a period of weeks or months for intensive treatment.

Although the types of treatment may not be so different from what you could seek as an outpatient, how often you see a psychotherapist, nutritionist, psychiatrist, and attend groups of all kinds is much greater, and you have food chosen or prepared for you with varying levels of your own participation. You're also temporarily removed from your typical work, school, home, and living environments and all of the most potent triggers and are completely taken care of in a nurturing, contained environment. Much deeper and lasting work can be accomplished in this kind of setting if it is recommended.

Of course, wherever you go, there you are, so the work must be aimed at enhancing your ability to support your own needs when you return home. In inpatient or residential settings, there's also an emphasis on educating and engendering the support of those who are important in your life so that they may also aid in your sustained recovery.

You may be thinking, "Isn't this like rehab?" In some ways, yes, but it would be a mistake to think that it's the magic bullet. After all, if all it took were being away from the things you and others are addicted to, be it drugs, alcohol, food, or any other stimulation to the pleasure centers of the brain, wouldn't that be enough to accomplish the task? Surely you've noticed that addicts who attend rehab must be in some form of supportive environments for life or the chances of relapse are exponentially higher and more frequent.

It takes time for long-standing, entrenched behaviors and mechanisms to no longer be your primary reflex. We cannot make this point loudly enough or too many times. It's key to the premise of this entire book.

To see if such a setting makes sense medically, financially, logistically, and therapeutically, first and foremost, you'll need to consult with eating disorder professionals to determine if you may be a candidate for this type of treatment. Some of the questions to consider together include

- Have the activities of daily life (ADLs) become more than I can handle? Am I unable to function because of my disordered eating?

- Am I on the verge of a serious, life-threatening health crisis that may permanently damage my body?

- Are my eating behaviors and overall mental functioning putting my job and/or other responsibilities at risk in a way I am unable to address or change in an outpatient setting?

- Do I have the time and the means to essentially be lifted out of my life for one-to-three months or more?

- Have I truly exhausted all other treatment options at my disposal?

If you answered yes to any of these questions, it may be time to talk to your doctor or any treating professional that you're seeing about more intensive treatment. Don't wait if you believe that you're in danger and need additional help.

Part III
Getting Well: The Team Approach to Recovery

Time/Meal	Food/Amount	Before the Meal Hunger Level/Emotions	After the Meal Fullness Level/Emotions	What would you do differently?
8 am Breakfast	Medium bowl cheerios, low-fat milk, 1/2 banana	3 - kind of hungry, I don't feel any emotions, need to get to work	5 - full, on my way to work, not feeling emotional	Nothing
10:30 am, snack	Coffee with milk	3 - I feel like snacking but know that I am not very hungry, just tired	4 - I'm glad I had a coffee, I feel more awake	Nothing
2 pm, lunch	Sandwich - turkey, lettuce, tomato & mustard on rye, baby carrots with light ranch dressing	2 - I am so hungry! Lunch is an hour late because of a meeting.	5 - I feel better but still a little hungry	Nothing
3 pm, snack	1 slice chocolate cake	5 - my coworker's birthday party had cake that smelled so good. I hate myself for not being able to say no!	5 - I feel guilty and embarrassed that I couldn't stop myself. Now I want to keep eating because I already messed up. I am going to focus on work and try not to beat myself up.	I would have eaten my apple instead. Or not had anything. I wasn't even hungry.
7:00 pm Dinner	One chicken breast, two scoops couscous, green beans. and side salad with light balsamic dressing, watermelon	2 - Very hungry. It was hard not to snack while I was making dinner. Proud that I didn't let myself start to binge after the cake!	5 - comfortably full. Still feeling a little guilty about the cake, glad that I didn't keep eating.	Nothing

Find suggestions for healthy eating at www.dummies.com/extras/overcoming bingeeating.

In this part . . .

✔ Meet the many types of professionals — and regular folks with binge eating disorder (BED) — who can help you through every step of your recovery.

✔ Use cognitive behavioral therapy (CBT) techniques to break bad habits and institute new ones. Coupled with psychological counseling, CBT can be a very practical and effective treatment option.

✔ Adopt healthy eating habits to help combat the urge to binge. Following a food regimen helps you beat the battle of the binge.

✔ Consider the benefits of medications and supplements. Taking medications and/or supplements that ease the symptoms of BED and additional or co-occurring ailments can help smooth the path to recovery.

✔ Seek support from family and friends. Not everyone is a candidate for your confidences about your eating disorder, but finding folks who can help you weather the storms can help keep you secure in your recovery.

✔ Reassess after a relapse. The reality is that most BED sufferers relapse. Recognize that a relapse isn't cause for despair; it's merely an opportunity to adjust your recovery plan to better meet your needs.

Chapter 9

Is Binge Eating an Addiction? (Well, if it Walks Like a Duck . . .)

. . . .

In This Chapter

▶ Understanding the biology of binge eating

▶ Recognizing addictive behaviors across the spectrum

▶ Knowing about other addictions that may go hand-in-hand with bingeing

. . . .

*A*s binge eaters emerge from the shadows, researchers are starting to figure out what happens in the brain and body of a binge eater before, during, and after a binge that makes the behavior so irresistible and compelling.

Binge eaters often describe their longing for food using the language of addiction. In common parlance, binges become *benders* and the morning after binge eaters suffer from *food hangovers.* The urge to binge is so strong that, like alcoholics and other addicts, a binge eater feels a biological drive to overeat even though she knows her desire isn't driven by physical hunger.

Because you can live without alcohol, drugs, gambling, and the object of some other addictions, the goal of treating them is total abstinence. But you cannot survive without eating, and that's why addictions related to food are some of the hardest to recover from. You must have a relationship with the very substances that have been the object of both your pleasure and torture.

Surprisingly, many people don't think of binge eating as an addiction because it's not an addiction to a substance. But people become addicted to behaviors as well as substances, which leads to gambling addicts, sex addicts, and binge eating addicts to name a few.

Furthermore, in May 2013, the American Psychiatric Association's fifth edition of the *Diagnostic and Statistical Manual of Mental Disorders (DSM-V)* included binge eating disorder (BED) as a condition separate from other eating disorders. By formally recognizing BED, patients, healthcare and mental health professionals, and the general public can begin to think about this disorder in a new, more productive way, and insurance providers may cover more of BED sufferers' treatment costs.

Most experts agree that binge eaters behave with food the same way alcoholics do with alcohol or drug addicts do when they take their drug of choice. Even more significantly, advances in brain science show that when binge eaters think about food or eat certain trigger foods, the pleasure circuits in their brains light up in the same way that the brains of other kinds of addicts do. In fact, in the past few years, Nora Volkow, Director of the National Institute on Drug Abuse, has been researching and making discoveries about the neuro-biology of binge eating and the ways in which the addictive pathways in the brains of binge eaters are similar to those of drug addicts.

In this chapter, we explore what's happening behind the scenes in the brain and body of a binge eater. We also talk about what makes an addiction an addiction, and we look at other addictions that can make bingeing worse and more difficult to stop.

Understanding Addictive Behaviors

To understand what addiction means, you first have to understand how a non-addicted brain works. When a person eats, drinks, has sex, or experiences any other type of pleasure or reward, the pleasure centers of the brain flood with chemicals, especially dopamine, that create a sense of satisfaction and well-being.

Human beings have evolved so that we continuously seek out the kinds of rewards that keep us alive — food and water — and that allow our species to survive — sex. Relatively recently, scientists have become aware that other substances and behaviors that our earliest ancestors never dreamed of — alcohol, drugs, shopping, and gambling among many others — light up the brain's pleasure circuits as well as the necessities of life.

No matter what the substance or behavior, the brain reacts to every type of pleasure in similar ways. Your reaction may be more or less extreme depending on the stimuli and whether you're addicted to those stimuli.

For the non-addicted brain, eating and drinking produces a temporary sense of satisfaction that's a combination of the physical sensation of a full stomach and the release of pleasure-causing chemicals into the neural pathways of the brain. Although the pleasure system in the brain never really turns off, even in the non-addicted brain, if you're not a binge eater, the drive to eat diminishes until you begin to get hungry again or until it's time for the next meal.

In the addicted brain, rather than revving up and then powering down, the pleasure centers are always revved up. Most of the time, the addicted brain works on overdrive, and it's nearly impossible for an addict to tell the difference between wanting something and needing it. Often the desire for the object of addiction becomes so overwhelming that it overshadows almost everything else in an addict's life including social contact, relationships, and other responsibilities. Even thinking about whatever fuels the addiction sends the addicted brain into overdrive.

Over time, any kind of addiction can significantly change the brain and the way that it responds to pleasure. The pleasure circuits become desensitized from frequent and often extreme bursts of chemicals from overuse of the addictive substance. To achieve the same levels of satisfaction, pleasure, and happiness, an addict must feed her addiction more often and in greater quantities.

The pleasure circuits also become attuned to certain kinds of rewards and desensitized to others. An addict may find it difficult or impossible to fill the pleasure void when he abstains from his substances or behaviors of choice. For example, if you're an alcoholic, the fun and enjoyment of seeing friends pales in comparison to the satisfaction you find from drinking alone. Over time, nothing else compares to drinking, and you may find yourself turning away from activities and people you once enjoyed.

Showing signs of addiction

Although every addiction has its own hallmarks, many addictions share the same symptoms. The following signs apply to all kinds of addictive behavior, including binge eating:

- ✔ **Focus:** Professional activities, friends, and social life all become a part of the addiction. Anything or anyone who stands in the way of feeding the addiction may fall by the wayside — especially someone who may call attention to how serious the problem is.

- ✔ **Lack of control:** Feeling powerless when faced with the addictive substance or behavior is one of the hallmarks of addiction no matter what you're addicted to. If you're a binge eater, you may not be able to control when the urge to binge strikes or how strong it is. Neither can you control the duration and depth of the actual binge.

- ✔ **Preoccupation:** If you suffer from any addiction, it's hard not to think about when you can get the next fix. You may spend every waking moment thinking about, planning for, or trying to resist your next binge. Just as you can't control the bingeing, neither can you control your obsessive thoughts about it.

- ✔ **Tolerance:** The more often an addict experiences his drugs or behaviors of choice, the more he needs to achieve the same kind of high. When you first start to binge, maybe once a week is enough, but as time goes on, you find yourself wanting and maybe needing to binge more often or for longer periods of time in order to get the same relief from depression, anxiety, boredom, loneliness, or other uncomfortable feelings.

- ✔ **Withdrawal:** If you're forced to stop the addictive behaviors for whatever reason, you may experience mild, moderate, or severe physical and/or emotional side effects. Your untreated depression or anxiety may worsen, and/or you may experience the effects of blood sugar instability, hormone levels, or other new physical sensations.

Treating addictions across the spectrum

One of the most compelling arguments for thinking of binge eating as an addiction comes from looking at how binge eaters recover. Like other addicts, many binge eaters benefit from specialized treatment from a team of clinical professionals. Also, when appropriate and recommended, binge eaters find value in participating in Overeaters Anonymous (OA) or Eating Disorders Anonymous (EDA), 12-step programs based on the principals of Alcoholics Anonymous (AA).

A *12-step program* includes a set of guiding principles as well as the support from a group or community, all meant to help promote recovery from addictive behaviors. Twelve-step programs have been one of the cornerstones of addiction treatment and recovery for decades, and although they may not work for everyone and/or may not be enough for everyone, many addicts across the spectrum of addiction find them a useful and important part of treatment and recovery.

More than 200 12-step programs for substance abuse and behavioral addictions exist worldwide, including Narcotics Anonymous and Gamblers Anonymous among many, many others. Most address very specific addictions, and all focus on the emotional, physical, and spiritual recovery of their members.

The 12 steps, as applied to overeating and binge eating, are

1. **We admitted we were powerless over food — that our lives had become unmanageable.**

2. **Came to believe that a Power greater than ourselves could restore us to sanity.**

3. Made a decision to turn our will and our lives over to the care of God *as we understood Him.*

4. Made a searching and fearless moral inventory of ourselves.

5. Admitted to God, to ourselves, and to another human being the exact nature of our wrongs.

6. Were entirely ready to have God remove all these defects of character.

7. Humbly asked Him to remove our shortcomings.

8. Made a list of all persons we had harmed and became willing to make amends to them all.

9. Made direct amends to such people wherever possible, except when to do so would injure them or others.

10. Continued to take personal inventory and when we were wrong, promptly admitted it.

11. Sought through prayer and meditation to improve our conscious contact with God *as we understood Him*, praying only for knowledge of His will for us and the power to carry that out.

12. Having had a spiritual awakening as the result of these Steps, we tried to carry this message to compulsive overeaters and to practice these principles in all our affairs.

Overeaters Anonymous offers daily or weekly meetings in locations around the world. Although the principles that govern OA and all 12-step programs have a spiritual component, OA meetings are non-denominational and include people of all faiths and backgrounds.

For many binge eaters, a supportive OA community forms a crucial part of recovery. In general, OA recommends every member have a guided or supervised eating plan. Without providing specific requirements for an eating plan, OA suggests consulting a qualified health care professional, such as a physician or dietitian, for a meal plan that fully meets your nutritional needs and cravings.

For more information about Overeaters Anonymous, visit their website at www.oa.org.

Looking at What the Research Says

If you're a binge eater, you may have heard over and over again that if you just had more discipline, resolve, or self-control, you'd be able to get a handle on your binge eating. You've probably heard yourself incorrectly described as lazy or weak for not being able to stop. This is simply not so.

It's important to want to stop enough to see that the benefits to stopping far outweigh the perceived, temporary benefits for staying with the addictive behaviors. But other forces are also at work, and advances in brain science offer new ways to understand the triggers and the drive to binge from a neurobiological perspective. By looking at images of the brain, scientists have begun to understand that processes similar to those that drive other addictions are what compel binge eaters to overeat.

Although the science is not yet conclusive, new information about how the brain works is changing the way experts think about binge eating and addictions in general.

In the same way that most people now consider alcoholism and drug addiction medical conditions that result from biological, hereditary, and environmental factors, current research suggests that binge eating may also eventually be understood in the same way.

Decoding the studies

Most of the studies regarding binge eating and addiction focus on what happens in the brain when someone binges. Brain-monitoring tools including PET scans and functional MRIs consistently show that the parts of the brain that light up when addicts abuse alcohol, drugs, or other substances are the same as during an eating binge.

Over time, the urge to binge and binge eating itself ultimately change the way the brain works in the same ways that the neural pathways of a drug or alcohol addict are often altered. These changes ultimately make professional intervention that includes, medical, psychological, and nutritional treatment necessary to slow and eventually stop the behaviors and cravings.

Both PET (positron emission tomography) scans and MRIs (functional magnetic resonance imaging) measure brain function, but because PET scans are quite costly and use a small amount of radioactive material, almost 95 percent of brain studies are now conducted with functional MRIs. Currently, these imaging techniques are used only for diagnosing neurological conditions, but with advances in neurobiology, they may someday also be used to diagnose other disorders and conditions that have an impact on the brain.

Mapping the body's response to binge eating

When you binge, your body has true physical responses that stimulate the brain's pleasure and reward centers in the same way that alcohol, drugs, or other addictive behaviors might. Just the urge to binge itself can set off a cascade of physiological events so that even without food, your urge to binge gets stronger.

Your brain on bingeing

Eating in general stimulates the brain's pleasure and reward centers. But for a binge eater, just thinking about food and eating is enough to flood the brain with the hormones and chemicals that can set a binge in motion. Often seeing or smelling something can also bring on a binge, referred to as *mouth hunger* rather than actual physical hunger. And once a binge is underway, stopping it is almost impossible. Not only can a binge eater not stop, she may not even want to.

When someone chronically binges, the pleasure centers in the brain receive frequent and strong stimulation, causing a cycle of emotions, reactions, and a motivation to binge. If you're a binge eater, you experience a constant and overstimulated hormonal cascade that affects your physiological hunger and your emotional state. As part of this round-the-clock hormonal imbalance, the urge to binge can be debilitating and impossible to break without professional help.

One of the key hormones that sparks a hormonal reaction chain is *ghrelin,* the primary hunger-generating hormone. It's secreted from the stomach and circulates until it reaches your brain, where it has receptors in the pleasure-and-reward center. The stomach secretes ghrelin not only in response to true physical hunger but also when you think about food, see food, or smell food. For binge eaters, the urge to binge can also trigger the release of *ghrelin,* which tells the brain that it's time to eat although ghrelin's true function is to alert the brain to actual physical hunger. When the stomach regularly releases ghrelin this way, the pleasure and reward center ends up causing a cycle of urges to binge, followed by actual bingeing, post-bingeing depression and guilt, and then the desire for pleasure, which starts the cycle all over again.

Binge eating disorder can stimulate the production of what are commonly known as stress hormones including cortisol, growth hormone, and noradrenaline. These hormones are usually released in higher concentrations at periods of high stress and can lead to sleep problems, feelings of anxiety, depression, and panic. These negative emotions may lead, in turn, to more bingeing, creating a deep psychological cycle that's difficult to break.

Because of stress hormones, you can actually gain weight and create a false sense of hunger simply by worrying too much about everything — including what to eat and not eat because of a fear of weight gain. A vitally important step is recognizing the need to calm the mind and body — not only so you require fewer addictive behaviors, but also so that your body does not secrete extra, unwanted hormones in response to your internal stress.

Your body on bingeing

Although not always, binge eating typically leads to *obesity,* defined as having a body mass index (BMI) above 30. *BMI* is a ratio of height to weight, and a BMI over 30 is known to promote health complications and reduced life expectancy. Obesity causes many medical complications such as high cholesterol, diabetes, heart disease, gallstones, gout, and certain types of cancer. Obesity also causes insulin resistance and the development of type 2 diabetes, which encourages the build-up of body fat, thus making it even harder to lose weight.

One of the reasons obese people gain weight at a faster rate, especially in the abdomen, is due to *leptin,* the fullness hormone. Leptin is secreted by fat cells, then circulates throughout the blood to the brain where it triggers a sense of fullness. In obese people, the brain becomes less sensitive to leptin, so even though you may have a lot of fat cells secreting leptin, your brain doesn't respond to it. This is a double whammy because ghrelin, the hunger hormone, is simultaneously working on overdrive stimulating hunger. The result is an overproduction of the hormone that triggers hunger and an inability to use the hormone that triggers fullness. If you're a binge eater and already obese, your body is programed to feel hungry rather than full, which leads to more weight gain and more difficult weight loss. The good news is that this process can be reversed, and you can lose weight as you reduce and eliminate your binge eating addiction. How long it will take you to lose weight is impossible to predict as weight loss is different for every individual, but because binge eaters rarely stop cold turkey, weight loss is generally not fast or consistent every week. Those in treatment working to reduce their binge eating behaviors may need weeks or even months to have a noticeable weight loss.

You may be disappointed by this news if you're hoping for a quick fix for your binge eating. And you're not alone because for people who need to lose weight for medical reasons, weeks or months without a noticeable change may actually trigger depression. But don't despair. Even before you lose weight, you'll probably experience noticeable and measureable changes in other areas. For example, you may lose inches before you lose pounds, reduce your percentage of body fat, and notice an improvement in your mood and in your overall sense of well-being.

Discovering a new normal

Betina first began her eating disorder treatment weighing 230 pounds. For years, she'd bounced between starving herself and then binge eating as a reaction to extreme hunger. Though she tried diet after diet, all of them left her hungry, and eventually she'd find herself bingeing again. When her husband suggested she try a different approach, she decided it was worth a shot.

She jumped into treatment with a psychotherapist, a dietitian, and a weekly support group meeting, and she expected immediate weight loss. Three months in, Betina's bingeing had decreased dramatically from five to six times per week to one to two times per week. However, even with this radical change, she still weighed the same as when she started. Although Betina initially stopped gaining weight, and even though she was no longer bingeing with the same frequency, she was still bingeing enough to prevent weight loss. It was only after months of treatment and no bingeing for several months that she finally noticed measurable weight loss. Two years later, Betina has successfully lost 35 pounds. It's taken longer than she hoped, but with slow and steady progress, Betina is finally in control of her food and urges to binge.

The most effective form of treatment for binge eating is to slow and then eventually stop the binges. In many cases, BED treatment results in weight loss but that's not, by any means, the only objective. The bigger picture is about not having to constantly think and plot and plan to actively avoid binges throughout your waking hours. Just imagine how much time you'll have when this is not a primary preoccupation.

Overlapping Addictions

Statistics show that if you're a binge eater or suffer from any other kind of eating disorder, you're more likely to have *co-occurring addictions* (additional, simultaneous addictions) and to come from a family with addictive tendencies.

Alcohol addiction is prominent among people suffering from eating disorders, particularly binge eaters and bulimics. And the lion's share of people with eating disorders of all kinds also come from families in which there are one or more alcoholics.

The combination of an eating disorder and alcoholism shows up in many ways, but one of the most distressing is *drunkorexia*. Though not a true medical diagnosis, it's not uncommon to find drunkorexics on college campuses where young women starve themselves all day to offset the calories they take in from binge drinking at night. Of those who suffer from eating disorders, drinking to excess, often followed by binge eating, affects bulimics most often, but it's also a problem for others on the eating disorder spectrum.

The little amount of data on drug use among binge eaters makes it impossible to know for sure if drug use is common among binge eaters or not. Studies on the relationship between other behavioral addictions such as gambling and shopping and binge eating haven't been done. But conventional wisdom leads many therapists to be aware of the possibility that binge eating may be tied into other addictive behaviors.

According to the National Comorbidity Study, up to 30 percent of people with binge eating behaviors have a related alcohol abuse or dependency issue. Furthermore, over 20 percent of individuals with binge eating behaviors were reported to have a coexisting condition of illicit drug abuse or dependency. Additional preliminary studies are also being conducted on binge eating behaviors and other behavioral addictions and impulse control disorders such as gambling and shopping. Thus far the researchers have found several similar character traits found to overlap binge eating with other behavioral addictions."

If you're seeing a psychotherapist about binge eating, he may also ask about your history of abuse or other trauma. It's quite troubling, but not surprising, that the majority of women with eating disorders report or discover that they have been abused. Many binge eaters also discover or report one or more traumas during their lives. *Trauma* can refer to many different kinds of events, but the event itself is less important than the perception and experience of having lived through it.

Chapter 10

Seeking Out Professionals and Support Groups

* *

In This Chapter

▶ Understanding all your treatment options

▶ Finding the best team for you

▶ Connecting with a dietitian

▶ Reinforcing your treatment with a support group

* *

As you work on moderating the symptoms of binge eating, you also need to think about why you may be doing it in the first place. We won't lie. Unraveling the reasons can be a complicated process, but it's the key to putting binge eating behind you and living a healthier life.

The first thing to understand is that there's no one-size-fits-all reason why people get trapped in the cycle of bingeing, gaining weight, dieting, and bingeing again. But it's important to remember that even though it's not easy to do, you can break the cycle and not have it dominate so much of your life.

To do that, you need to get to the heart of the matter. Unfortunately, when low self-esteem, depression, anxiety, childhood trauma, ADHD (attention deficit hyperactivity disorder), or other psychological conditions come into play, they can set off a chain reaction that may trigger binge eating. That's why finding experienced, compassionate professionals who specialize in treating disordered eating makes understanding and interrupting your binge eating much more likely.

Understanding and changing years of disordered eating takes time, patience, honesty, and a compassion for yourself that you may have not cultivated for some time — if ever. You may hope to avoid dealing with the root cause of your binge eating, but taking care of your overall psychological health is an essential part of reaching your goals and living a fuller, freer life.

In this chapter, we dig into the why's of binge eating and outline the psychological, biological, and social conditions that sometimes go along with it. We also show you how to translate knowledge into action with concrete tips and advice on who to call for help and which treatments may be best for you or someone you love.

Understanding the Most Effective Treatment Options

Finding the right treatment team, including a psychotherapist specializing in eating disorders and the right form of treatment is a little like love at first sight — you don't know why it works, but when it does, something clicks.

Even though there are some differences in education and therapeutic orientation among various mental health professionals, remember that one of the most important parts of successful psychotherapy is to find someone you trust and with whom you can develop a productive, truthful relationship. So, in addition to expertise and experience, you need to take personality into account as you consider your choices.

Depending on where you live, you may have lots of treatment options or not very many at all. Either way, as you do your research, know that you'll have to look at the personal connection you have with potential therapists as well as investigate credentials. Be flexible and trust yourself to pick the right person for you and your situation. And if at first you don't succeed, try, try again with someone else.

Not every type of therapy works for every person who suffers from binge eating disorder, but be assured that everyone can find a treatment that works best for him or her.

Good therapists have a whole bag of tricks with a variety of therapies based on years of experience working with those who suffer from eating disorders. An experienced therapist can develop a therapeutic plan based on each individual, and most importantly, is flexible and knowledgeable enough to make changes as the patient recovers or circumstances change.

If you're medically stable, look for a psychotherapist who can help you get to the driving forces behind your binge eating quickly. Be reasonable about your expectations. Maybe individual therapy is your best option, but you can often accelerate your progress by participating in a therapeutic support group as well.

In an ideal world, a patient who binge eats is seen frequently and regularly by a specialized team including a physician, a psychotherapist, and a nutritionist — among others. In the real world, managed care, limits on the time you can devote to treatment, and sometimes reluctance on the part of the binge eater, determine the frequency and type of care she receives. Not every treatment may be covered by your insurance plan nor will every treatment appeal to you. That doesn't mean you won't be able to get the care you need. It just means that you have to understand the ins and outs of your healthcare plan and know all your options — and being creative and flexible doesn't hurt.

Talk therapy

No one path to recovery is right for every person who seeks help for binge eating, but some time during your journey to health, you'll probably participate in traditional psychotherapy.

Talk therapy is the process of exploring your past, present, and future by talking through patterns you may or may not be aware of and discussing feelings and thoughts that may have an impact on binge eating.

You may see a therapist one or more times per week, either individually or in a combination of individual and group sessions. Over time, the therapist evaluates your progress by assessing your overall mood, weight changes, functionality, social involvement, motivation, behavior, and more.

Good therapy should not go on forever, but change does take time. After all, you didn't get this way overnight, and the long-term changes you're seeking won't happen overnight either. However, if you don't see measureable improvement, you and your therapist can evaluate together whether you need a different type of therapy in addition to or instead of what you're doing.

It can be costly to see a psychotherapist, a nutritionist, and the team of other eating disorder professionals you may want to see to recover from binge eating. This may or may not involve any medical/behavioral insurance you have. Keep in mind that if you are stable and seeing steady improvement, therapy groups run by a psychotherapist can be a cost-effective alternative to individual therapy when both are not possible.

Psychotherapy may bring up difficult memories and experiences, but identifying and understanding longstanding reasons you binge is as important as learning practical techniques for stopping the binges on a day-to-day basis.

If you're looking to tackle some of the reasons that lead you to binge, it's not enough to talk about feelings and family without talking about why and how food became your defense or weapon of choice, so to speak. You can't deal with one without sorting out the other.

Cognitive behavioral therapy

Cognitive behavioral therapy (CBT) is a goal-oriented approach that focuses on identifying and hopefully changing some of the links between thoughts, feelings, and behaviors. CBT is a focused, structured process that prioritizes concrete solutions and usually lasts a specific number of sessions or cycles. Like talk therapy, CBT depends upon a good relationship between patient and psychotherapist even though this type of therapy perhaps incorrectly has a reputation of being somewhat unemotional, detached, or formulaic. (We explore CBT in more depth in Chapter 11.)

For binge eaters, the goal of CBT is to become more self-aware about the feelings and thoughts that may trigger a binge. By recognizing the thoughts that typically come before a binge, you can eventually retrain your brain to think different thoughts, and therefore, to stop the binge before it starts.

As you know, it's not enough to tell yourself that you have to stop bingeing without having a plan to replace the binges with healthier behaviors. Try not to lose sight of the fact that ending your binge eating is a process of developing new ways of thinking, new habits, and new ways of dealing with stress, anxiety, and other negative feelings. Those changes are not easy. If they were, you probably wouldn't need this book!

Using CBT or CBT techniques integrated into more traditional talk therapy, you can discover how to

✔ Monitor your eating habits so that you understand exactly how much you're eating and when you tend to binge. In fact, it's often a shock to see exactly how much you eat when you keep a record for several days. It's important to be honest and non-judgmental. After all, this is why you're engaging in the process to begin with.

✔ Develop the coping skills you need in order to eat regular snacks and meals and head off the hunger or cravings that may trigger a binge. During the time you've been alternating between the extremes of restricting and bingeing or overeating in some way, you may have gotten so used to swinging back and forth between two extremes that eating regularly can bring on negative and potentially paralyzing emotions. At first, your dietitian and therapist may ask you to "eat on the clock" just to establish new patterns, but ideally you eventually find out how to recognize physical cues about your hunger and satiety and to eat in a more intuitive way.

> ✔ Avoid situations that may cause bingeing or find ways to eventually integrate them back into your life but in less triggering ways.
>
> ✔ Plan for ways to manage stress and anxiety that don't involve food.

Using food to address emotional hunger probably seemed like a really good idea at one time — whether this was a conscious choice or not. Overcoming your impulses to binge will take time and patience.

Although CBT has been extremely effective in treating binge eating and other forms of chronic overeating, a creative psychotherapist ultimately knows how to combine CBT, talk therapy, and many other techniques into an effective plan for each patient.

Dialectical behavior training

An offshoot of CBT, *dialectical behavior training (DBT)* utilizes many of the elements of cognitive behavior therapy together with a focus on mindfulness and self-acceptance.

DBT was originally developed by Dr. Marsha Linehan to help self-harming patients with borderline personality disorder (BPD). It has also proven quite effective for people who have difficulty regulating their emotions in other situations, including those who suffer from eating disorders.

As part of a treatment plan utilizing a variety of approaches, DBT places a particular emphasis on being present in the moment, despite any perceived discomfort in that moment, and experiencing the world around you. So often people go through life in a numb, less aware, or even dissociative state. If you're a binge eater, DBT helps you to eat more mindfully with full awareness of your own hunger and fullness cues, and an awareness, rather than an avoidance, of how food tastes, smells, and feels as you eat it.

As with other therapies, DBT works best in conjunction with complementary treatments. A good therapist integrates the right elements of DBT with other therapies to create a tailor-made plan that can help you confront the specific reasons that contribute to your binge eating.

Mindfulness training

Mindfulness training expands on the idea that being in the present moment and becoming more self-aware can help you stop binge eating. One of the most important principles of mindfulness training is eating only when you're hungry. Easy to say; hard to do. Even though it seems obvious, you may have gotten out of touch with your body's signals during months or years of binge-ing. Mindfulness training is one way to reconnect with your physical self.

Sometimes you eat more than you realize — everyone does — because you're paying attention to other thoughts, feelings, or activities. For binge eaters, this problem is much more dramatic.

Mindfulness training comes from the idea of *intuitive eating,* the practice of responding to cues your body sends to signal that you're hungry and should eat. Although it takes time to clear away years of dieting behaviors, negative thoughts about food, and body image issues, intuitive eating aims to restore a healthy relationship between food, your body, and your mind.

Mindfulness training focuses on stripping away all the confusing and often contradictory thoughts in your head and the impulses to binge eat. It is also a way to prime a person to use alternate coping strategies or other ways to deal with stress than eating.

Alternate coping skills

When binge eaters use food to cope with stress, anxiety, depression, or other triggers, one strategy clinicians employ is to teach alternate coping skills or how to deal with the inevitable ups and downs of life without using unhealthy food or perhaps without using food at all.

Although it seems counterintuitive, stopping a binge does not mean not eating at all. Quite the contrary — if you create unrealistic, restrictive, and unhealthy rules about food, you often end up swinging back and forth again and again between "never eating again" and binge eating.

In fact, eating healthy foods in response to hunger and in manageable and per-haps more frequent and smaller portions is important to heading off binges. If you are face-to-face with an uncontrollable urge to eat, what you eat, how much, and the way you eat it determines whether you head straight into a binge or cope with the urge by eating something within a controlled setting.

You may be thinking right now, "Yeah, but you don't understand. There is no such thing as portion when I'm on a tear. There is never enough." That percep-tion leads to a thought ("I must have more"), a feeling ("I'm uncomfortable, I'm upset, I'm frustrated, I'm lonely,"), and then inevitably to a behavior — the binge. The binge results in only temporary calm or high. That's why the key to overcoming this condition is to create a different path from perception to thought to feeling and, ultimately, to behavior.

A couple of strategies to forestall a binge are

- ✔ **Have a pre-planned snack.** The secret is to eat something that precedes, anticipates, or feeds the urge in a healthier way. If you have urges to binge on ice cream and cookies, then baby carrots dipped in fat free dressing probably won't do. However, instead of ice cream, mix a cup of fat-free Greek yogurt with two cups of berries. You can top it with some honey or other sweetener of your choice. Here's the secret — make it ahead of time and freeze it!

  When you just can't stop yourself from bingeing, go for this healthier but similar snack. You take the edge off of your urge to binge by eating something similar to what you're craving, and you won't feel bad about it. Without the extreme guilt that comes after bingeing, you're more likely to keep up with your healthier behaviors.

- ✔ **Substitute healthier, more productive behaviors.** In many cases, this is easier said than done, but again, the trick is to stay one step ahead of the urge to binge by having a plan. Some alternatives to bingeing include

  - Set a timer and postpone the binge for 15 minutes. During that time, try to distract yourself with TV, music, knitting, reading, or anything else you can become fully engaged in. This delay may short circuit the binge altogether. No, this is not just busy work. It's truly an attempt to short circuit the urge. It may return, but it is staved off for now.

  - Brush your teeth, paint your nails, and/or take a shower or bath.

  - Leave the environment that is triggering you. Go to another safe place. (Be aware of time of day, weather conditions, and other safety considerations.)

  - Call or reach out to someone who can be supportive.

  - Try relaxing with deep breathing and/or music. Take a deep breath in for six counts, hold for six, and blow it out for eight counts. Do four to six sets.

  - Let out your aggressions in a physical but safe way such as punching a pillow or boxing bag. Allowing yourself to cry can also be a relief.

  - Go for a walk, jog, swim, or bike ride if physical activity is sanctioned or monitored by your physician or other healthcare professional.

Over time, you may need to experiment until you find the strategy that works for you. The goal of developing alternate coping strategies is not to eliminate all negative feelings — that's unrealistic for pretty much everyone — but rather to develop new ways to confront stress, anxiety, and sadness without doing yourself additional harm.

Finding a Therapist who Specializes in Eating Disorders

If you're a binge eater, finding a psychotherapist with expert training in eating disorders is an important part of your journey because a specialist

- ✔ Can perform a comprehensive assessment and, as part of a multi-pronged treatment plan, get you medical help right away if your health is threatened.

- ✔ Knows how to talk about food-related issues and behaviors in ways that are less likely to trigger the disordered behavior you're trying to eliminate.

- ✔ Has training in a variety of therapies and techniques relevant to eating disorders.

- ✔ Understands the vital importance of how a team approach works and can refer you to appropriate specialists when necessary.

Recovering from an eating disorder is a highly personal process that takes time and may require counseling and help from a variety of different treatment providers over a period of months or years. This may seem like a long time, but it took longer to get where you are now and there will also be motivating benchmarks along the way. Relying on a group of professionals with different specialties is the best way to slow down and eventually to stop binge eating.

You can go about finding a therapist in any number of ways, and technology makes it easier than ever to find an experienced, reputable professional who can help. Try any or all of these methods:

- ✔ **Search the Internet.** Several national, accredited organizations can make referrals to professional therapists in your area, although those therapists may or may not specialize in treating eating disorders. Other organizations can steer you in the direction of eating disorder specialists in particular. Some of the organizations we recommend include

    - • Academy for Eating Disorders (www.aedweb.org)

    - • Binge Eating Disorder Association (www.bedaonline.com)

    - • Eating Disorder Hope (www.eatingdisorderhope.com)

    - • National Eating Disorders Association (www.nationaleating disorders.org)

    - • Something Fishy (www.something-fishy.com)

- ✔ **Talk to your physician.** Ask for a recommendation. If your doctor can't make a recommendation of someone who treats eating disorders specifically, get the name or names of psychotherapists or psychiatrists she likes and trusts. Call one or two, explain your situation, and ask again for a more specialized recommendation. Hopefully, you'll have several possibilities to consider.

✔ **Get a referral from a friend or family member.** Reach out to someone who's struggled with the same or similar issues. Explain that you're looking for help and see whether that person can refer you to someone.

✔ **Check with local universities, hospitals, or treatment centers.** Find out if the psychotherapist at the university health center can help you make a match with the right therapist. See if the local hospital has someone on staff who can help guide you. Call a psychological treatment center of any kind and explain what you're looking for.

The more people you talk to, the more likely it is that one of them can make a connection for you through her professional network.

Making a Match with the Right Dietitian

A psychologist or social worker works with you to investigate the reasons why you binge eat; a registered dietitian (RD) or nutritionist excels at the practical, concrete side of recovery by helping you develop routines, strategies, and techniques to keep the bingeing in check.

First and foremost, a RD or nutritionist develops a meal plan and asks you to keep a food journal detailing your daily routine. Even more importantly, if you have a setback of any kind, an experienced RD or nutritionist can help you deal with it in a productive way. Not only can a well-trained RD identify and deal with any number of mental, emotional, or physical conditions, she can also recognize and help you change the thought processes and feelings that can interfere with your recovery.

Just as with other therapists, it makes a world of difference to work with a RD or nutritionist who specializes in eating disorders. Only someone who has worked in this area can truly understand what recovery from binge eating is like. And on top of that, an RD or nutritionist who understands binge eating can reassure you every step of the way that a slow and steady recovery is the best approach for long-term success.

Seeing a registered dietitian as part of an overall recovery plan gives you a foundation for forming new, healthier eating habits. The right person not only has a combination of experience and eating disorder expertise but also puts you at ease and creates an atmosphere of trust and communication.

You also have to think about how seeing a dietitian fits into your budget. Most insurance plans don't cover visits to a nutritionist, so you have to pay out-of-pocket. However, if you, like many binge eaters, have been diagnosed with diabetes, high cholesterol, high blood pressure, or another condition that makes it medically necessary for you to change your eating habits, you may find that your insurance covers visits to the dietitian.

Deciphering mental health professionals

If the alphabet soup trailing after some therapists' names confuses you, you're not the only one. Making sense of the various degrees and training can leave anyone's head spinning. In the following list, we try to clarify the differences and help you figure out which type of professional will be a good fit for you:

✓ A **psychiatrist** has received a Doctor of Medicine (M.D.) and is a medical doctor with training in assessment, diagnosis, treatment, and prevention of mental illness. That matters to you because, with the exception of a few states, psychiatrists are the only mental health professionals who can prescribe medication. You may not know yet if you need medication, but even if you're not seeing a psychiatrist, psychologists and other non-prescribing therapists, especially those who see patients with eating disorders, work together with psychiatrists if they feel prescription medication might be beneficial.

✓ A **psychologist** is trained in assessment, diagnosis, and treatment of mental health conditions; however, psychologists have a Doctor of Philosophy (Ph.D.) or a Doctor of Psychology (Psy.D.) and are not physicians. They use various forms of psychotherapy but do not prescribe medication.

✓ **Clinical social workers** (LMSW, LCSW, CSW, MSW) receive training similar to psychologists in the assessment, diagnosis, and treatment of mental health conditions. To receive an MSW, social workers must complete a minimum of two years graduate training and must pass a licensing exam to receive an LMSW, the first level of licensure by examination. LMSWs can only work in a supervised clinical agency or setting. An LCSW is the next level of licensure by examination available after having completed three additional years of supervised clinical work. LCSWs may work in independent practice or in clinical settings after receiving LCSW credentials.

✓ A **master of art/science** has usually received one to three years of post-graduate (after a bachelor's degree) study, including an internship if the degree is in a counseling area, and the therapist or counselor is aiming for licensure. Once licensed, the letters LPC (licensed professional counselor) may also appear after their name in some U.S. states.

Depending on where you live, you may also have access to other credentialed mental health professionals including those that have received masters in psychology, who must work in supervised clinical settings, licensed marriage and family therapists (LMFT), licensed mental health technicians (LMHT), and licensed professional therapists (LPT).

Finding a dietitian

Many people use the terms *dietitian* and *nutritionist* interchangeably, but the two professions are not the same:

✓ A **registered dietitian (RD)** has completed an accredited program that includes the study of dietetics and nutrition as well as anatomy, food science, and other subjects related to understanding nutritional needs. A RD has also received hands-on training, has passed an accreditation exam, and must fulfill continuing education requirements yearly. Registered dietitians are regulated by the Academy of Nutrition and Dietetics.

✔ **Nutritionists,** on the other hand, are not regulated. Although some people may have advanced degrees and extensive training, anyone can call himself a nutritionist without meeting any standards whatsoever, so it's difficult to know what kind of education and experience a nutritionist has.

Although some nutritionists may be qualified to treat binge eaters, look for a RD first. By choosing a RD you can be confident that you're working with someone who has the education, training, and experience to help you with binge eating.

Researching RDs and insurance

One of the best places to start if you're thinking about visiting a dietitian is to figure out what's covered under your insurance. Though it may take several phone calls, e-mails, or visits to your provider's website, knowing which dietitians are on your plan and how many visits you can make can be a deciding factor when choosing a dietitian.

If you have already been diagnosed with diabetes, high blood pressure, high cholesterol, or another condition that makes weight loss medically necessary, ask for a referral from your physician and make sure to discuss your medical history with your insurance provider.

Just as you can search your insurer's website for a doctor, most insurance providers make it easy to search for a dietitian by specialty.

If you're a binge eater, it's important to look for a dietitian who has experience working with all types of eating disorders. Some other factors to consider include

✔ **Being a smart consumer:** Even if your insurance website says a dietitian works with clients who suffer from eating disorders, do your own research on every RD you think about seeing he. Check out practice websites, read client reviews, and make sure that the dietitian's philosophy rings true for you.

✔ **Expanding your search area:** You're better off finding a RD that's qualified and has experience working with eating disorders than staying close to home and working with someone who doesn't. Even if you have to travel to work with an RD who's experienced with BED, the extra effort is worth it to get the tools you need to follow a meal plan and deal with your bingeing more effectively than you might be able to with an RD who's not familiar with bingeing. Remember, an RD with experience offers advice that has been tested and proven effective, which may be the edge you need to stop bingeing. If you had a brain tumor, would you go to a gastroenterologist? Think of RD's in the same way. They're trained in specialty areas, and BED is one of them.

✔ **Thinking about convenience:** Office hours, parking, and proximity to public transportation may make or break your experience. Try to find a situation that makes it easy to keep your appointments. And of course, if you work full-time and need to meet with someone in the evening or on the weekend, double check that the dietitian sees patients at those times.

Using the Internet to find a dietitian

If you've asked other therapists you're working with for referrals, interviewed dietitians, looked at your insurance provider's website, and still not found someone you like or who you feel would be a good fit, you can go online to find a RD in your area who works with clients who binge eat.

A number of national organizations and online communities provide listings of eating disorder professionals across the spectrum of specialties including the following:

✔ **Academy of Nutrition and Dietetics (AND)** www.eatright.org: The world's largest organization of food and nutrition professionals with over 75,000 members, AND's website offers a <u>Find a Registered Dietitian</u> button that allows you to search by zip code and by specialty.

✔ **International Association of Eating Disorder Professionals (IAED)** www.iaedp.com: The IAED provides education and training to health-care providers who treat the full spectrum of eating disorders. The <u>Find a Therapist</u> link on their website allows you to search not only for therapists but also for other health care professionals such as registered dietitians specializing in eating disorders.

✔ **The National Association of Anorexia Nervosa and Associated Disorders (ANAD)** www.anad.org: ANAD is a national, non-profit organization committed to the prevention and treatment of all eating disorders. Its website allows you to search for treatment centers, therapists, dietitians, and support groups.

✔ **Something Fishy** www.somethingfishy.org: Something Fishy is a worldwide nonprofit dedicated to raising awareness about eating disorders. Its website contains listings from more than 1,800 therapists, dietitians, treatment centers, and other professionals treating eating disorders. Its listings are fully searchable by type of treatment, country, state, area code, name, services, description, or zip code.

Making a personal connection

Trust and connection are the foundation of a successful working relationship between a client and dietitian. If you feel good about the dietitian and have a good rapport, you go a long way toward advancing your recovery regardless of the dietitian's experience with eating disorders or whether she's covered by your insurance.

That said, if you can, it's always better to choose someone who's familiar with the challenges of binge eating and other eating disorders and who has experience working with patients along the eating disorder spectrum. Before you commit to a dietitian, set up a 15-to-20-minute phone conversation to figure out whether she will be a good match by asking

- ✔ What is your nutrition philosophy? ·
- ✔ Can you give me examples of how you have worked with other clients?
- ✔ How often will I come to see you?
- ✔ What should I expect during the first several appointments?
- ✔ How do you do meal planning?
- ✔ Will I need to count calories or measure food?

Even if you love the first person you talk to, take the time to interview several dietitians so you feel confident about your choice. You can also get a sense of the different strategies and techniques that dietitians use so that you can be an educated participant in your own nutrition counseling. Also, if worse comes to worse and you don't end up liking the person you choose, you know you have other options.

Working with a team player

Recovering from binge eating is a complex, holistic, long-term process that includes medical evaluations and interventions, psychological support, nutrition counseling, and alternative therapies along with patience and time.

If you're seeing a psychotherapist or doctor you like and trust who has an established relationship with a registered dietitian, seriously consider working with that RD and his entire team of integrated providers who hopefully are experts in treating eating disorders.

Working with a team of healthcare providers is the foundation of a healthy, productive recovery. Even if your dietitian isn't part of a network, make sure she's willing and capable of regular communication with your other health care team members.

Paying for nutrition counseling

If you've searched your insurance provider's website and can't find what you're looking for, you may need to consider whether you can afford to pay to see a registered dietitian even if you can't use your insurance to pay for those visits.

The unfortunate truth is that many highly specialized RDs, including those who treat patients with eating disorders, do not take insurance. That leaves you to weigh the options and decide how to fit visits to a dietitian into your overall recovery plan.

The upside to this dilemma is that you may get more for your money when you pay out-of-pocket. More convenient office hours, better location, extended appointment times, and individualized meal planning are just a few of the perks you get when paying a fee.

If you're thinking about going with a RD who doesn't accept insurance and you're worried about what you can afford, ask about a *sliding scale fee,* a discounted rate usually about 15-20 percent below the full fee for clients who can't afford the higher rate.

You may also be able to claim out-of-network benefits that pay for a portion of the visits or that reimburse you after you've met a deductible. Most RDs are familiar with the paperwork and can help you make your claims — assuming that nutrition counseling qualifies for benefits.

Finding Community in Support Groups

If you're a binge eater, support groups can be one of the most important pieces of the recovery puzzle you and your therapist put together. Unlike group therapy, which is led by a psychotherapist, support groups are usually led by group members themselves or by someone who has herself recovered from binge eating.

Support groups can be a lifeline for socially isolated binge eaters. If you've spent months or years feeling alone or ashamed because of your binges, seeing that other people think or feel like you do can be healing and transformative. A nonjudgmental environment where everyone shares the experience of bingeing and can talk about it openly is one way to find companionship and encouragement as you recover.

Which group is right for you?

Just like finding the right psychotherapist, physician, psychiatrist, and nutritionist, finding the right support group involves some trial and error. There's not just one way to figure out which group works for you because everyone's different. It all depends on where you feel comfortable.

One option is to seek out the 12-step programs offered by Overeaters Anonymous and Eating Disorders Anonymous. These are free of charge, and there tend to be many in most geographical areas.

You can find other community-based and free-of-charge group resources at Health At Every Size (www.haescommunity.org) and the Binge Eating Disorder Association (www.bedaonline.com). When you are looking for the right support group, some of the issues you may want to consider are

- ✔ **Neighborhood:** Some people prefer the convenience of attending support groups close to home while others seek out the anonymity of groups further away.

- ✔ **Time of day:** Do you work full-time and need a group that meets in the evening? Do you prefer a meeting during the day while the kids are in school? Or do you need a group that meets on the weekend? Consider your schedule when determining which group works for you.

- ✔ **Is it a closed or open group?** Open groups don't have restrictions on who attends or how frequently. Closed groups are the opposite and require a membership commitment.

Why go to a support group?

Whether you've been bingeing for a short time or for most of your life, you know the shame and isolation that binge eating can bring on. Even worse, the thoughts and feelings that trigger your binges can be as bad as the binges themselves because they make you feel worthless and leave you wondering if there's a place for you in the world.

A support group is a wonderful opportunity to see that you are definitely not alone. Not only can you learn from your peers about how to change the patterns that lead to binge eating, but support groups can also give you a much needed opportunity to meet friends and to talk with like-minded, non-judgmental people in a confidential and safe environment. People in support groups are there because they want to help themselves and also want to help others in an open setting.

Chapter 11

Using CBT to Replace Damaging Behaviors with Healthy Ones

In This Chapter

▶ Understanding the principles of cognitive behavioral therapy (CBT)

▶ Applying CBT to the treatment of binge eating

▶ Mastering the practical skills behind CBT

*I*f you've done any research about treatments for eating disorders, then you've probably come across the term *cognitive behavioral therapy,* or CBT. Originally developed primarily for treating depression and anxiety, over the past several decades, CBT has become one of the cornerstones of helping binge eaters and anyone on the eating disorder spectrum reframe negative thoughts and behaviors and replace them with healthier and more constructive ones.

CBT takes a practical, commonsense approach to problem-solving by breaking down the damaging assumptions and attitudes you may have about yourself and the world around you.

In this chapter, we explore the basics of CBT and show how the principles of CBT apply to binge eating. We also break down some of the practical skills you and your therapist may consider using during your treatment and show you how CBT can be useful not only in psychotherapy but also when approaching your nutrition and food plan.

Breaking Down the Basics of CBT

At this point, you may be asking yourself, "What the heck is CBT anyway?" The basic answer is that *CBT,* or *cognitive behavioral therapy,* is a logical, scientific approach to understanding and managing certain psychological problems. Using journaling, a variety of other techniques, and workbooks that teach you how to break down your daily life into discrete moments, you can use CBT techniques to track your feelings, behaviors, and actions in order to discover patterns and then change those patterns as necessary.

Explaining the CBT method

CBT is a goal-oriented psychotherapeutic technique that involves setting specific weekly objectives in order to move toward resolving whatever issues lead you to seek treatment. In traditional psychotherapy, a patient and therapist may work not only on the actual unwanted behaviors but also on trying to locate their original sources such as traumatizing events in the past. Although this approach can be quite valuable, cognitive behavioral therapy is a more present and future-focused treatment that centers on the direct connection between perceptions, thoughts, feelings, and behaviors. Put simply, perceptions lead to thoughts, which lead to feelings, which lead to behaviors. CBT offers ways to interrupt the cause-and-effect relationship among these four elements by breaking down and analyzing each one as you're experiencing the behavior you're trying to slow or eliminate.

CBT uses the scientific method to identify, verify, and possibly refute your beliefs about the world around you, to explore your perceptions about yourself, and, if you're a binge eater, about food and eating in general. If you're someone who's always loved science or are just rather organized, you'll probably find the recordkeeping and data gathering part of CBT quite fascinating. And if you aren't, you'll probably still find CBT interesting and useful as the subject of this experiment is none other than *you.*

Using CBT, you realize that your perceptions about yourself and the world around you influence how you think, feel, and act, whether or not those beliefs are based in reality. Make no mistake, whatever you believe is very real to you and your life, but if you're willing, you can sometimes see things in an entirely different light — through a different lens or filter, if you will.

Much of the information you gather and use comes from worksheets and activities you do between therapy sessions. (We talk about both later on in this chapter.) You review the information during your meetings with your therapist.

By writing down what you think and how you feel and act in real time, rather than after the fact, you can see what seems rational or irrational and what thought patterns and habits you may need or want to change. Sometimes, the mere recording of thoughts and actions effects change in the moment.

And because CBT is an action-oriented therapy, after you have a clearer idea of what needs to be different, the focus of both your psychotherapy and nutrition sessions isn't just to think about what changes you might make but also to experiment with and practice concrete new ways of doing things. It is both customary and beneficial to carefully track your progress week by week.

Changing the way you think

You may be saying to yourself, "If stopping my binges were as easy as just changing the way I think, I would have taken care of this already." But changing the way you think isn't always a piece of cake (metaphor alert!), mostly because the way you think is based on what you believe to be true about the world around you.

Changing the way you think starts with understanding the way you think, and CBT's very specific framework is a critical part of making changes. The CBT system involves

- ✔ Defining the problem
- ✔ Tracking your thoughts and feelings about the situations and individuals troubling you
- ✔ Recognizing room for change in your perceptions
- ✔ Testing new ideas and behaviors
- ✔ Making permanent changes

Much of the work of CBT therapy is done between therapy sessions in workbooks or on worksheets based on the CBT methodology. Your therapist can recommend a book that's a good fit for you or may give you weekly exercises and homework based on your weekly progress.

Introducing the ABC's of CBT

One of the first steps to using CBT is to become familiar with what's called the *ABC Model of CBT.* You use the ABC's to identify and understand the specific problems you'd like to take on with cognitive behavioral therapy.

The ABC Model breaks your problem into three segments:

- ✔ **A:** A is the *activating event* or the *trigger* — an event that you anticipate will happen in the future or a memory of something that has happened in the past. In an ABC worksheet — one is shown in Figure 11-1 — you write down the exact circumstance or situation that's a source of difficulty for you in the A column.

    In the case of binge eaters, an activating event is generally something that has triggered a binge, particularly if the same type of event triggers bingeing or overeating on a regular basis. Even if you can't initially identify a pattern, regularly tracking the events, however large or small, that precede a binge is an important strategy when you're trying to understand and change your habits and attitudes toward food, eating, and yourself.

✔ **B:** B represents your beliefs about the activating event(s) or at least your perceptions when it (they) occurred. No thought or reaction about an A event is too big or too small to include on your worksheet when analyzing your in-the-moment thoughts at the time the precipitating event(s) occurred.

For a binge eater, it's important to document your thoughts and beliefs about the event that occurred and how you feel about it. It may not be easy at first to articulate the feelings associated with a triggering event, particularly because many binge eaters report that in the time leading up to the binge, they feel overwhelmed by many conflicting emotions.

Start small, identify whatever you can in the moment, and resolve to work with your therapist on being both increasingly aware of your emotions as they're happening and able to distinguish one emotion from another.

✔ **C:** C refers to the consequences, both physical and emotional of your various feelings. It's important to separate out emotions and behaviors when you write about consequences on your worksheet. In other words, you want to record

- How you acted. Don't judge or critique yourself; simply record the facts.

- How you felt. Be accurate but compassionate.

By visualizing your thought processes, you can begin to change or reframe your interpretation of your past experiences, rethink the origins of some of the negative emotions holding you back, and find ways to positively affect future actions or behaviors.

If you're seeing a psychotherapist for binge eating, it's fair to say that your goal is to slow and/or stop bingeing. Using the ABCs is one way to try to figure out some of the triggers and patterns around your binge eating and change the pattern in a way that supports your goals.

Denise is a divorced, 35-year-old woman who's seeing a therapist because her bingeing has gotten out of control in the year leading up to her sister's wedding. Denise's ABC form about her most recent binge is shown in Figure 11-1.

If you're curious about what other CBT record sheets and exercises look like, you can go into any bookstore with a self-help section and find CBT workbooks. Although these books may not be specific to eating disorders or to binge eating, they can give you an idea of the kind of questions and psychological work CBT involves.

A: Activating Event	B: Belief at the Time	C: Consequences
My mother called me to tell me that my sister ordered her wedding dress and that we must choose my dress for the wedding soon since I'm in her bridal party.	I'll never be in another relationship again, and I'll definitely never get married again because I'm too fat. Even if I did get married again, no designers make dresses large enough for me. And I'll ruin my sister's wedding pictures. She should really choose someone else to be her maid of honor.	Actions: I stopped at the grocery store on the way home and bought three gallons of ice cream. I ate most of all three. Emotions: I felt ashamed when I bought the ice cream and lonely while I sat at the table by myself eating it. I also felt hopeless because I didn't understand why I simply had to eat when it made me feel so sick and didn't actually change anything.

Figure 11-1:
Denise's
filled-in
ABC form.

As you can imagine, there's an infinite number of possible thoughts and interpretations that can lead to a binge, but the idea is to identify and then intervene with the most common triggers and/or beliefs that consistently end in binges *for you*. Keeping consistent and truthful records of your binges helps take some of the guesswork out of figuring out the underlying reasons why you binge. Only by understanding the ABCs of your bingeing can you start to identify the faulty beliefs that underlie your binge eating and start to change them.

Using CBT to Treat Binge Eating Disorder

Although it's possible to find a psychotherapist who uses cognitive behavior therapy exclusively, it's more likely that the eating disorder professionals you seek out will incorporate CBT into an individualized treatment program that includes a variety of different therapeutic tools and techniques.

Because CBT is a measurable approach, your therapist will probably ask you to keep a detailed record of your thoughts, feelings, and behaviors, much in the way you may have already started to keep track of what you're eating in a food journal. (We talk about keeping a food journal in Chapter 12.)

If you're struggling to stop bingeing, the obvious and immediate goal of CBT is to work on reducing the frequency and eventually stopping your binges. Although examining the root psychological causes of why you binge is essential, your psychotherapist may simultaneously use CBT while continuing the exploration of the driving forces because it can help you make the measurable and more immediate short-term progress needed to stay motivated for the long haul.

Using CBT techniques, you can interrupt a hurtful chain of events by adopting realistic and flexible thoughts and beliefs. That way you can react in more productive ways to the ups and downs of everyday life. If you're a binge eater, you may also be able to put to rest some of the fear and anxiety that brings about your binges and establish new patterns that help you make better choices more consistently and with greater ease for the rest of your life.

Your therapist may use CBT to focus on the false or irrational thoughts and feelings that may precede a binge. Or he may bring in CBT when asking you to track the triggers that lead you to binge. Often CBT is one part of a comprehensive psychotherapeutic approach that you and your therapist can use to address and correct specific undesirable behaviors.

CBT is generally a very structured therapeutic technique that you tackle issues in stages. Because CBT is a measurable approach, your therapist will probably ask you to keep a detailed record of your thoughts, feelings, and behaviors, much in the way you may have already started to keep track of what you're eating in a food journal. (We talk about keeping a food journal in Chapter 12.)

There's no one size fits all approach to recovering from binge eating. Your eating disorder therapist pulls an array of goodies from her bag of tricks depending on your specific set of issues. She may combine CBT with traditional psychotherapy, dialectical behavior training (DBT), mindfulness techniques, and a variety of alternate coping skills — all in an effort to help you establish a new set of reactions or reflexes to the pressures and difficulties in your life. (We talk about DBT and other treatments in Chapter 10.)

Of course, your long-term goal is to slow down and eventually end your binge eating, but many people feel overwhelmed at the thought of tackling the whole set of issues all at once. By using CBT, you and your therapist break down your binge eating into smaller, bite-sized pieces (hang on, folks — just another food metaphor — they're hard to avoid!), so that you can work on them slowly and individually without feeling that you have to change everything all at once. By contrast, feeling that you have to solve all the problems that lead you to binge eat right away is typical of the all-or-nothing thinking that probably got you here. Treatment must be in manageable portions. (Yet another food metaphor — we warned you!)

Filling in CBT worksheets

Although it's tempting to dive right in to actual problem solving, scientific methodology and recordkeeping are the foundations of CBT. Using worksheets, you record exactly when and where you binge, exactly what you binge on, and exactly what was happening at the time or earlier that may have triggered your binge. Your triggers may not always be clearly identifiable, but even just making your best guess provides great data that you and your team can use to try to figure them out. As you move forward, having this information on paper, in black and white, can help you methodically understand and interrupt the patterns that lead you to binge eat.

Sometimes recording all this information seems hard because you're afraid your team will judge you. Rest assured that you yourself are likely the only judge and jury. The eating disorder professionals you're seeing have heard and seen and helped other people who are binge eaters or who overeat in other ways. Their interest is in helping you recover. By being as honest and forthright as you can about your unique triggers and experiences, you help your team come up with an individualized plan that will work for you.

During this phase, your team may talk about what binge eating disorder is and about the consequences of binge eating on your emotional and physical health. This is called *psycho-educational training*. You may already know many of these facts, but the disconnect between what you know and what you do may be part of what's kept you from being able to stop your binge eating.

Establishing regular eating patterns

Many binge eaters restrict their food intake during the day only to find themselves starving by the end of the day and bingeing at night. You may have been eating like this for years. Because one of the goals of treatment for binge eating is to establish new habits, one of the first steps is to begin eating in a way that stabilizes your appetite and diminishes your urge to binge.

Banning *always*, *ever*, and *never*

When you say, "you *always* do that" or "I'll *never* get well," it destroys all possibility of transformation or self-improvement. There's no future, no hope, no reconciliation. It reinforces the idea that whatever's going wrong is bad and always will be. Lots of relationships have broken up over the use of "always, ever, and never," not to mention the people who've been left without hope from hearing or thinking those words over and over.

Change begins when you can make a distinction between the person and the behavior. They are not the same. It's one thing to say "when you do this, I feel that way." It's called "the use of I statements" — I'm feeling a particular way

and wish to let you know that in order to effect a change.

It's another thing entirely to say "You are an idiot" rather than "this (behavior you do) is not okay." What's even worse is when it turns into indictments like, "you *always* do that" or "I'll *never* get well." Once again, little hope is left for possibility or change.

If you find yourself using *always*, *ever*, and *never*, it's a clue that you may be trapped by the kind of all-or-nothing thinking that can keep you from seeing the potential in other people and in yourself. Nobody is perfect, and no one is all bad — the challenge is to believe it and to put your new understanding in practice.

Your dietitian can help you decide on exact times of day to eat your three meals and one to two snacks. (Chapter 12 helps with meal planning.) The goal is to eventually be able to easily and reliably recognize physical hunger and fullness cues on your own. By eating on the clock to start, you learn to reset and regulate the rhythm of your eating so that bingeing and over-sized portions become much less likely.

If you haven't eaten breakfast or lunch in years, you can gradually phase in full meals in the morning and midday, but don't let more than three or four hours pass without eating something. And, of course, use written records to track what, when, and where you ate and how you felt before, during, and after your meals.

Challenging your thinking and replacing irrational thoughts with rational ones

You may be on your way to figuring out the circumstances, both past and present, that trigger binge eating for you. As you begin to look forward to the next phase of your life and consider how you can put binge eating in the rearview mirror, it's time to confront some of the irrational thinking that may make your bingeing worse.

Using some of the records you've kept about your binges, you can look back and see what kind of thinking contributed to both the urge to binge and the binges themselves.

It's crucial not to judge your binges or their triggers. What you want to do is merely notice them; treat them simply as information.

Binge eaters report all kinds of beliefs and thoughts that spur them on, but some examples include

- ✔ If my boss doesn't say good morning to me, that means she doesn't like me or value my work.
- ✔ My boyfriend hasn't called me from his business trip. This must be his way of breaking up with me. It's probably over.
- ✔ I've already had three cookies, so I'm a failure. I might as well eat the whole bag and the pint of ice cream in the freezer, too.

You may recognize some of your self-sabotaging thoughts in these examples, but even if you don't, you can probably remember some of the negative thoughts or beliefs that have come before your binges. In the moment, they may even have seemed rational, reasonable, or accurate, but when you sit down to think them over more carefully, you may see cracks in what seemed like sound reasoning.

Different psychotherapists take different approaches after you've identified consistent beliefs and thoughts that bring on bingeing. Some may ask you to do written exercises; some may help you devise real-life experiments to test your theories and beliefs about the world. If the beliefs you're discussing are directly related to food and eating, your therapist may even encourage you to face your fears and anxieties head on, with much support of course, and eat some of your forbidden foods in a predetermined and well-planned setting.

Whatever you and your therapist decide is the best tactic for you, understanding and debunking some of the sabotaging ideas you have about food really matters for long-term success and is one of the foundations of your recovery.

Developing alternatives to binge eating

When you're feeling relaxed, even while in a therapy session, write down a list of activities, other than binge eating, that you can use to calm yourself when you feel the urge to binge. Consider including pastimes that fully engage you and lead you to think, "Wow! Where did the time go?"

Your list may include going for a walk, painting your fingernails, cleaning out a closet or drawer, taking a shower, calling a friend, painting, doing photography or other arts and crafts projects, or anything else that can provide a healthy distraction until the urge to binge passes.

Journaling or writing is an especially helpful activity. Your writing need not be edited, legible to anyone other than you, or grammatically correct. It's just a download of everything in your head onto the page. Just put down whatever's on your mind until you've said all you need to say. It's at once cathartic and distracting. Journaling reduces the overwhelming amount of chaotic thoughts and can provide some great material for your next treatment session.

You may want to try actually carrying the list or a cheat sheet with you so that when you feel the urge to binge, you can take it out and begin to try calming activities as needed. Hopefully you'll be able to head off the binge and move on with your day. But even if you don't succeed the first several times, try again until you do. You probably just need a little more practice and a lot less self-judgment.

As always, keep track of your progress by noting when the urge to binge came on, what activities you tried to keep from bingeing, how long it took for the urge to pass, and how you felt as you tried to keep yourself from losing control. Keep in mind that sometimes just writing things down can help keep you from bingeing.

Building problem-solving strategies and taking stock

There's no timetable for working your way through the steps that can help you stop binge eating, so take your time and slowly build your confidence and coping skills at each stage of the CBT process. When you're ready, you can take a step back and get a sense of your progress, the work you've done, and the work you may still need to do.

This is a great time to use the records you've kept over the weeks or months you've been in treatment. Looking at all of the information you've gathered can tell you what's working for you and how and when you've had success. It can also reveal the situations and feelings that may still be challenging for you.

Although you've probably been using various therapeutic techniques in working with your therapist, this may be the moment when you address some of the emotional or psychological issues from your past and present that may be holding you or your recovery back. You can also work on developing a general problem-solving technique that you write down, carry with you, and use whenever a difficult situation arises.

Addressing Food Issues with CBT

If you're a binge eater, facing the way you perceive food and eating may be your greatest challenge but also the most obvious way to dive right into your recovery and begin making progress.

Using CBT, you and your therapist and dietitian work toward a new way of eating and a healthier relationship with food because CBT principles and techniques can apply directly to nutritional therapy. *Nutritional therapy* within the context of CBT involves changing your thoughts and then actions specific to food and bingeing. In this way, your dietitian functions much like a nutritional therapist.

Focusing on specific foods

In this section, you take yourself through a step-by-step evaluation to establish or reestablish a healthy way to think about a specific food. Get a pen and paper, and answer the following questions in order:

1. **Choose one food that you perceive as bad.**

   For example, Gomez can't see pizza on a menu without wanting to order a large pie all for himself.

   Remember that context is everything — if you were stranded on a deserted island, no food would seem bad.

2. **Record your first emotional experience with this food.**

   For Gomez, the first time he binged (at the time he didn't even realize he was bingeing) was on a whole pizza. He ordered the pizza with the intention of having two pieces and saving the rest for later, but once he started eating, he couldn't stop himself from finishing the whole pie.

3. **Explain what makes this food bad?**

   What qualities about this food are bad? Is your experience with this food generally negative or bad? Do you associate negative emotions with this food only in certain amounts or portions? What makes it irresistible? Really delve into this this last question — there's a lot of data to mine here.

Gomez understands that pizza is not an inherently bad food, but for him whenever he eats it, he binges because he can't stop at a reasonable portion size. Extreme negative feelings of guilt and shame follow the binge. Therefore, in the context of Gomez's life, pizza is bad.

4. **Identify at least one new positive way to think about this food, and write it down.**

   Don't write down something you think you should feel, but rather a thought that makes sense to you.

   Gomez focuses on his memories of pizza day from his high school lunch. At the time, he could eat pizza without bingeing; pizza was simply a treat and one of his favorite foods. He reminds himself that if pizza was not a trigger food at that time in his life it can be it can be an acceptable food in his life again.

5. **Repeat this positive thought to yourself daily, even if you're not near or eating the food.**

Changing the way you think about food does not happen without effort or overnight. In adjusting your relationship with food, you must gently replace negative, destructive, or judgmental thoughts with positive, healthy ones.

If you're on the eating disorder spectrum, you may be used to telling yourself over and over again how bad or wrong you are or how insufficient your efforts are. Over time, you may have come to believe these things about yourself even if they have no basis in reality. These negative patterns become ingrained and hinder your recovery. So, even though it may seem artificial at first, repeat positive thoughts or affirmations to yourself in difficult moments. Eventually, you can rewire your brain so that these positive, encouraging, kind, and compassionate thoughts come to you automatically in times of stress.

Setting attainable goals for nutrition

When it comes to applying CBT to nutrition, your first priority is to change the food thoughts that lead you to binge or that get you off track when you're following your eating plan. One way to start is to begin to challenge common food myths.

A *food myth* is an irrational belief about a food or food group that has no basis in scientific fact. You may hold onto food myths because you're afraid of gaining weight. One common food myth is "Pasta is bad because it makes you gain weight."

You may know that a little bit of pasta isn't actually going to lead to instant weight gain, but you still can't get over the idea that you shouldn't eat pasta. You may also worry that eating a few bites will trigger a binge that you can't stop. But you may also know that forbidden foods also tend to become trigger foods, all the more reason that you shouldn't say that you'll never eat one food or another.

You can use CBT to unravel what's true and what isn't around food and eating by following these steps:

1. **Challenge the irrational belief.**

   Continuing the pasta example, it's not pasta that makes you gain weight, it's eating too much pasta and other foods when you binge that actually causes the weight gain.

2. **Validate the food myth.**

   Strong beliefs often form as a reaction to a fear about a food. If pasta is a trigger food for you, you feel like you can't stop at a reasonable portion when you eat it and thus trigger a binge. In this case, your fear of pasta is valid, and you should recognize that and make plans for when you're served pasta. At the same time, you need to realize that pasta in and of itself is not bad and does not cause weight gain.

3. **Create a different experience with the myth, fear, or food.**

   You can do this in a number of ways that you can plan in detail with your dietitian and your therapist. Continuing with the pasta example, you could eat pasta in a controlled setting, either with a friend or in a restaurant, so that you can't binge. Another idea is to share a pasta dish with a friend or a nutrition group (some dietitians or nutrition groups have meals together) so that you eat a moderate amount of pasta without feeling overwhelmed or guilty about it.

Challenging a food myth and succeeding in changing your experience can be an accomplishment that you build upon as you work to transform other perceptions, thoughts, feelings, and behaviors with and around food.

Tracking your thoughts about food

In the next chapter, we discuss food journaling, otherwise known as writing down what you eat, when you eat it, how hungry you felt before and after, and what your emotional state was once you finished eating. If you're using CBT as part of your therapy and nutrition plan, you may need to take food journaling a step further. Your psychotherapist and/or dietitian may also ask you to record any and all thoughts you have about food during the day.

Although it may seem fairly straightforward, tracking your positive and negative thinking about food can be a critical part of slowing and eventually stopping your binge eating. The important part is to get your thoughts down on paper without censoring yourself or judging anything you're writing. It may be that seeing you own internal dialogue about food in black and white is all you need to start to change.

Consider this actual entry in a client's food journal:

> If I eat the salad, I will feel good about myself and lose weight. No one wants to see a fat person eating a burger and fries; if I eat that my coworkers will see what a pig I am. Not that it matters anyway, they are probably judging me and talking about everything I eat anyway. So why should I care? I may as well get the burger and fries. Then since I will have already screwed up for the day, I will stop and pick up a pizza for dinner.

In the moment, this woman felt that she was being perfectly rational, but when she put her thoughts on paper, she saw she was talking herself into a binge. After applying the principles of CBT, her journal might look like this:

> I need to eat lunch, and I know that I need to eat something that will fill me up and not trigger me to eat more. The salad is my go-to diet food, and I know it will not fill me up. The burger and fries is my go-to binge food that I know will lead to a bigger binge later. Neither option is good for me and at one point or another will lead me to binge.

In this case, the client could choose a turkey-and-cheese sandwich with avocado, lettuce, and tomato and a banana on the side. Choosing a completely different lunch and evaluating how you feel about it is a way to start changing thoughts, which leads to feeling differently about food, and eventually changing the choices you make.

Chapter 12

Nourishing Your Body with Proper Nutrition

*I*f you've decided you want to stop bingeing, you may be wondering what you're going to eat and when you're going to eat it. A registered dietitian (RD) or nutritionist can reintroduce you to the fun and function of food as well as give you concrete plans to start eating differently and more healthily than you may ever have. (Go to Chapter 10 for tips on finding an RD.)

In this chapter, we discuss the myths and realities of emotional eating and offer tips on how to use meal plans and journaling to keep binge eating in check. We also give practical suggestions on how to eat with friends and family on holidays, special occasions, and every day.

Seeing Food in a Whole New Light

If you've been bingeing for a while, you may have developed a love/hate relationship with food and eating. But now that you're on the road to recovery, you've probably already discovered that you're going to have to figure out new ways to nourish and sustain yourself, both with and without food.

One part of that process is learning more about nutrition and healthy eating, but the other part is discovering more about you, your habits, your feelings, and the way food factors into your life. Understanding the relationship between your body, your mind, and your meals, and tracking your feelings is one way to start.

Another is to follow a meal plan developed by you and your RD and to record what you eat and information about your eating habits, so you can get a full, unbiased picture of what's working and what isn't. That way you can see your success and learn from missteps and setbacks along the way. Keeping a food-and-feelings journal can also help the team of eating disorder specialists guiding you toward healthier eating and living.

What is emotional eating?

Everyone emotionally eats sometimes, from finishing a whole bag of chips out of boredom to downing cookie after cookie while cramming for a big test. But if you find yourself eating emotionally again and again — especially without realizing it — it can quickly turn into binge eating.

Instead of eating to satisfy true physical hunger, when you eat emotionally, you use food to deal with complicated feelings and emotions. And binge eaters tend to eat emotionally on a frequent and regular basis. Making the connection between eating and feelings is a crucial piece of treatment and recovery from binge eating.

One of the biggest myths about emotional eating is that it's always prompted by negative feelings. Yes, people often turn to food when they're stressed out, lonely, sad, anxious, or bored. But emotional eating can be linked to positive feelings, too such as sharing dessert on Valentine's Day or having a birthday feast.

Only by understanding what drives your emotional eating can you take the necessary steps to change it. A dietitian trained to work with patients suffering from eating disorders can help you tease out the difference between positive, healthy emotional eating and unhealthy emotional eating that leads to bingeing.

Figuring out whether your hunger is physical or emotional

Being able to recognize your body's signs of true, physical hunger is one of the major milestones on the path to recovery from binge eating. Over the months or years, you may have confused wanting to eat for emotional reasons and needing to eat for physical reasons. One of the skills you can develop as you work with your RD is knowing when you need to eat to nourish yourself and when you may be using food to fulfill your emotional needs.

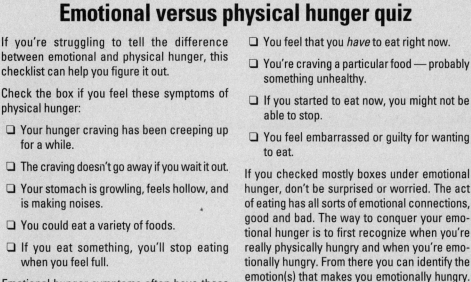

Emotional versus physical hunger quiz

If you're struggling to tell the difference between emotional and physical hunger, this checklist can help you figure it out.

Check the box if you feel these symptoms of physical hunger:

❏ Your hunger craving has been creeping up for a while.

❏ The craving doesn't go away if you wait it out.

❏ Your stomach is growling, feels hollow, and is making noises.

❏ You could eat a variety of foods.

❏ If you eat something, you'll stop eating when you feel full.

Emotional hunger symptoms often have these characteristics:

❏ The craving comes on quickly and is generally coupled with a negative emotion.

❏ You feel that you *have* to eat right now.

❏ You're craving a particular food — probably something unhealthy.

❏ If you started to eat now, you might not be able to stop.

❏ You feel embarrassed or guilty for wanting to eat.

If you checked mostly boxes under emotional hunger, don't be surprised or worried. The act of eating has all sorts of emotional connections, good and bad. The way to conquer your emotional hunger is to first recognize when you're really physically hungry and when you're emotionally hungry. From there you can identify the emotion(s) that makes you emotionally hungry. Then you can take steps to tackle those emotions in ways other than eating.

The subtle difference between physical hunger and emotional hunger is tricky, but distinguishing between them is all about identifying what's going on in your physical body and in your emotional mind at the same time.

Physical hunger is your body's true need for food. Emotions, whether positive or negative, do not affect true hunger.

Some signs that you're physically hungry include

✔ The hungry feeling builds up gradually over several hours.

✔ The sensation comes from below the neck — a growling or gurgling stomach, for example.

✔ Your hunger isn't accompanied by a sense of compulsion.

✔ The feeling doesn't go away when you try to wait it out.

✔ You notice it several hours after a meal.

✔ You experience a feeling of satisfaction after eating.

Some signs that you may be emotionally hungry are

- ✔ The urge to eat comes on suddenly.
- ✔ You feel it above the neck, and often the hunger is specific, meaning that you want a particular food or taste.
- ✔ You feel that you must eat right now; you have a sense of urgency.
- ✔ The urge to eat occurs right after a meal.
- ✔ It doesn't matter what you eat, you just want to eat.
- ✔ The feeling goes away when you wait it out.
- ✔ You feel guilty and ashamed after eating.
- ✔ You have an urge to eat in secret.

Meal planning to stop binge eating

Planning when and what to eat is the first step toward establishing normal eating patterns and beginning to eat for health and hunger. No one meal plan works for everyone. Some people may love cooking, some may feel that cooking is too risky and can trigger bingeing. Some people like eating early and some late. No matter what your preferences, the right meal plan provides a balance between flexibility and structure so that you can eat the right kinds and amounts of food in a way that suppresses and hopefully eventually ends the urge to binge.

To keep food cravings, which may trigger binge-eating episodes, at bay, a successful meal plan includes regularly timed meals and snacks. Ideally, you should eat three meals and one or two snacks per day to balance your blood sugar and keep you full. Some other factors to consider

- ✔ Meal plans should be flexible. You should have multiple options for each meal, so you can stick to the plan and be successful.
- ✔ Meal plans may require weighing and/or measuring food.
  - • The amount you weigh and measure your food depends on the meal plan you create with your RD. For some binge eaters, weighing and measuring foods feels too much like a diet and is a trigger to binge. In that case, you can use a meal plan with a more general portion guide that doesn't require measuring.
  - • For some binge eaters, weighing and measuring food is very helpful. It guides the binge eater to eat the proper portion without feeling guilty.

- Knowing exactly how much to eat is crucial to healthy meal plans. Many times binge eaters tend to eat way too much then attempt to eat too little, which then sets in motion a binge. Having a sense of how much to eat is key so the binger can avoid the trigger of being overly physically hungry.

✔ Initial meal plans should avoid trigger foods. Eventually you can plan ahead for trigger foods and situations as part of the meal planning process.

  - If you know that eating one cookie leads to eating 20 cookies, then your meal plan should avoid cookies, at least in most situations.

  - If your office has donut Fridays that send you into a binge every weekend, plan strategies and alternate foods to help you stay on your meal plan and avoid bingeing.

The initial goal of a solid eating plan is normalizing your eating patterns, not losing weight. Trying to lose weight before controlling your binge eating is a disaster waiting to happen. Be patient, and know that you are setting yourself up for long-term success and eventual weight loss when appropriate. Also, in many cases, you may lose weight as a natural byproduct of stopping the binges.

There's no one-size-fits-all meal plan because everyone has different nutritional needs as well as preferences, schedules, and triggers. Although every meal plan is different, Table 12-1 shows a sample one-day meal plan to give you an idea of the kinds of food you might eat and the specificity of the plan. Together, you and your RD can figure out what foods and routines keep you on your plan and in control.

Realistic meal planning for health

Keshia has struggled with an eating disorder her entire adolescent and adult life. Since the age of 14, she has been either dieting or bingeing. The constant cycle allowed her to maintain a normal weight for most of her 20s. At 30, she started a new, stressful job, which triggered the most severe bingeing she has experienced. This time was different because Keshia was not able to immediately redirect her bingeing to dieting, and over the course of one year, she gained 50 pounds.

She worked with a dietitian in an effort to get control over her bingeing and normalize her eating. The focus was to become a healthy, normal eater and avoid a diet (something she knows would only lead her to more bingeing). During the first five months working with her RD, Keshia lost 15 pounds. This may sound disappointing considering a 50-pound weight gain, but Keshia lost 15 pounds without dieting. Her more normalized eating alone has been enough to start the weight-loss process and to help her understand her triggers. In the long term, what Keshia learns about herself and her food habits will allow her to maintain a healthy weight and have a positive relationship with food.

Table 12-1		One Day Sample Meal Plan	
Time and Meal	*Menu*	*Portion*	*Preparation*
9 a.m. Breakfast	Cheerios with blueberries	1 cup Cheerios 1 cup skim milk 1 cup blueberries	Top cereal with milk and blueberries.
1 p.m. Lunch	Chicken and hummus romaine wrap with cantaloupe	¼ cup hummus 4-ounce chicken breast, diced 2 teaspoons avocado ½ cup shredded carrots 1 small cucumber, sliced Romaine leaves 1 cup cubed cantaloupe	Dice chicken small. Mix the hummus, finely diced chicken, avocado, and carrot. Place a dollop of the mixture on each romaine lettuce leaf and roll the leaves around the filling. Serve the sliced cucumber and melon on the side.
3 p.m. Snack	Cheese wrap and apple	1 low-fat cheese stick one wrap small apple	Put the cheese stick in the wrap. Apple on the side.
6:30 p.m. Dinner	Turkey-stuffed baked potato and orange	6-ounce potato 6 ounces ground turkey 2 tablespoons sour cream ½ cup diced onion ½ cup diced pepper Medium orange	Wrap the potato in a moist paper towel and microwave it on high for 6 to 8 minutes until it's soft. Brown the turkey with the diced onions and peppers. Add salt, pepper, oregano, and garlic for taste. Open the potato from end to end and fill with the turkey mixture; top with the sour cream. Fruit on the side.

Keeping track of what you eat

They say knowledge is power, and knowing what you eat, when you eat, and how you feel when you eat helps you understand your current habits and patterns so that you can make necessary changes and see your successes right before your eyes.

Keeping a detailed food journal allows you to track not only your food but also your sense of hunger and fullness before and after a meal. Getting used to identifying the difference between physical hunger and emotional hunger can help you keep binges in check, and understanding what it feels like to be appropriately full is one way to start eating and enjoying your meals without the worry that you'll get out of control.

Writing down more than what you ate

Food journals also keep you honest and accountable — it's all there in black and white for you and your dietitian to discuss each week. At each appointment, you'll review the entries and compare them against your meal plan if you have one, celebrate your successes, and strategize for your difficult times with food.

Aside from the foods you eat and beverages you drink, the key elements to record in your food journal are

- ✔ **Feelings/Thoughts:** Take a second at mealtime to figure out how you feel. Are you anxious, happy, bored, busy? Comments about emotions can be detailed or just a few words, but keeping track of your state of mind can help you and your RD figure out your triggers and further your recovery.

- ✔ **Hunger/Fullness Level:** Use the hunger/fullness scale in the next section before and after each meal to get in tune with how your body feels and to connect with your true physical hunger.

- ✔ **Meal/Amount:** Include as much detail as you can about what you ate and how much. If you're weighing and measuring your food, be specific about quantities. With portions, you can keep more general notes.

- ✔ **Time:** When you eat affects your blood sugar levels, and you should be eating every couple hours. You and your RD can figure out the meal times that work best for you.

Figure 12-1 shows a sample food journal to give you an idea of how to make and keep your own.

Time/Meal	Food/Amount	Before the Meal Hunger Level/Emotions	After the Meal Fullness Level/Emotions	What would you do differently?
8 am Breakfast	Medium bowl cheerios, low-fat milk, 1/2 banana	3 - kind of hungry, I don't feel any emotions, need to get to work	5 - full, on my way to work, not feeling emotional	Nothing
10:30 am, snack	Coffee with milk	3 - I feel like snacking but know that I am not very hungry, just tired	4 - I'm glad I had a coffee, I feel more awake	Nothing
2 pm, lunch	Sandwich - turkey, lettuce, tomato & mustard on rye, baby carrots with light ranch dressing	2 - I am so hungry! Lunch is an hour late because of a meeting.	5 - I feel better but still a little hungry	Nothing
3 pm, snack	1 slice chocolate cake	5 - my coworker's birthday party had cake that smelled so good. I hate myself for not being able to say no!	5 - I feel guilty and embarrassed that I couldn't stop myself. Now I want to keep eating because I already messed up. I am going to focus on work and try not to beat myself up.	I would have eaten my apple instead. Or not had anything. I wasn't even hungry.
7:00 pm Dinner	One chicken breast, two scoops couscous, green beans. and side salad with light balsamic dressing, watermelon	2 - Very hungry. It was hard not to snack while I was making dinner. Proud that I didn't let myself start to binge after the cake!	5 - comfortably full. Still feeling a little guilty about the cake, glad that I didn't keep eating.	Nothing

Figure 12-1:
Record
emotions
and hunger
levels in a
food journal.

Finding your place on the hunger/fullness scale

The hunger/fullness scale isn't clear cut like counting calories. It takes practice to use. Focus on your body's signals, and over time it gets easier to figure out where you fall on the scale before and after each meal.

- 1 = Starving, shaky, and lightheaded

- 2 = Very hungry, you have to eat soon

- 3 = Moderately hungry, you feel you could eat a meal

- 4 = Neutral, neither hungry nor full

- 5 = Moderately full, comfortable

- 6 = Somewhat uncomfortable, your stomach feels overfull or uncomfortable

- 7 = So stuffed you can't take another bite

Use these tips to get the most out of using the hunger/fullness scale:

- Try staying between 2 and 5.

- Never allow yourself to get down to 1. Have healthy snacks planned in advance and eat one if you fall below 2. Try not to let more than three or four hours pass without eating.

- Stop eating at 5. Eat slowly because your brain needs 20 minutes to know that your stomach is full.

- Ask yourself if you're actually hungry before you eat anything. Tune in to the physical sensations you experience. If you are hungry and it's time to eat on your meal plan, go ahead. If not, you may be eating in response to emotions or stress.

Eating with a group

Sitting down to eat with others should be a happy, pleasurable experience, but when you're a binge eater, it can be full of stress and anxiety. At the beginning of your recovery from binge eating, it may be difficult or impossible to eat with others, and you may avoid, as best you can, the combination of eating with friends and family.

But eating alone for the rest of your life isn't realistic or desirable. Life is full of situations when eating with others is the only choice. And it can be a good, fun, happy choice if you approach social situations that involve food with smart strategies and meal options in place.

Sitting down to dinner with the family

Your family may be the source of your eating disorder (ED), or it may provide the supportive environment you need in order to recover. In either case, chances are you'll benefit from setting some ground rules for yourself — and your family — so you're better able to keep your eating in check and ward off triggers that may occur.

An open and honest discussion is the best way to create realistic expectations. For instance, if pasta is a trigger and your spouse is Italian, it may not be realistic to outlaw pasta as a dinner option. You may, however, be able to plan to have pasta on a specific night of the week. If you know in advance, and plan with your RD accordingly, the pasta trigger is much more manageable.

Other family ground rules may include

- ✔ **No food talk at the dinner table:** It's common to talk about the meal you're eating, the last meal you ate, and even the dinner you're going out to tomorrow, but food talk can be a trigger if you have binge eating disorder, are a compulsive overeater or an emotional eater. And food talk is often a metaphor for other things that may be occurring in the home. Although families certainly do not cause disordered eating, family dynamics can sometimes unwittingly contribute to an eating disorder. (We talk more about family dynamics in Chapter 22.)

- ✔ **Avoid family-style meals:** Ask your entire family to serve themselves directly from the pots and pans used to prepare the meal. Don't bring the entire dish to the table and leave it there while you eat. If someone wants a second helping, let her get up and get it.

- ✔ **Slow down your eating time:** You can stretch your eating time in many ways ,but first, determine how long you're going to eat. If your household is busy and the kids have to get back to their homework, a 20-to-30-minute meal may be all you have time for. If you're having dinner with your extended family and expect to be sitting at the table for an hour, you need to have a different plan in place. In general, 30 minutes of actual eating time is ideal. This is because it takes about 20 minutes for your fullness hormones to register fullness in specific parts of your brain.

Socializing and food

There's no escaping social eating. Inevitably, you'll attend a birthday dinner, a work lunch, or holiday feast. But know that social eating does not have to be a gateway to bingeing. With a solid food plan and your long-term goals in mind, you can reduce your urge to binge, control bingeing, and have a good time. Use these tips:

✔ **Plan ahead:** If you know you're going out to eat, check out the restaurant ahead of time, and, together with your RD, choose a meal that is appetizing and filling but that also provides you a sense of healthy control. If you're attending a gathering in someone's home, ask what food will be served and/or offer to bring a dish.

✔ **Eat only one plate of food:** It's better to have even one large plate of food than to go back and forth multiple times and not have any idea what or how much you ate.

✔ **Don't go to an event overly hungry:** Saving up calories or food is a set-up for bingeing. Stick with your meal plan all day, and even plan to have a snack before you go out. You're much more capable of making reasonable food decisions when you're not starving.

✔ **Don't take home leftovers:** Having extra food often triggers bingeing. It doesn't matter if the food is healthy or if you're taking it for your lunch tomorrow. Bringing home leftovers is a habit that must be broken. Declining leftovers is a way for you to say no to food and to take back control.

✔ **Don't completely avoid the foods you love:** If your cousin Sally has ice-cream cake, and you *love* ice-cream cake, you may not want to avoid it completely. Avoiding foods you enjoy denies you healthy emotional eating and sets you up to feel deprived, which often leads to bingeing.

✔ **Find a buddy:** Ask a friend or family member you trust to sit next to you at the table, or have that person check in with you sometime during the party. This can help keep you grounded around the food. It also provides a sense of accountability. Taking responsibility for your choices and how you handle social situations keeps you focused on eating and not bingeing.

✔ **Write in your food journal:** It doesn't matter if you have no clue how much you ate, what exactly the food was, or how it was prepared, writing down everything you ate, how you felt emotionally, and your levels of hunger and fullness can help keep you from bingeing. If you're at a party or restaurant, you're probably not able to openly write in your journal, but you can make very specific mental notes and record them in your journal after the meal when you get home or jot them down when you take a bathroom break. It may not be ideal, but it's better than not keeping track.

If you have a smartphone, use the notes section and jot down your food, then transfer the information to your journal later. At the time, it'll look like you're simply texting.

Chapter 13

Considering Medication and Dietary Supplements

*E*ven if you're on the path to recovery, years of binge eating may have taken a toll on your body that new habits can't overcome right away. You may also be dealing with psychological issues that contribute to your binge eating disorder and affect how you overcome it.

Most nutritionists and physicians take a *food first* approach to getting the vitamins and minerals the body needs to thrive, meaning they advise getting your nutrients primarily from food. But, at times, dietary supplements give a nutritional boost that you may not be able to get directly from foods.

If you're seeing a dietitian but still finding it difficult to eat your meal plan as prescribed, it may be time to consider oral supplements. Adding certain vitamins and minerals to your meal plan can not only improve your overall health but may also bridge the gap between your nutritional needs, which are affected by factors such as stress levels, aging, heredity, environment, and what your food intake provides in addition to your binge eating.

The same is true for medication to treat psychological conditions that make binge eating worse. Medication is not for everyone, and many people go out of their way to avoid taking it. But sometimes, without it, you can do all the right things to get better but still feel as if something is getting in the way. By working with a psychotherapist and a psychiatrist, you can tackle the many factors that may be preventing you from achieving the results you hope for and deserve.

Even if medication and/or supplements are the right tools for you, no magic pill, no matter how effective or helpful, can replace the long-term benefits of good nutrition, counseling, and your continued efforts toward recovery.

In this chapter, we start by highlighting several psychological conditions that may be complicating your recovery and review medications a psychiatrist may recommend as part of an overall treatment plan. We also discuss what nutritional supplements are and the various symptoms that may lead a dietitian to recommend them. We also decode labels on supplements and teach you to figure out what's safe and what may not be.

Considering Medication for Underlying Conditions

With binge eating, as with any eating disorder, there's often more to both the cause and treatment of symptoms and behaviors than meets the eye. As you begin to make progress with decreasing or stopping binge eating altogether, your team of eating disorder professionals may recommend that you consider uncovering or addressing previously undiagnosed psychological conditions that may be contributing to your urges to binge.

Three conditions that often go hand-in-hand with binge eating include ADHD or attention deficit hyperactivity disorder, anxiety disorders, and various types of depression. In these cases, it's not always clear whether binge eating triggers these conditions or vice versa — or both. In the end, it doesn't really matter. If you suffer from undiagnosed ADHD, anxiety, depression, or any other related conditions, you must address these issues to keep your recovery moving forward.

Some symptoms of these conditions overlap with those of other psychological conditions, and you may well suffer from more than one disorder. Nevertheless, your team of medical professionals and counselors (we talk about them in Chapter 10) should be able to do a full assessment and determine whether medication is needed and which type may be best for you. It may take time and experimentation with the correct drug and dosage, but if you need medication, it's an important part of establishing your psychological well-being and putting an end to binge eating.

The purpose of prescribing medication as part of your plan is to ease some of the binge-eating triggers based in your brain. By identifying and addressing some of the neurobiological factors that may lead to or exacerbate bingeing and other unhealthy behaviors, medication can be an important part of learning to manage the behaviors and habits that have developed over months and years.

Attention Deficit Hyperactivity Disorder (ADHD)

If you believed everything you watched on the news or saw on television, you might think that just about everybody suffers from ADHD. These days, ADHD is something you hear about all the time, either as a way to describe yourself when you're distracted or as the punch line of a joke about not being able to focus. But real, diagnosable ADHD is no laughing matter and can make recovering from binge eating extremely difficult.

Looking at symptoms

If you suspect that ADHD may be a part of what leads you to binge, consider the most common symptoms of the disorder:

- ✔ **Trouble concentrating and staying focused:** One of the first and most obvious signs of ADHD, this is more than getting distracted every once in a while. If you suffer from ADHD, you may find yourself unable to pay attention when other people are talking or to finish most tasks, no matter how small or seemingly manageable.

- ✔ **Disorganization and forgetfulness:** Are you always late? Are your car and your house a total mess? Do you spend lots of time looking for things? Do you procrastinate about everything? If these are chronic problems for you, it may be a sign that ADHD is keeping you from a larger sense of organization and routine in your life.

- ✔ **Emotional difficulties:** If you have ADHD, life seems to be too much to cope with most of the time, and even the smallest things really get to you. You don't feel good about yourself, and you can't seem to get motivated to change. Sometimes you're moody and irritable, and other times it's even worse than that, and your temper gets out of control.

- ✔ **Impulsivity:** You just can't control yourself. You say and do things you know you shouldn't, and if you're a binge eater, that includes eating foods in quantities that aren't good for you. Consequences don't matter to you even if you know what they are.

If you're a binge eater suffering from ADHD, the impulses, boredom, and lack of ability to concentrate often leave you standing in front of the refrigerator or pantry looking to graze. Not being able to achieve or maintain routine and order may be getting in the way of being completely successful with your eating plan and the new habits you'll need to develop for a healthier, binge-free life. For you, treating the ADHD at the same time you're working on ending the binges may be essential to recovery.

What is ADHD?

In the simplest terms, *attention deficit hyperactivity disorder (ADHD)* is the inability to focus during the activities of daily life. If you're suffering from ADHD, whether you know it or not, you may have noticed that you have trouble paying attention to other people and to the tasks you need to perform at home or at work. For some, this inability to stay focused can cause significant problems in personal relationships and/or in social, academic, or work environments. Often the symptoms of ADHD appear before the age of 7, and the most common ones include:

✔ Difficulty maintaining attention

✔ Becoming easily distracted or bored

✔ Frequently misplacing items

✔ Being disorganized

✔ Daydreaming

✔ Restlessness

✔ Risk-taking

✔ Being overly talkative

✔ Impatience with people and situations around you

Before 1994, the term ADD was often used to describe people who had symptoms of inattention without any hyperactivity, but since then, the *Diagnostic and Statistical Manual for Mental Disorders (DSM)* has officially used the term ADHD with the specification of three different subtypes: predominantly inattentive (ADHD-I), predominantly hyperactive-impulsive (ADHD-H), and combined type (ADHD-C).

Considering treatment options

Although there's no specific test per se for ADHD, your psychotherapist or psychiatrist can assess the likelihood that you're suffering from one of these conditions. And if you're diagnosed with the disorder, several medications — both stimulants or non-stimulants — can be prescribed to treat it.

The good news is that if you've spent your whole life suffering from ADHD without knowing it, using medication in a gradual, cautious way can bring about extraordinary relief and focus. Though the medication won't magically end your binge eating, it can be a great help as you address the habitual, self-soothing behaviors — including binge eating — you developed to cope with a lack of focus.

Psychiatrists commonly prescribe a class of drugs called psychostimulants to treat ADHD. Psychostimulants help those with ADHD to focus their thoughts and better manage distractions, and they're effective for most patients. However, stimulant medications used to treat ADHD sometimes have mild and short-lived initial side effects. The most common stimulant side effects include decreased appetite, weight loss, sleep difficulties, headaches, and jitteriness. In most cases, your psychiatrist can help you relieve any side effects by changing the medication dosage or choosing a different medication that you tolerate better.

Common stimulant drugs to treat ADHD include:

- ✔ Adderall and Adderall XR
- ✔ Concerta
- ✔ Daytrana
- ✔ Dexedrine
- ✔ Focalin and Focalin XR
- ✔ Metadate CD and Metadate ER
- ✔ Methylin and Methylin ER
- ✔ Ritalin, Ritalin SR, Ritalin LA
- ✔ Quillivant XR
- ✔ Vyvanse

In cases where stimulant medications are not a good choice for any of a variety of reasons, nonstimulants can help. Strattera (atomoxetine hydrochloride), Intuniv (guanfacine), and Kapvay (chlonidine hydrochloride) are commonly used nonstimulant medications used for children, adolescents, and adults. Intuniv (guanficine) is also used for children and adolescents to young adults.

Anxiety

Everyone feels anxious or worried from time to time. Concerns about upcoming work deadlines, having enough money, finding the right life partner, or getting into college — to name just a few — are a normal part of everyday life. But when anxiety begins to dominate your thoughts and controls every decision you make, it's time to consider that you may be suffering from a diagnosable anxiety disorder.

There's no one way to define anxiety. Just as a binge eater binges because of a set of triggers and circumstances unique to that person, the reasons people suffer from anxiety are different from person to person.

Some of the most common symptoms of anxiety include

- ✔ Generalized persistent and excessive worries about everyday situations, both real and imagined.
- ✔ Insomnia.

> ✔ A sudden and almost unexplainable sense of overwhelming panic, also
> called *panic attacks,* that may include nausea and/or dizziness, muscle
> tension, shortness of breath, cold or sweaty hands and/or feet, or
> numbness or tingling in the hands or feet.

If you're a binge eater suffering from anxiety, overeating may be a way to
help keep it at bay and calm the panic and distress of those seemingly uncontrollable feelings. However, if you want to stop bingeing, it's important to also
address the underlying causes so that you won't fall back on the same habits
you're trying to break.

If you and your psychotherapist or treatment team decide that therapy for your
anxiety isn't enough, you may be referred to a psychiatrist or *psychopharma-
cologist* (a pharmacist expert in psychoactive drugs) for further evaluation.
You'll be asked to talk about your medical history and when and how your
anxiety manifests itself. The evaluation includes questions about how much
your anxiety interferes with everyday life.

Your treatment team may suggest medications as well as certain nutritional
herbs and/or supplements meant to calm some of the panic enough for you
to deal with the underlying causes by taking the edge off. Be sure to tell
everyone on your treatment team that you're taking a new medication to
help prevent drug interactions and ask those closest to you to watch for any
changes in your behavior.

Antidepressants were developed to treat depression, but they help people with
anxiety as well. Antidepressants, antianxiety medications, and beta-blockers
are the most common medications used for anxiety. Your psychiatrist or
physician will generally prescribe antidepressants at low doses and increase
them over time, if necessary.

Prozac, Zoloft, Lexapro, Paxil, Celexa, Effexor, and Wellbutrin are some of the
most commonly prescribed medications for treating anxiety symptoms. Your
doctor chooses a particular medication depending on which symptoms are
most prevalent. These include generalized anxiety disorder (GAD), panic disorder, obsessive compulsive disorder (OCD), posttraumatic stress disorder
(PTSD), and social phobia among others.

Depression

Like other forms of mental illness, depression comes in all shapes and sizes.
Having a bad day can leave anyone feeling mildly depressed, but some people

suffer chronic depression for years due to some combination of brain chemistry, genetic predisposition, and physical or emotional trauma. Whatever the reason, trying to escape or soothe depression can be a persistent trigger for binge eating and must be addressed as part of your recovery.

If you suffer from depression or other forms of mental illness, binge eating probably began as a way to distract you from the feelings of sadness and distress you felt. Initially, your binges may have helped calm a persistent sense of helplessness or hopelessness, but now that you want to stop binge eating, you also have to deal with your feelings as well.

As you progress toward recovery, your team of professionals may notice that you're showing signs of depression, whether it's something recent or something you've experienced your whole life.

To get started with treatment, you visit a psychiatrist who does a thorough physical and psychological assessment looking for symptoms such as

✔ Difficulty concentrating, remembering details, and making decisions

✔ Fatigue and lack of energy

✔ Feelings of guilt, worthlessness, and/or helplessness

✔ Feelings of hopelessness and/or pessimism

✔ Insomnia, frequent awakenings, or excessive sleeping

✔ Irritability, restlessness

✔ Loss of interest in activities or hobbies once pleasurable, including sex

✔ Persistent aches or pain, headaches, cramps, or digestive problems that do not ease with treatment

✔ Persistent sadness and feeling of emptiness

✔ Thoughts of suicide or even suicide attempts

Some of these symptoms overlap with those of other psychological conditions, and the fact may be that you're suffering from more than one condition. Nevertheless, your team should be able to do a full assessment and determine whether medication is needed and which type may be best for you. It may take time and experimentation with the correct drug and dosage, but if you need medication, it's an important part of establishing your psychological well-being and putting an end to binge eating.

There are several classes of antidepressants used to treat depression and conditions that have depression as a component, such as anxiety disorder.

Antidepressants improve symptoms of depression by increasing the availability of certain brain chemicals called *neurotransmitters,* which can help improve emotions.

Major classes of antidepressants are:

- **Selective serotonin reuptake inhibitors (SSRIs):** A newer form of antidepressant and the most commonly prescribed antidepressants. They ease symptoms of moderate to severe depression, are relatively safe, and generally cause fewer side effects than other types of antidepressants. SSRIs alter the amount of a brain chemical called serotonin.

  Common SSRIs are citalopram (Celexa), escitalopram (Lexapro), fluoxetine (Prozac, Prozac Weekly, Sarafem), paroxetine (Paxil, Paxil CR, Pexeva), sertraline (Zoloft), and fluoxetine combined with the atypical antipsychotic olanzapine (Symbyax).

- **Serotonin and norepinephrine reuptake inhibitors (SNRIs):** Another newer form of antidepressant medicine, SNRIs treat depression by increasing availability of the brain chemicals serotonin and norepinephrine.

  Common SNRIs are duloxetine (Cymbalta), venlafaxine (Effexor, Effexor XR), and desvenlafaxine (Pristiq).

- **Tricyclic antidepressants (TCAs):** Some of the earliest antidepressants used to treat depression, TCAs primarily affect the levels of two chemical messengers (*neurotransmitters*), norepinephrine and serotonin, in the brain. Although these drugs are effective in treating depression, they have more side effects, so they are much less frequently chosen.

  Common tricyclic antidepressants include amitriptyline, amoxapine, desipramine (Norpramin), doxepin, iipramine (Tofranil, Tofranil-PM), maprotiline, nortriptyline (Pamelor), protriptyline (Vivactil), trimipramine, and surmontil.

- **Monoamine oxidase inhibitors (MAOIs):** Another early form of antidepressant, MAOIs are most effective in people with depression that doesn't respond to other treatments. MAOIs usually aren't the first medicines given for depression because they have serious side effects when combined with certain foods and/or medicines. Current research suggests that MAOIs work better than other antidepressants in those who have depression with uncommon symptoms such as sleeping and eating too much.

  Common MAOIs are isocarboxazid (Marplan), phenelzine sulfate (Nardil), tranylcypromine sulfate (Parnate), and selegiline (Emsam).

Talking with Your Team about Dietary Supplements

More than half the population of the United States uses dietary supplements on occasion. Canadian supplement use isn't far behind with Statistics Canada saying use of vitamin and mineral supplements is 47 percent among females and 34 percent among males. Although nutrition and medical professionals generally take a food-first approach to achieve sufficient nutrition, some professional bodies, including the Academy of Nutrition and Dietetics as well as the International Network of Integrative Mental Health (INIMH) and the Institute for Functional Medicine (IFM), recognize that dietary supplements play a role in improving nutrient intake and supporting health and wellness. Surveys show that many health professionals use dietary supplements themselves and also recommend dietary supplements to their patients or clients.

With so many dietary supplements on the shelves, choosing the best one (or combination) may feel overwhelming. Your dietitian is the best person to advise you on which dietary supplements may help you as you progress through recovery and stabilize your eating patterns. Your doctor is also an excellent resource; however, dietitians are typically more educated on the dietary supplement industry and may know best how to match your needs with the best product. Remember to consult with both a dietitian and a doctor before starting to take any supplements.

Even if your doctor isn't an expert on dietary supplements, never take any supplement without letting her know. Some supplements interfere with certain medications, and your physician can advise you about what's safe and what may not be, given your health and the medications you're already taking. It's also important that your doctor and dietitian know the exact quantities of vitamins you take because fat-soluble vitamins — A, D, E, and K — can build up in your body and produce toxic effects. Your doctor can order blood tests to check on your current vitamin levels to determine whether you have any specific vitamin or mineral deficiencies. The next section offers more advice on putting safety first when taking supplements.

Taking supplements safely

If you've discussed taking supplements with your dietitian and your doctor and received their approval, it's still important to be careful and to take supplements safely. You need to be sure you know what you're getting in your supplements and that the supplements you take don't interfere with other medications.

Being sure about what you're getting

Canada has tough standards for the manufacture of supplements, but in the United States the responsibility is on the supplement manufacturer to produce safe products; the Food and Drug Administration (FDA) does not certify or regulate dietary supplements. Manufacturers adhere to manufacturing standards on a voluntary basis. In the United States you can't be sure that manufacturers are checking their products for overall quality, safety, potency, and purity.

Supplements manufactured in the United States have been found to contain traces of lead, arsenic, mercury, and a whole host of other contaminants. And unless you purchase a supplement from a company that follows Good Manufacturing Procedures (GMPs), or subscribes to an independent verification program, there is no guarantee that the product has been tested or deemed safe for consumption.

Before you buy any supplements, be sure to follow these two important suggestions to ensure you are buying a quality product and not overdosing:

✔ **Look for a USP label.** The USP (United States Pharmacopeia) is a dietary supplement verification program. It's a voluntary testing and auditing program that ensures the quality of supplements for consumers. Seeing the USP verified mark on a label indicates that the dietary supplement product has been tested and meets industry standards. The USP specifically tests to ensure that the supplement

  • Contains the ingredients listed on the label in the declared potency and amount

  • Doesn't contain harmful levels of specified contaminants

  • Will break down and release into the body within a specified amount of time

  • Has been made according to FDA current good-manufacturing practices using sanitary and well-controlled procedures

✔ **Follow the recommended dosage.** There's no reason to spend extra money on mega vitamins or lots of different vitamins. A dietitian can guide you on what supplements may benefit you, if any. When you choose a supplement, aim for one that supplies the Recommended Dietary Allowance (RDA) and not more. You can tell this by looking at the back of the bottle at the percent of daily value. If the value exceeds 100 percent, choose another supplement.

You can search specific brands, ingredients, and references on the United States National Library of Medicine website database at `http://dietary supplements.nlm.nih.gov/dietary/glossary.jsp`.

Being smart about drug interactions

Knowing how a supplement interacts with your current medication is critical to your mental and physical health. All supplements are not created equal, and many have dangerous side effects if taken in combination with certain medications. Unfortunately, the risks are not always clearly labeled.

Don't assume that just because a supplement has claims of being all natural that it is safe for you to take.

The first and most important step before taking any supplement is to check with your doctor and/or dietitian. Don't take any supplement without discussing it with your healthcare professional. Many people rely on the advice of the salesperson at the health food or vitamin store. Remember that they are salespeople and generally not trained, licensed professionals fully qualified to dispense advice on your medical health and well-being.

Do research on the supplement you're considering and the medications you currently take to determine whether there are any contraindications. Although your treatment team looks out for anything that may not be in your best interest, you may pick up on an important consideration your team overlooked or that you forgot to mention. By playing an active role in your health care you will be setting yourself up for success.

Among the best and most reliable resources is the National Institutes of Health Office of Dietary Supplements Fact Sheet at `http://ods.od.nih. gov/factsheets/list-all`.

Explaining dietary supplements

A *dietary supplement* may be anything from vitamins, minerals, or herbs to *botanicals* (plant or plant parts used for medicinal or therapeutic properties), amino acids, and other substances such as organ tissue and *metabolites* (intermediate molecules part of a larger metabolic function that can help to start or stop that function). You find supplements in many forms including tablets, capsules, softgels, gelcaps, liquids, and powders. Whatever their form, dietary supplements are not considered food, and all must be labeled as dietary supplements.

The U.S. Congress defined the term *dietary supplement* in the Dietary Supplement Health and Education Act (DSHEA) of 1994. The DSHEA was created to amend the Federal Food, Drug, and Cosmetic Act as a way to establish standards with respect to dietary supplements. It defines dietary supplements as food and not drugs. Under DSHEA, the supplement company is responsible for determining that the dietary supplements it manufactures and distributes are safe and that any representations or claims made about them are substantiated by adequate evidence to show that the claims are not false or misleading. Only after a supplement has been reported to cause adverse health effects does the FDA (Food and Drug Administration) perform an investigation.

Dietary supplements are not regulated by the U.S. Food and Drug Administration (FDA) in the same way that prescription medications are. Instead, the safety of each and every supplement is determined by the company that makes and sells it. That means that if you're in the United States, you should never take a supplement without doing research, getting a recommendation from your dietitian, and checking with your physician.

In contrast to the lack of regulation in the United States, Canada requires products to be licensed prior to market entry by the Natural Health Products Directorate (NHPD), a branch of Health Canada. To be legally sold in Canada, all natural health products must have a product license, and the Canadian sites that manufacture, package, label, and import these products must have site licenses. To get product and site licenses, specific labeling and packaging requirements must be met, good manufacturing practices must be followed, and proper safety and efficacy evidence must be provided.

If you're worried about getting enough vitamins and minerals, taking the right supplements better insures that you get the essential nutrients you need. For binge eaters working on developing new eating habits, it can be reassuring to know that you have backup in the form of supplements as you plan your meals and confront the challenges of slowing and eventually stopping the binges.

Dietary supplements aren't a replacement for a varied diet rich in healthy, nutrient-dense food, and you should never consider supplements a substitute for healthy eating.

Looking at supplements for everybody

Most people, not just binge eaters, can benefit from taking a few standard supplements. Regardless of your bingeing history, whether you binge daily or haven't binged in five years, these supplements are considered safe and may help you stay healthy. However, it's always good to check with your healthcare provider to make sure these are appropriate for your particular case:

- ✔ **Multivitamin:** A daily multivitamin is a potent combination of vitamins and minerals. If you're deficient in particular vitamins or minerals, a general multivitamin can make up some of the difference between what you need and what you're not getting in your food. A multivitamin can help fill in the gaps.

Dosage: You can take a multivitamin as often as once daily or even just a few times per week.

✔ **Omega-3 fatty acids:** The standard American diet contains very little omega-3 fatty acids, which are found in oily fish such as sardines and salmon and in flaxseed. Omega-3 fatty acids are important for the relaxation and contraction of muscles, blood clotting, digestion, and fertility among other bodily functions.

Dosage: The usual dose is 600 to1,000 milligrams daily taken with a meal for best absorption. Side effects of taking too much omega-3 may include a fishy taste in your mouth or fishy breath (if your omega-3 is made of fatty fish), upset stomach, loose stools, and nausea. Often, switching to another form of omega-3 alleviates these side effects. One alternative is a flaxseed omega-3 supplement. Taking more than 3,000 milligrams of fish oil daily may increase bleeding and extend bleeding time in people who are already taking anticoagulants or blood thinners.

✔ **Probiotics:** Probiotics are strands of bacteria that help maintain the natural balance of your digestive system. Binge eating can upset the balance of your body's good bacteria and can lead to infections. A probiotic can help to get your digestion back on track after one binge episode or prolonged bingeing.

Dosage: There is no one-size-fits-all when it comes to probiotics. Take the probiotic as recommended on the label as some say to take with food and some say to take it on an empty stomach, depending on the strain. Different brands and types of probiotics vary in dosage and number of capsules or pills. Your digestive functioning and symptoms will determine what probiotic is best for you.

If you're considering taking a probiotic, ask your doctor or dietitian for a specific recommendation. She'll be able to advise you on which probiotics are best for the symptoms you experience. For example, probiotics that tend to be effective in treating prolonged diarrhea include bacteria strands *Lactobacillus GG* and *Saccharomyces boulardii*.

✔ **Vitamin D3:** Vitamin D is crucial for the absorption and metabolism of calcium and phosphorous, which have various functions, especially the maintenance of healthy bones. It supports the immune system, and adequate vitamin D levels are linked with healthy weight.

Vitamin D deficiency is more common than you may expect. People who don't get enough sun, especially people living in northern climates, are at risk. Vitamin D deficiency also occurs in sunny climates, possibly because people are staying indoors more, covering up when outside, or using sunscreen more consistently these days to reduce the risk of skin cancer.

Dosage: The recommended daily allowance (RDA) for adults is 600 IU (international units) with an upper limit of 4,000 IU per day. For most adults, 1,000 to 2,000 IU per day is adequate.

✔ **Calcium:** Most individuals get about half of the calcium they need from food, which means they are lacking. Women are especially at risk, and calcium deficiency can lead to osteoporosis.

Dosage: For women 1,200 milligrams (mg) daily and for men 1,000 milligrams daily. Take in 500 to 600 mg doses with food for best absorption.

✔ **Glucosamine and chondroitin:** The body naturally manufactures glucosamine and chondroitin, both of which promote joint health and support healthy joint movement. Glucosamine is thought to promote the formation and repair of cartilage, and it's believed that chondroitin helps prevent the breakdown of cartilage. Glucosamine supplements are derived from shellfish shells; chondroitin supplements are generally made from cow cartilage. Because binge eaters have an added risk of joint damage from carrying excess weight, glucosamine and chondroitin can both be helpful in restoring joint health and preventing further damage.

Dosage: Take as recommended on package with food/meals. Different brands and types vary in dosage and number of capsules or pills. There's no RDA for glucosamine but well-conducted research studies have seen benefits with no reported side effects with a standard dose of 500 mg in the form of tablets or capsules taken three times daily. For this reason, most practitioners recommend that adults older than 18 take 1,500 mg daily, regardless of weight. It may take up to three months for maximum benefits to be realized.

Recognizing the false promise of weight-loss supplements

If you're a binge eater, you may be looking to supplements for more than just help with living a healthier lifestyle and adopting better eating habits. Many people believe that supplements can cure binge eating or help with rapid weight loss. However, no magic pill can substitute for doing the work of psychotherapy and developing an eating plan for putting an end to the binges.

No matter what you've heard, not a single weight-loss supplement has been proven to be effective in the long term.

You can purchase a variety of weight-loss supplements through online sources, at vitamin stores, at your local grocery store — almost anywhere.

Some of these supplements are harmless, some are marginally beneficial (though often not for weight loss), and some of them are downright dangerous (for example, ephedra-caffeine was banned in the United States because of potential effects on the heart). And, we say it again: None of them has been shown to have a lasting effect on weight loss.

If a weight loss supplement seems too good to be true, it probably is. The bottom line: Avoid supplements that promise a quick fix, and never take a dietary supplement that hasn't been approved by your doctor and your dietitian.

Supporting a healthy mind with supplements

Although there are no weight-loss supplements that work in the long term, you may be wondering if there are any to help with mood or the urge to binge. Experts have not reached a complete consensus, and there needs to be more research to figure out if and what supplements may help with mood and ultimately the urge to binge.

If you suffer from severe mood fluctuations, you must see a doctor before you reach for supplements. There are no supplements to cure or fix depression, anxiety, OCD, or other psychological conditions. Therapy and medication should be the first line of treatment.

Even though all the data isn't in yet, some supplements have shown potential to improve moods. These supplements may help keep your brain functioning at its best — in the long run, this can help improve your emotional state, which helps to keep the urge to binge in check.

- ✔ **St. John's wort:** St. John's wort is commonly used for sleep disorders, anxiety, and mild to moderate depression. Data from clinical trials show that St. John's wort may not help those with more severe forms of depression.

    St. John's wort may also have the potential to reduce symptoms of anxiety, premenstrual syndrome (PMS), or perimenopausal mood changes.

    Available as capsules, tablets, liquid extracts, and teas, a typical dose of St. John's wort ranges from 900 to 1,200 milligrams a day, and it needs to be taken for at least one to three months to see the best effect.

    St. John's wort has the potential for serious interactions with a wide variety of prescription drugs including birth control pills, antidepressants, HIV medications, and blood thinners. It can also interact with other herbs or supplements. Mainly, it may lower the effectiveness of certain medications. Never take St. John's wort without first consulting your physician.

✔ **SAM-e (S-Adenosyl-L-Methionine):** SAM-e occurs naturally in the cells of plants, animals, and humans. Because the body produces less SAM-e with age, some people think that SAM-e may be a helpful supplement for some conditions such as depression and osteoarthritis.

Although current trials are inconclusive, some studies show that improvements were comparable to conventional antidepressants such as the class of medications called tricyclic antidepressants. SAM-e is particularly helpful for those with a type of depression that produces low energy. The exact mechanism by which SAM-e works is unknown. It may affect levels of neurotransmitters, which are chemicals produced naturally in the body that promote communication between nerve cells in the brain and nerve cells in the rest of the body.

The dosage is 400 to 800 milligrams daily, depending upon need or tolerance. The dose most often used for depression in clinical studies is 800 to 1,600 milligrams daily for up to six weeks.

Although SAM-e doesn't usually cause side effects, use caution if you have diabetes, low blood sugar, or an anxiety disorder or other type of psychiatric disorder. SAM-e is not recommended for those with bipolar disorder as it tends to worsen manic symptoms. Gastrointestinal problems, headaches, fatigue, and skin rashes are the most common side effects.

✔ **Dehydroepiandrosterone (DHEA):** DHEA is a hormone produced by the adrenal glands that the body uses to make male and female sex hormones. DHEA levels peak when you're in your mid-20s and steadily decline as you get older, leading researchers to wonder whether DHEA could work as an anti-aging treatment.

In older people, lower-than-normal levels of DHEA have been associated with osteoporosis, heart disease, memory loss, and breast cancer, but there's no proof that low levels of DHEA cause these conditions or that taking DHEA can help prevent them.

DHEA supplements vary widely in quality. Many products tested don't have the amount of DHEA the label says they do. DHEA supplements can also have side effects: They may lower levels of HDL cholesterol (good cholesterol), and in women they may raise levels of testosterone as well as estrogen.

Because DHEA in supplements is a synthetic hormone, talk to your doctor before taking it. Your doctor may want you to have a blood test before you start taking any synthetic hormone.

In a few clinical studies of people with major depression, DHEA improved symptoms compared to a placebo. However, the results aren't entirely clear, and researchers don't know what the long-term effects of taking DHEA may be. More research is needed. Don' t try to treat depression by yourself. People with depression need medical care.

✔ **Vitamin B12 (cobalamin):** B12 is one of eight B vitamins, all of which help the body convert food (carbohydrates) into fuel (glucose), which produces energy. These B vitamins, often referred to as *B-complex vitamins,* also help the body use fats and protein. B-complex vitamins are needed for healthy skin, hair, eyes, and liver. They also help the nervous system function properly. All B vitamins are water-soluble, meaning that the body does not store them, and therefore they're considered safe, non-toxic supplements.

Vitamin B12 is an especially important vitamin for maintaining healthy nerve cells, and it helps in the production of DNA. Vitamin B12 also works closely with vitamin B9, also called *folate* or *folic acid,* to help make red blood cells and to help iron work better in the body. Folate and B12 work together to produce S-adenosylmethionine (SAM-e), a compound involved in immune function and mood.

Although these supplements may help with symptoms of depression and anxiety, if you're on any medications for anxiety, OCD, depression, or any related illness, it's absolutely essential that you check with your doctor and/or psychiatrist before you begin taking any supplements. Some supplements may be contraindicated in combination with prescribed medicines. Be sure to always check before you begin taking a supplement.

Chapter 14

Enlisting Family and Friends

*N*o man or woman is an island, and as you become more invested in your recovery from binge eating, you may begin to tell your friends and family about your successes and confide in them about the challenges you're facing.

Hopefully, you have people in your life who accept, love, support, and encourage you in all of your endeavors. If you don't have a supportive community around you, now is the time to consider how to create one.

You may be one of the many unfortunate binge eaters who has someone — or even several people — in your life who've made you feel bad about yourself over the years, whether they meant to or not. Close friends and relatives may have judged you or been critical, either openly or more subtly. One of the challenges you now face is how, or even whether, to include these people in your recovery.

As you begin to figure out whom to ask for help, you may want to leave out anyone who hasn't been really positive. You can always include those people later when your recovery is underway and you feel more confident about your ability to face criticism without backsliding or bingeing.

You'll always face people who are negative or unsupportive, so at the beginning, focus on friends and family who can lift you up and help launch your journey to better health.

In this chapter, we talk about the various roles friends and family can and should play in your recovery. We point out the limits of what other people can do for you, and we give you a checklist to help you decide who to tell about your attempts to stop binge eating and who not to tell. Finally, if you're the friend or loved one of a binge eater, the sidebars in this chapter offer tips on how you can be most supportive and helpful and what to do and not to do. (Chapter 21 also addresses how to help a recovering binge eater.)

Asking for Help from Friends and Family

Friends and family can be a crucial part of your recovery from binge eating. The people who love you most may have been patiently waiting for years for you to be ready to seek help. Over time, they may have realized that you yourself needed to find the reasons for a change and that their best option was to support and love you just as you are.

Whether you jumped wholeheartedly into treatment or are getting a slower, more moderate start, you may not have told many people about beginning therapy, your visits to your physician and/or dietitian, or why you may have been busier than normal. As you imagine a new life for yourself and begin to manage your binge eating, you'll probably want to slowly widen the network of people who can support you and help you make significant changes now and into the future.

Looking to your inner circle

Having a network of supportive friends and family who know you're in treatment for binge eating, and can support you as you recover, can be extremely helpful as you move forward. You may already have at least one go-to person who has encouraged you up until this point. Now more than ever, you may want to turn to that person or to others you meet on the way for support in a variety of ways.

If you don't have someone like that in your life, it's time to figure out who can play that role for you. When you're trying to decide who the right people might be, ask yourself three questions:

- ✔ Who do I feel safe with?
- ✔ Who doesn't judge me?
- ✔ Who has supported me through both my successes and challenges?

Though the obvious first choices may be close friends or family, think carefully about whether or not the support person(s) you consider have been helpful in the past. Keep in mind that someone may be helpful one minute and hurtful the next without even knowing it. That's why taking extra time to be thoughtful about each potential support person is so important.

Take a piece of paper and make three columns: positive, neutral, and negative. Without thinking too much, separate your friends and family members into each of these categories. Hopefully, when you finish, you'll have a few good choices in the positive column!

Someone who has been critical, judgmental, frustrated, or who makes you feel anxious every time you see them, isn't the right friend or family member to include in your treatment plan. Over time, you may have the confidence to ask for the exact help you need from these people, but at the beginning, you may want to limit your support circle to those you're sure you can count on.

Focus on who can help you the most. This is about your recovery, you don't need to tell everyone you're close to at the beginning, and you certainly don't have to worry about hurting someone's feelings by not including him. Even if you know a loved one doesn't mean to be critical or negative, there's no need to spend valuable energy coaching and cajoling that person into being someone different.

For example, if your sister is your best friend and number-one supporter but also happens to be a marathon runner who simply can't understand how you "let yourself go," it won't matter that she loves you so much or that she wants the best for you. If she inadvertently says things that feel unsupportive, she's probably not going to be a good person to talk with about this yet.

Finding new friends and supporters

You can look beyond the people around you for support and find someone who may be on the same journey. Three possible sources of support include

- ✔ **Therapy groups:** If you're not already in a therapy group about binge eating or disordered eating, now's the moment to seek one out. After you find a group you're comfortable with and get settled, hopefully you'll meet someone who makes you think, "she sounds just like me." And even if you don't find another person who's facing the exact same challenges you are, you may connect with someone who can help you with ideas and encouragement at the same time you're helping her.

- ✔ **Overeaters Anonymous (OA):** OA can be another regular source of friendship and community in an informal setting. If you like, you can be paired with a sponsor either in person or online. That person will likely have more experience in recovery than you and can help you with challenges you face as well as introduce you to others in the group.

OA also runs telephone meetings and online meetings for people who can't or don't want to go to face-to-face meetings. Depending on your personality, one of these options may be a good fit for you. However, keep in mind that getting out and seeking help in person may be quite important if you're someone who has typically isolated yourself at home to eat.

✔ **Chat rooms and other online communities:** Even though you're not face-to-face with other binge eaters, chat rooms can serve as a highly valuable way to connect with people going through the same experiences you are. Online communities give you a far wider reach than in-person groups and can provide an opportunity for you to ask questions and share information that you might otherwise be nervous or embarrassed to tell someone face-to-face.

There are several different options for finding community and support online. Some sites maintain open, 24-hour chat rooms for people in recovery, and some have either closed or open groups moderated by a therapist that you can join on a regular basis.

Most chat rooms and online communities have their own guidelines that members must follow. Most of these rules have to do with common courtesy (respect others, no personal insults, no swearing, and so on), but others concern privacy, safety, confidentiality, anonymity, and interactions among members. Many groups, particularly those for binge eaters and others who may participate in addictive behaviors, have specific rules designed to keep participants from triggering each other by discussing certain subjects.

Some examples of guidelines that might be part of a binge eating chat room include

- Please do not discuss numbers such as weight, calories, measurements as they may be triggers for others.

- Please do not talk about specific foods or restaurants as these too may be triggers.

- Please don't bring up dieting tips or weight-loss strategies.

The point of online support groups is not necessarily to lose weight. Most binge eaters probably already know about every diet in the universe, and talking about dieting may trigger bingeing.

As with in-person therapy and groups, meeting and talking with people online is most helpful when it's focused on the feelings and actions that underlie and trigger the binge behaviors, how not to be alone in your thoughts and shame, and/or how to find alternate coping methods.

Wherever you're looking for support, remember to treat others just as you would like to be treated, and you'll likely attract and meet people who can assist you along just as you help them.

Don't forget to share your positive experiences at the same time you're looking for guidance yourself. Helping and supporting others in their recovery from binge eating can be healing for you and a way to celebrate your successes in a productive way.

If you search online even for a few minutes, you find out that many sites exist for binge eaters and people with other forms of eating disorders. Some of our favorite, most useful, sites are

- ✔ **Binge Eating Disorder Association (BEDA)** (www.bedaonline.com): BEDA Online offers a members-only section of the website with resources including bulletin boards and other online resources for binge eaters. If you're a student, it costs $20 to join BEDA. Otherwise, it's $50 for individuals.

- ✔ **Body Positive** (www.bodypositive.com): Body Positive, a site maintained by Health at Every Size (www.haescommunity.org), includes a list of online resources including websites, chat groups, newsgroups, mailing lists, and "other cool stuff." The site focuses on how to feel good about yourself, and it contains resources for therapy, children and weight, books, and many other subjects.

- ✔ **Something Fishy** (www.something-fishy.com): Something Fishy maintains two websites. In addition to other information on addiction and therapy, this site has links to online therapy groups.

- ✔ **Something Fishy** (www.something-fishy.org): The more extensive of the two sites, Something Fishy has a wealth of its own online resources including chat support, bulletin boards, instant messaging support, and a whole section for family and friends of people with eating disorders. In addition, this site has an extensive directory of other online resources that includes chats and forums, e-mail lists, newsgroups, and positive, inspirational sites.

Knowing Who to Tell and Who Not to Tell

As you settle into the routine of treatment and feel a sense of improvement and success, you may be tempted to tell everyone you know about your progress.

Your closest supporters may already know because they've been with you every step of the way. They may have even helped you by gathering information about psychotherapists, groups, and dietitians or by going with you to your first appointments.

But you may not yet have told anyone who's been less than supportive over the years, and your instinct to protect yourself and your newfound attempts to live a healthier life is probably the right one. You may also find yourself dodging questions from the friends who were fellow overeaters in the past. Even though you want to share your success with them, it's important not to fall back into undesirable behaviors in order to maintain relationships or to keep someone else from feeling bad.

Finding the right support for the right time

As you progress in your recovery, you may want to widen your circle of support. One place to start is by identifying people who can help you during the parts of your day when you typically binge. Maybe your roommate or spouse keeps you on track if you binge at home, maybe you have a work buddy if you binge after lunch or when you're under a lot pressure on the job, maybe a friend at OA can help you if the weekend is your prime bingeing time, or perhaps there's someone you check in with online after dinner if you feel vulnerable then. Whether or not these are new or old friends doesn't matter. What matters is that they are loving, non-judgmental, and focused on your recovery.

As you discover more about what you need to successfully recover, remind those closest to you about specific ways they can help. If, for instance, you always binge on sweets after lunch at work, ask your friend in the next cubicle to take a quick walk with you every day at 1 p.m. If one of your trigger foods is ice cream, ask your roommate not to keep it in the freezer. Most often, a simple, direct and specific request is easier to respect and fulfill than a bigger, more general appeal for help.

Neutralizing your detractors

Though it may seem obvious, the people you don't want to include in your recovery are those who have been toxic to you in the past. Choosing not to spend time with acquaintances or friends who have been unsupportive, hypercritical, or impatient is quite doable, but creating some separation from family members can be considerably more difficult. It's simple to say that you won't engage anymore with people who trigger you to binge, but if one of those people is a parent, grandparent, sibling, or other close relative, then getting away may be easier said than done.

If, for instance, your grandmother tells you how fat you are every time she sees you, maybe you should see her as little as possible until you develop a strategy with your team or group about how to deal with her. If you and your brother binge together on Sunday nights after family dinner, perhaps you should plan to see a movie or take a walk instead (with him or with someone else) or to leave before dessert.

You can't avoid everyone who's ever triggered you to binge, but you can, over time, figure out ways to neutralize the negative feelings that lead to the behaviors.

As you gain more knowledge about your triggers, you also gain a greater understanding of which people and situations are more likely to bring on a binge.

You may not be able to avoid everyone who has ever seemed unsupportive to you, but you can use the following tips to help lessen the negative impacts:

✔ **Make a direct request.** Though it may take time to work up to being direct, it's much easier for you and the listener if you use "I" statements. For example, instead of saying, "you always make me upset when you do that. You're such a …," say something like, "when that happens, I feel …." You're not accusing. You're commenting on the behavior rather than the person and taking responsibility for your own feelings. At the same time, you're also modeling how you'd like to be spoken to.

✔ **Avoid people who have insulted or judged you in the past.** This can mean literally breaking up with some people. To avoid other negative influences, it's a matter of changing routines to minimize contact with the person who insults or judges you. For instance, if you have a coworker who always makes rude comments about your lunch, talk with your boss about taking a different lunch time.

✔ **Enlist a trusted friend or family member to help you calm down at events or in situations that have triggered binges in the past.** You've probably noticed that someone saying, "calm down" generally doesn't create calm. In fact, it can make things worse. What may be more helpful is to have a secret signal that means "can we get out of here for a few minutes?" Then, take a short walk or just go into another room or area to breathe deeply and catch up with your feelings.

Can you get someone to enter treatment?

If you know and love someone who's a binge eater, you already know that the simple answer to this question is no. Just like other people who behave destructively, a binge eater has to decide to stop for herself. Pressure or criticism just makes things worse (and likely triggers bingeing) even if you have loving intentions.

The best you can do before someone decides to seek help or treatment is to be non-judgmental and supportive. It's also not a good idea to bring up the binge eating unless the person you'd like to help brings it up first. Then, and only then, do you have a chance to jump in and start a conversation about what you can do and what she might like her life to be in the future.

Dealing with overeating friends

It's natural that you may have a group of friends who binge or even just overeat with you. Many very overweight people end up with overweight friends who don't judge them and who make bingeing seem like the norm.

If you've begun treatment, figuring out what to do with these friends can be challenging. At first, you may still want to spend time with them because you love them and because you don't necessarily have other friends to turn to. But if what you do together is eat, it's probably not a good idea in the long run to keep up these relationships unless you participate in activities that do not involve food.

Although it's difficult, try to put some distance between yourself and friends who may also be binge eaters. Don't go to your weekly dinners, and try to avoid the situations and places where you binged together. Suggest other activities, but if these friends don't want to change, you may have to allow the friendships to fall by the wayside. In time, you'll develop other friends who share the same interests, goals, and the healthier habits you're trying to cultivate.

Being realistic about what others can and cannot do for you

Chances are, your friends and family want to do as much as they can to support you. At times, they may even be more enthusiastic and hopeful about your treatment than you are. On bad days, you may find their relentless good cheer as much annoying as it is helpful.

But at the end of the day, you're the one who needs to be your own best friend in this. If you find yourself going to treatment to please others or if you tend to blame others for your setbacks, it's time to regroup and focus again on your own reasons for wanting to establish a healthier life as well as the power of your own role in initiating change.

Dining Do's and Don'ts

Support from friends and family can take many different forms, but sometimes even the best intentioned people don't know quite what to do to help. One of the simplest and most direct ways to ask for help is to make a list of what to do and what not to do at the dinner table or in any dining situation.

Having a clear-cut list can make eating with friends and family much easier because your expectations are clear, and the people who support you know *exactly* what to do or not to do to help. You can start with a general list that you can apply to most, if not all, meals. Then you can work to refine your do's and don'ts for particular situations.

✔ Do keep my water glass filled.

✔ Do plan to share dessert when it is offered.

✔ Don't discuss the calories or fat content of the meal.

✔ Don't eat diet foods — they only make me feel deprived.

Your dining do's and don'ts may be different depending on the situation. You need different help at a party than you do when you're dining out. You may have a completely different set of do's and don'ts for a restaurant than you do for a family holiday with a buffet-style meal. It's important to be flexible and to understand that you may have to develop several sets of rules for yourself and others as you move forward.

You can make itemized lists of do's and don'ts for various dining situations on your own or with your treatment team. The following list includes common problem areas and sample do's and don'ts:

✔ **Buffet-style meals**

- Do have Jessica sit next to me and help me not go for second or third helpings.

- Don't avoid all the foods I love to eat.

✔ **Family meals**

- Do make a side dish to bring that's safe for me to eat.

- Don't sit next to Uncle Scott, he always seems to say things that upset me and make me want to eat.

✔ **Parties**

- Do enjoy a piece of my favorite pie, which Jen will cut for me.

- Don't take home leftovers.

✔ **Romantic meals with your special someone**

- Do let Jim order an appetizer for both of us to share.

- Don't talk about food at the meal.

✔ **Restaurant dining**

- Do share dessert with Sam, he knows how to cut it right down the middle, so I don't feel tempted to eat more than half.

- Don't eat from the breadbasket. Ask the server to remove it from the table right away.

✔ **Vacation meals**

- Do stick with eating only at meal time.

- Don't order dessert every night.

Post your dining do's and don'ts in your kitchen or dining room, and share them with the people you're relying on to help you stick to your rules. Keep your lists with you before, during, and after mealtimes to remind yourself of the small steps you can take toward your larger goal.

Make sure to review your list on a regular basis with your support crew. If something's not working, make adjustments and try again.

If you set guidelines and boundaries for yourself before you jump into tricky situations, it can be easier to stick with your food plan and avoid the triggers that might lead you to binge.

Chapter 15

Relapsing and Reassessing: It's a New Day

*N*o one likes to talk about the possibility of relapse, and you may dread or deny the possibility that you may binge again. Since you've begun your journey, be it in direct treatment or in other ways, you've probably started to feel hopeful about the future, but maybe you've also worried about the possibility of falling back on bingeing behaviors. Unfortunately, looking both at the research statistics and at your own personal history, you probably already know that it's highly likely that binge eating could creep up on you again some time in the future.

Both the good news and the bad news is that recovery isn't an all-or-nothing proposition for most people. As you probably realize, knowledge is power, but it's also not enough to know what you have to do to recover. If that were the case, you'd have stopped bingeing long ago. Now that you're making changes in your life, you have to give yourself time to heal and a chance to practice your new coping skills and strategies. The same thinking that may have launched you into the cycle of dieting-bingeing-gaining weight is the kind of thinking that can make relapses more frequent and more intense.

If you binge during recovery, all is not lost. Far from it. A relapse — or even multiple relapses — is an opportunity to make changes to what you're doing and adjust according to what you're learning about yourself, your body, and your emotional well-being. Perhaps the most important goal of recovery is not letting a relapse turn into a long series of relapses. Be gentle with yourself and remember that anger, frustration, and doubt only prolong the behaviors you want to stop.

Relapsing in response to stress

Michelle had been in treatment for binge eating for more than a year, and she hadn't binged for several months. She was feeling more positive, confident, and optimistic about her future. One Thursday, she went to work only to find out during a morning meeting that half of her office was going to be laid off and that on the following Monday morning, her supervisor would announce exactly who was being terminated. The fear, anxiety, and unpredictability of her future sent her into binge mode. She couldn't think of anything else but food — what to buy, where to buy it, and how to eat it. She used to binge in front of the television, something she hadn't done in months, but in her current predicament, she couldn't imagine distracting herself any other way. She binged all weekend and went to work on Monday morning with a food hangover. Thankfully, she found out she was not being laid off.

It hit her then that she was still susceptible to the urge to binge. Had she thought that by bingeing she could change the outcome of events at work? Had she thought that by numbing herself she would not have to think about anything unpleasant? But all was not lost. Though the relapse was quite costly for Michelle — physically, emotionally, and financially — she learned a very valuable lesson, and the weekend became a seminal event in her journey. She was able to see clearly that the costs of bingeing outweighed the benefits, if there ever were any, and that especially when her anxiety went sky high in response to things out of her control, bingeing wasn't the way to cope.

In this chapter, we tackle the reality of relapse in a way that furthers your journey towards recovery. We talk about how to cope with the disappointment of bingeing again in positive ways. We break down how to figure out why you relapsed, and show you how relapse is a bump in the road rather than the end of the line

Preparing for the Possibility of Relapse

Even though no one in recovery for binge eating wants to talk about relapse, it's important to be honest with yourself about the fact that it can and likely will happen at some point. Most people who were chronic binge eaters have at least one relapse on the road to recovery. You may be horrified to read that sentence, but studies and personal stories from patients suggest that it's the truth.

Whenever you began bingeing, at whatever age that was, you started because it seemed like a good idea at the time and was an effective way to soothe yourself, whether you consciously knew it or not. When binge eating stops working and the risks and negative feelings outweigh the benefits, you're forced to find new and healthier ways to calm yourself. Those changes take time. After all, you didn't develop the binge behaviors and all that goes with them overnight, nor will you replace them all overnight.

Being realistic about relapse

Some people say that planning for relapse is pessimistic, but because it tends to be the norm for most people, think of it instead as a proactive, preventive, and realistic approach to treatment and recovery. As far as relapses are concerned, you have two choices

- ✔ You can passively wait for a relapse to happen (not recommended).
- ✔ You can be aware and alert that relapse is a possibility while you learn how to be more gentle and non-judgmental about your own behaviors.

If you choose the second option, please be assured that talking about relapse isn't what makes it happen. A relapse occurs when a change or several changes happen in your life that you haven't been able to anticipate. Even though everyone recognizes that you can't plan for everything, when the unexpected occurs, your fallback response is to revert to the old comfortable habit of your automatic, maladaptive coping methods. This is to be expected. However, with proper guidance and some kindness toward yourself, relapse binges become much, much less frequent, shorter in duration, and less intense than when you binged more regularly.

Defining a relapse

Just as binge eating varies from person to person, every relapse is different. Even if you haven't binged on as much food or for as long as when you binged more regularly, you may know for yourself that you've slipped.

Watch for these common signs and thoughts:

- ✔ Negative self-talk that becomes like the devil on your shoulder, convincing you that you're entitled to binge, that you deserve the break, and that it's only one time.
- ✔ Taking chances with foods that have historically been triggering or set off binges. For instance, buying one of those foods when grocery shopping and telling yourself, "I won't binge on this. It's really for my family."

✔ Skipping meals, especially for several days in a row, knowing full well that being ravenous when you do finally get to eat will create a binge rather than eating a meal.

✔ Not being protective of your sleep and allowing the irregularity of your rest to confuse your cues about hunger, thirst, and fatigue.

✔ Just a general sense that "uh-oh, my switch has been flipped again, I feel like a bottomless pit" when, in fact, the question you may want to ask yourself at that moment is "what am I really hungry for?" (It may not be food — check out the upcoming "Understanding the reasons for the binge.")

Rebooting after a Relapse

If you relapse, it's important to pick yourself back up again and get on with your journey to restore your physical and emotional health. It may feel like the end of the world, especially after you've worked so hard and not binged for a while, but relapses happen, and the easier you are on yourself and the better you deal with it, the more quickly you can move forward.

Sometimes relapse is unavoidable, especially when you're faced with situations, people, or feelings that you haven't addressed yet in therapy or that you're having trouble figuring out how to handle.

No matter what the reason, never underestimate how positive an episode of relapse can be. You may be wondering how the words "relapse" and "positive" can even exist in the same sentence, but the reality is that a relapse lets you know that something in your plan isn't quite working. It may be that you're not eating enough, not getting enough rest, or not developing strategies that work for you during those difficult emotional times when you're faced with all sorts of triggers.

The main thing to take away from a relapse is how to use it to develop new plans and strategies and to be stronger next time you are facing a triggering situation.

Putting the binge in perspective

Before you beat yourself up and throw in the towel on your recovery, remember that not all binges are created equal. Think back to a time before you found help and take a moment to remember what your binges looked like when they were a regular part of your life.

Now, take a slow, deep breath, and try to take an objective and non-judgmental look at what just happened. Even though it's difficult to separate fact from fiction in the heat of the moment, when you're calm enough to think rationally about your most recent binge, you may notice it's not like what it used to be.

Consider these factors for comparison when working through the aftermath of a relapse binge:

✔ **Quantity of the binge:** Okay, you binged. There's no denying that. Look at how much you binged on. Was the amount different? How does this binge compare to others you've experienced?

It's common for a relapse binge to include significantly less food, although that's not always the case. If your relapse binge was comparatively smaller, that's an important distinction. The fact that your binge may be a third or even half of the amount you typically binged on is a direct result of the improvement in your coping skills overall.

✔ **Amount of time spent bingeing:** What time of day did your old binges start? How long did they last? Hours, maybe even days? When you're figuring out how to move forward after a relapse binge, take into account both the timing and the length of this most recent binge.

Say you used to start bingeing at 9 p.m., and the binges generally lasted until you went to bed at 11:30 p.m. If your relapse binge started at 9 p.m., but you were able to stop by 10 p.m. (probably having eaten less along the way), you have reason to be proud. While bingeing isn't ideal, take some satisfaction from the fact that you used some of your new coping skills to stop the binge from going longer.

✔ **Guilt and other negative emotions associated with the binge:** Being calmly and gently aware of the emotions you experience after a binge can help put relapses into perspective. As you probably know, the buildup of negative or judgmental feelings after a binge only makes matters worse, generally leading to more of the very bingeing for which you're feeling shame or self-loathing. How you handle yourself now, and how you choose to cope with the relapse has a great impact on when and if you will binge again.

Understanding the reasons for the binge

When the relapse binge ends, you may be left wondering why it happened in the first place, especially if your resolve is strong and you've been on the right track up until now. Maybe you're so wrapped up in feelings of shame and guilt that you can't even think about how or why it happened. No matter what the situation, understanding why you binged is important and avoiding self-recrimination and blame is essential. Beating yourself up never ends well and, in fact, is likely to perpetuate the slip. Being your own cheerleading squad always feels a whole lot better in the end.

By and large, a relapse can usually be traced back to feelings of deprivation. Perhaps you feel like you don't have enough love, enough money, enough respect from family or friends, or you're just suffering the sensation of missing something. Chances are it's not a lack of food, and trying to fill the void with food sets a relapse in motion. Part of retracing your steps and understanding your most recent binge is figuring out how to make sure that the sense of deprivation doesn't sneak up on you and sabotage your steady progress forward.

Even though it can be difficult, honesty is the best policy when you relapse. Telling the truth about the binge — most importantly to yourself — is the best way to get to the bottom of what triggered your relapse in the first place. You may be worried about what your support system — be it clinicians you're working with, trusted loved ones, or a support group — will think, but don't. Their job is to not judge you but instead to help you figure out which strategies you're using aren't working and find ones that do.

Examining the emotional reasons

You may know right away why you binged, and the reason may be little or big. Although it's tempting to imagine that only a catastrophic event such as a death, divorce, or job loss could trigger you now that you've been stable for a while, the reality is far more complicated and much less clear-cut.

A relapse can occur for many reasons, some positive, some negative. Of course, an upsetting event or person can trigger you, but relapse may also happen because of something as simple as seeing an old friend who's now quite fit, which triggers jealousy and self-loathing on your part. Or perhaps even though you're given a promotion at work, you're convinced you've fooled them, they've made a mistake, and you're certain you'll fail at your new responsibilities.

When you relapse, even if you think you know and understand why, the first step is to take an inventory of how your life may have changed lately, and how you feel about it. Start by considering the following questions:

- ✔ What time of day was the binge? Was there a change in your schedule or did you wake up later than usual? Was your day much more hectic than usual? Did the pressure of your shifting schedule feel overwhelming?

- ✔ Was there a pattern to the time or duration if there were several binges? Recognizing binge patterns can tell you a lot about the role of your emotions. If you previously binged just on Friday nights but you have a series of relapses that last full weekends, you're probably experiencing strong emotions that you've not yet recognized or identified because the binge has numbed them out.

✔ Did something happen at work, with family, at home, or in one of your relationships that you didn't immediately associate with the need for self-soothing?

✔ Was there a big shift in the weather? Was there inclement or dreary weather for a longer than usual period of time so that staying indoors and feeling bored pushed the urges to binge over the edge?

✔ Were you feeling physically ill? How you feel physically can have a serious impact on whether or not you binge. Were you overly tired, in pain, or just plain sick with a cold or flu ? Any kind of illness can be a trigger, especially if you've been sick for several days in a row.

✔ Was it the anniversary of a traumatic life event? Does the reminder of a specific event or period of time lead to feeling upset, angry, or sad?

✔ Did someone say something to you that you may not have interpreted correctly or that you overreacted to? Did the comment make you feel inferior or inadequate in some way?

✔ Were you stimulated by seeing or smelling foods you've been avoiding? Does seeing others enjoy foods that you have binged on stimulate your urge to binge? Also consider the people you were with when you saw the triggering foods. Are they people that support you or people who tend to set off your binge triggers? Consider that it may not just be the food but the environment, as well.

✔ Was there a change in your financial situation? Financial stress is one of the most significant challenges you can face. Have you had a change in your pay, been laid off, or had your budget derailed by a large expenditure that was out of your control such as having to purchase a new car unexpectedly?

It's worth noting that your attitudes and reactions toward the subject of money often mirror your habits and reactions with food. See whether you can think of your own example of this. It's an interesting and common correlation.

✔ Is there some special event you're anticipating? Perhaps warmer weather is coming up, and the thought of wearing less clothing makes you feel uncomfortable. Or are the holidays approaching and you know you'll have to spend time with triggering family members as well as a lot of food?

✔ Have you been feeling deprived? ? This could mean feeling deprived in your food choices by restricting the variety of foods you eat and being "good." You can also feel deprived in other ways not directly related to food such as having to always put the needs of others first. When normal household or family responsibilities have to come first, it can leave you feeling deprived, which is a trigger to binge.

Considering food-related reasons

Even if you choose to, chances are you can't identify all the reasons you binged — at least not right away. If you have an eating plan and you're keeping a detailed food and feelings journal, you may be able to trace some of the concrete issues and emotions that may have triggered your most recent binge.

Although it's unlikely that your binge came on for one single reason, the most common nutritional triggers stem from a sense of deprivation. Restricting your food or starving yourself to offset your bingeing are often part of what brings on the relapses.

REMEMBER

Even if you're eating regular, nutritious meals and snacks now, your recovery is still a work in progress that requires flexibility and experimentation throughout the duration of your recovery and into the future. Although that may be difficult to accept, especially if you've just relapsed, you have to make adjustments to your nutrition plan as you go along to allow for the overall changes you're experiencing.

Just as foods can be seasonal, so are taste preferences. The natural shifts in your appetite and the flavors, textures, and quantities that satisfy you from season to season are one reason why making regular changes to your food plan is important. In the summertime, people eat lighter or cooler foods while in the winter we tend to want warmer, more comforting foods. In any season, there may be foods that you find triggering and that require you to adjust your meal plan in a strategic way. On the positive side, making changes to your plan allows you to feel greater personal freedom with food as your recovery progresses and lends itself to food experimentation including foods that may have been off limits in the past.

Although there are other explanations for relapse, the three most common food-based reasons for relapse binges are

✔ **You're not eating enough.** Hunger is probably the number-one physical trigger for binge eating. When you're overly hungry, it's hard to stop eating, and you may make unhealthy food choices.

When you were bingeing regularly, you may have tried to offset the binges by dieting or starving yourself. With your nutrition plan, you may not be as hungry now between meals, but it still takes time to overcome the feelings of panic, anxiety, and desperation that even a little bit of hunger may set off for you.

On the other hand, if you're regularly hungry, talk to your dietitian about increasing the amount of food in your nutrition plan. Bigger portions or additional food may counteract your impulse to binge and can keep you moving forward as you get back on track with your recovery.

✔ **You're not eating foods you enjoy.** Steering clear of your trigger foods is an important part of your recovery, but giving up trigger foods sometimes also means giving up the foods you love most.

And realistically speaking, you can't stay clear of all your favorite foods all the time. For example, if pizza is a trigger for you, and your office has Pizza Fridays, it's only so long before you feel left out and/or the aroma of pizza leads to a Friday night pizza binge.

Whatever the foods may be, you can work with your dietitian to integrate them into your food plan as part of a healthy routine. Absolutes don't work when it comes to ending binge eating, and staying away from any one food forever is almost guaranteed to complicate and slow down your recovery.

✔ **Your hormonal balance is upset.** Your hormones can get out of balance for reasons that encompass nutritional, genetic, environmental, stress-related, and menstrual causes. It's always a good idea to check in with your physician to see whether there are newly emerging potential triggers in this area.

If you've binged, let your treatment team know right away. No need to feel ashamed. It is to be expected. Make an appointment with your dietitian to rework your meal plan or come up with concrete ideas for how to deal with the urges that drove you to binge. In addition, talk with your therapist as soon as possible so you can identify what was happening in the moment, in your thoughts and/or in your world, and what thoughts, feelings, or reactions led to the binge. It's also helpful to journal about all of this so you don't have to rely on your memory in the time between the binge and when you next communicate with your team.

Ending the blame game

Part of your recovery game plan is to deal with the specifics of your regular routines and to establish healthier thinking and eating habits as part of gradual lifestyle changes. But no recovery can take into account every possible scenario, and as you progress, you'll inevitably come up against situations, people, and feelings that make you feel like bingeing.

If you relapse, it's normal to want to know whose fault it is. Your first response may be something like, "I can't believe Aunt Lisa made my favorite dessert! She knows I can't resist it!" or "It was bound to happen — things were going too well," or "It's hopeless; I'll always be a binger." You may want to blame others, and you'll probably be just as hard on yourself as you are on them. However, the sooner you can move on from the blame-fest, the more likely you are to contain the relapse and keep it from continuing.

Emerging with an emergency binge plan

After a long weekend of bingeing, on Monday morning Michelle realized that she was still at risk. While feeling confident and positive about yourself is a crucial and important part of the game plan, it's also important to not let your guard down. Michelle felt foolish now that she had binged so hard all weekend. "How could I have done that?" she kept asking herself even though she knew she had done it because she was faced with a situation that she was not expecting and that felt out of her control.

She decided to come up with an Emergency Binge Plan that included immediately going for a walk, calling her sister to talk about whatever had happened, and going to see a movie. That way, the next time a difficult situation came up, she would have something concrete to fall back

on if she couldn't rely on her new coping skills, positive self-talk, and confidence alone.

Michelle reviewed all the details of her binge with her therapist and support group. While this recent binge was similar in the amount of food and intensity as her former binges, in the past Michelle would have avoided work on Monday and kept bingeing. This time she was able to pull herself together, to go into work to learn the outcome of the layoff, and, most importantly, to call her therapist and make an appointment for Monday evening. This was her way of stopping the binge. When looking at the full picture, Michelle recognized that she had taken some very important steps forward and hadn't fallen back into all of her old bingeing habits.

The most effective ways to cope with a relapse binge without needing to lay blame include

- ✔ **Be curious, not furious.** Take time to notice the circumstances and details of your relapse. Even though you may be sad, frustrated, or angry that you've binged again, try not to judge what you've done. Instead, document the incident objectively, as if you were a scientist, so that you can figure out the who, what, when, where, and why of what happened.

- ✔ **Talk to yourself the way you would talk to a friend who came to you for help.** Chances are you wouldn't tell someone else who relapsed what an idiot she was, so don't tell yourself that either. When and if you find yourself saying harsh or judgmental things in your mind, test the words you're using. If you wouldn't say what you're saying to someone else, don't say it to yourself either. Be a gentle self-parent.

- ✔ **Turn to your support group.** Not only do you get encouragement from others in a group, but you also get practice talking to people with the same issues you have. Group members can share and remind you of useful, concrete skills that allow you to be more gentle with yourself. You should also figuratively take your group with you (unless they all actually fit in the car and have nowhere else to be) so that when you do something you wish you hadn't done, you can imagine what the group might say to you and how they might support and pick you back up.

Getting Back on Track

You can move forward, but you can't change the past. Once a binge has occurred, you might feel defeated or ashamed, but getting back on track is the healthiest option.

There are many ways to get back on track, and chances are you'll need to use several of them. Some involve adjusting your nutrition and some involve adjusting the way you live. No matter how bad the binge is or how bad it feels, remind yourself that moving forward is still the best option.

Real change is about progress, not perfection. Let us say that again: Perfection is never the object of the game; progress is. All-or-nothing thinking that demands perfection leaves you with little to work with when you can't meet that impossible standard.

You and your support system or treatment team can collaborate about what needs adjusting after a relapse. In the meantime, try the following

- ✔ Kindly and gently admit to yourself that the relapse occurred.
- ✔ Stop punishing or blaming yourself after a relapse.
- ✔ Go back to the basics and figure out what happened.
- ✔ Focus on all you've accomplished to date — not on all that you should've, would've, or could've done.
- ✔ Come up with a new plan to move forward and address what may have triggered your relapse.
- ✔ Whatever you do, don't give up. That's an old song that you've sung before, and it brings you right back to the original refrain. Don't waste the trip.

Keeping Triggers at Bay

Even though it's perfectly normal to relapse if you're in treatment for binge eating, you still want to take a proactive approach to preventing another relapse once you're back on track again.

Your current triggers probably aren't so different from the triggers that brought you to seek answers or treatment in the first place. Even though you have more emotional coping skills than you used to, be aware of the same-old, same-old situations that may push you to binge eat.

Now that you know more about the holes in your eating plan or the coping skills that still need work, it's crucial that you spend time getting yourself back into the groove. You may have to take a few steps back and create more structure for yourself so that the relapse doesn't trigger a downward spiral. You need to anticipate both old and new triggers and develop more effective strategies for dealing with them. Just remember, now is the time to protect yourself, your emotions, and your physical needs by acknowledging the reality of relapse at the same time that you strive for your best.

Saying goodbye to dieting

After a binge, your first instinct may be to restrict or diet for a few days to make up for it, but that's the absolute last thing you should do. Even though it sounds counterintuitive, dieting or swearing off any food forever eventually leads you back onto the same path that leads to bingeing. It's that inevitable pendulum swing from all to nothing, from restriction to bingeing, from bad to good, that promotes great loss and a sense of imbalance.

Dieting is one of the factors that probably started you bingeing in the first place. Although a relapse may get you down, lean on your new coping skills to avoid falling back on destructive ways of thinking.

If you developed a meal plan with a dietitian or other health professional, following it more mindfully may be a good option right now. You can keep a food journal, taking extra time to write about your feelings and emotions as well. Even plan your meals ahead, write them out and organize your kitchen accordingly. But don't cut back on what you need to be eating. Cutting back can leave you overly hungry, and hunger is a huge trigger for bingeing.

Managing day-to-day stress and anxiety

Bingeing is stressful, and a binge relapse is incredibly stressful. A relapse binge can make you feel as if the rug was pulled out from under you or that all your recovery efforts flew out the window. These types of feelings cause stress and anxiety. Both stress and anxiety are triggers, but if you find your anxiety level heightened after a relapse, remember the coping skills you gained in treatment and that we talk about in Chapter 10.

If you haven't already, now is the time to come up with some ideas on how to reduce stress. This may involve something simple like watching a movie, getting a massage, or taking a walk. At other times, it may be much more complicated, and you may need additional support from your psychotherapist or from any support groups you may attend.

One way to reduce your stress levels with regards to food is to plan ahead. Take some time to plan what you will eat for the next couple of days, then grocery shop and prepare lunches and dinners. Knowing what you will eat and having it prepared will not only reduce your stress about the food, it's also and excellent way to channel the stress you're feeling into something positive and productive for your recovery.

Planning shouldn't be its own trigger. If you over-plan or worry you are not planning the right foods, you're not contributing to your recovery. Be as gentle and balanced as possible in your approach. Lean into this as an act of self-support and comfort rather than as a have-to, so it doesn't add to your stress level instead of relieving it.

Being scared of your own success

As your recovery progresses, you may develop a brand-new trigger — fear of relapse. If you don't believe in yourself and you feel that everyone around you is just waiting for the inevitable return of your old habits, you may consciously or inadvertently set yourself up for yet another relapse.

Although it seems counterintuitive, another feeling that may crop up as you move forward is a fear of your own progress. Yes, that's right — fear of actually accomplishing the very thing you set out to do. If you're at a weight that feels more comfortable and if your binges feel more or less under control, you may worry that life is going too well and that it won't last — you're waiting for the other shoe to drop. This fear of success is more common than you think and can sabotage and jeopardize your success simply because you don't trust yourself not to go back to your old ways.

First things first: Talk to your psychotherapist, if you're working with one, in order to explore feelings of anxiety over doing so well. Together you can come up with some strategies to calm your fears and keep you on the right track. If you're not seeing a therapist one-on-one, a support group can provide essential aid as can some motivational self-talk.

An exercise to circumvent your fear of success is to ask yourself, "What will life look like if I achieve and maintain the results I've been striving for?" Then try to come up with one really good reason and remind yourself why you deserve to live in a healthy and balanced mind and body. You may notice yourself drifting to reasons that are solely your weight, shape, or size and how you look. And although your life may get easier in some ways if you lose weight and look better, for the purposes of this exercise, think about more emotionally driven reasons such as "I'm a good grandparent. I deserve to see my grandchildren grow up and have the ability to play with them," or "It's okay to achieve success. After all, I've done so in other areas of my life. Why not here too?" or "I don't need food or a larger body to protect me. I can count on myself. After all, I've taken care of others. Why not take care of me?"

Sleeping better and feeling better

Sleep forms the foundation of good mental and physical health and is a critical part of putting an end to bingeing.

If you're chronically sleep deprived, it can be hard to tell the difference between thirst, hunger, and fatigue. You may think you're hungry when what you really need is an extra hour or two of sleep every night.

That's because your body rebuilds and heals itself while you sleep, and if you don't sleep enough, your metabolism slows down and your hormonal cycles are disrupted, leaving your body completely out of balance. Sleep deprivation can contribute to some devastating long-term effects on your health including

- ✔ Cardiovascular disease and hypertension
- ✔ Diabetes and impaired glucose tolerance
- ✔ Hormonal shifts resulting in poor functioning of many organ systems
- ✔ Neurological and psychiatric disorders
- ✔ Endocrine imbalances
- ✔ Obesity in adults and children

A common cause for poor sleep, especially in people with obesity, is *obstructive sleep apnea,* or *(OSA),* a condition in which something — usually the tonsils — obstructs the breathing airway during sleep. Often characterized by loud snoring, OSA causes the brain to receive less oxygen at night leading to a slower metabolism, daytime fatigue, weight gain, and mood disorders. Consult your physician if you think you may have sleep apnea. If you do, getting it treated can make a world of difference in how you feel and how you eat.

Of course, getting adequate sleep not only helps the body, but it's also essential to a healthy mind. If you've gone without sleep for any period of time, you already know that not sleeping enough, particularly over a period of months and years, results in mood shifts, fuzzy thinking, poor decision making, and memory problems just to name a few problems. If you suffer from anxiety, depression, ADHD, or any mood disorder, sleep deprivation worsens these and makes the symptoms more difficult to regulate and manage.

Making sleeping well a habit

Going to sleep seems so easy, but the truth is that, just as you need to work to develop better eating habits, sleeping well requires planning and preparation. Having a routine and sticking to it over time helps you feel more relaxed and sleep longer and more deeply.

Most people need between seven and nine hours of sleep per day, but many sleep less than this and suffer the consequences. If you feel that you need to sleep more and sleep better, consider these suggestions for creating a more peaceful environment for rest:

✔ Go to bed and wake up at the same time every day. You may need to set an alarm in the morning until your body gets used to your new wake-up time.

✔ Make sure your room is quiet, dark, and that the temperature is comfortable — not too hot or too cold.

✔ Use your bed only for sleeping. Plan to watch TV, listen to music, eat, or do other activities in other areas of the house.

✔ Keep your bedroom free from electronics. Studies show that using backlit devices such as televisions, e-readers, cellphones, and other electronics within an hour before bedtime make it difficult to fall asleep.

✔ Avoid large meals, caffeine, or alcohol within a few hours of bedtime.

If you're still having trouble falling asleep, try these techniques for relaxing before bed:

✔ Take a warm bath an hour before bedtime.

✔ Plan to meditate (or use any relaxation technique that works for you) for ten minutes before you climb into bed.

✔ Exercise regularly (just not within three hours before you go to bed).

✔ Use sleep rituals to help you feel tired.

✔ Have a warm cup of caffeine-free herbal tea.

If you've relapsed, take another look at your sleeping habits and make a plan to get the amount of sleep your body requires in the weeks and months ahead. Getting enough rest is a key ingredient to your recovery but one of the first things you might give up when you get busy or feel overwhelmed. Take time to rest enough every day, and you'll ensure that you have the physical and emotional resources to keep moving forward.

Part IV

How BED Affects Special Populations and Biological Systems

Five Surprising Groups Affected by BED

- **Men:** In contrast to anorexia nervosa and bulimia nervosa, which afflict primarily young women, the incidence of binge eating disorder (BED) in men continues to rise.

- **Children:** Children, especially young girls, may fall prey to societal, parental, or peer pressure to look or behave a certain way. Binge eating may develop as a response. Many adult binge eaters remember their first binge occurring when they were youngsters.

- **Menopausal women:** With changes in hormones come changes in metabolism. Many women develop a different relationship to food and weight during their menopausal years and may develop BED.

- **The elderly:** Aging can produce unexpected physical and mental changes. Coping with the changes may trigger a variety of disorders, including BED.

- **People of normal weight:** Although many BED sufferers are overweight, you can maintain a normal weight and still be a victim of BED. In fact, the compensatory behaviors needed to maintain a normal weight can make recovery from BED even more difficult — but never impossible.

Visit www.dummies.com/extras/overcomingbingeeating for resources on a range of BED-related topics.

In this part . . .

✔ Realize that the incidence of binge eating disorder (BED) in men has been increasing steadily. Men face unique challenges in overcoming BED, not least of which is that they're often encouraged to overeat.

✔ Understand that even children can use food to self-soothe in response to pressures they're not equipped to cope with in healthier ways.

✔ Consider that women going through menopause can develop a different relationship to food, which may lead to BED.

✔ Recognize that BED and obesity often go hand in hand. To overcome BED, you may need to deal with the problems and symptoms of obesity as well.

✔ Recognize that the endocrine system plays a large role in regulating how you process food. Getting a handle on what you can do to help your endocrine system function well can aid your recovery from BED.

Chapter 16

Men Who Binge

Although most sufferers of eating disorders such as anorexia and bulimia are women, binge eating affects almost as many men as women. About 40 percent of people with binge eating disorder or who compulsively over-eat are men, and the numbers are growing. Whether or not more men suffer from binge eating than before is unknown, but the fact is that more men are coming forward to seek treatment.

It makes sense that bingeing is rising for both genders given the American food supply. As a society, we have easy access to tasty, convenient, and often low-cost food that may not be nutritious. In Chapter 9, we talk about how food triggers the pleasure center in the brain, especially high fat and sugary foods. A man's brain is just as responsive to food pleasure as a woman's.

For years, the eating disorder treatment community tended to focus on women because it seemed that they were more affected by body image concerns, trends, and fashion. But men also suffer from obsessive thinking about how they look as well as from the tendency to use food as a vehicle for self- soothing when suffering from stress and trauma. Although men often are socialized to be more stoic and hide their emotions, keeping a stiff upper lip in the face of life's ups and downs can lead to physical and emotional problems —for men and women.

Although binge eating can show up at any time in a man's life, most men tend to start bingeing later than women — usually in their mid-30s and beyond. It's then that the multiple stresses of young families, increasing work responsibilities, aging parents, and other pressures pile up. To make matters even more complicated, natural changes in men's metabolism and activity levels may also add to their changes in body size. Like women, men with poor coping skills can find themselves turning to food to deal with their stress, anxiety, and depression.

In this chapter, we talk about men who binge and why, and we get to the bottom of what men and women who binge have in common as well as what's different about the two. We'll also talk about the most effective treatment for men and how you can get the help you need.

The Rising Tide of Men Who Binge

In the past, because fewer men showed up in treatment programs, people assumed their absence meant that bingeing was less of a problem for them. Not true. Instead, if you're a man who binge eats, you may have trouble seeking help because eating disorders are often still considered to be a woman's problem.

For binge eaters, that couldn't be farther from the truth. Unlike other eating disorders, binge eating is almost as common in men as it is in women, and the available research to date proves it. Perceptions of what a binge eater looks like are changing, and if you haven't found treatment yet that's a good fit, the likelihood that you can and will is higher than ever before.

Men with eating disorders aren't so different from women with eating disorders, and both may

- Be overachievers and perfectionists
- Be eager to please others
- Suffer from psychological conditions such as anxiety disorder, obsessive-compulsive disorder, depression, or ADHD, among others
- Abuse drugs or alcohol or have other addictive tendencies
- Have self-esteem issues related to abuse or trauma

If you recognize yourself in the list above, you may be relieved to know that you've come to the right place after not understanding and not knowing what to do about your binges before this. And even if none of the characteristics above rings true for you, it doesn't mean you're not a binge eater. People of all shapes and sizes and all walks of life binge eat, and just because you may not fit into the neat, but general, categories doesn't mean you can't benefit from taking time to figure out what's going on with your life and with your eating.

Comparing Men and Women Who Binge

The reasons men and women binge aren't that different from one another, but the world has historically ignored overweight or obese men while focusing a great deal of attention and disapproval on overweight or obese women who seem as if they might overeat. For men, the standards have always been somewhat different, and the sense that you may be able to get away with eating to excess may be part of what's sabotaged you all these years.

A number of cultural norms sometimes make it okay for men to binge or to be obese:

✓ In Western cultures, and elsewhere, it's more culturally acceptable for a man to be overweight or obese than it is for a woman. Even though some communities of men (athletes, gay men, and others) place great importance on weight and body image, the vast majority of men don't necessarily experience the same level of social pressure about their physique that women do.

✓ Men are often praised when they finish a big meal, and to a degree, eating large amounts of food may be considered masculine.

One powerful example is *Man v. Food*, a popular television show, which follows a man literally eating his way across the United States. He goes to restaurants known for serving huge portions and challenges himself (or another man) to eat the entire meal. In each episode, the host explores big-food offerings from different cities before facing off against a pre-existing eating challenge at a local restaurant. If you've ever seen the show, a bunch of onlookers cheer on the host as he eats vast amounts of food that would qualify as a binge in most cases.

Even if you know that your bingeing is out of control, the fact that no one else has noticed or seems to feel you need help may allow you to pretend that you don't really have a problem. Just because you have no diagnosis and others haven't acknowledged your binge eating doesn't mean that all is okay. If you've had a health scare or you've just reached a point when enough is enough, there are treatment programs for you.

As you move forward toward change and recovery, remember that binge eating isn't really about food. It's about using food as a way to soothe yourself when you don't have sufficient coping skills to deal with day-to-day stress or traumatic events from the past or present.

If you've been bingeing for some time now, you might have been able to convince yourself that it's normal, that it's just about being hungry and not about anything else. Both men and women who binge eat tend to be out of touch with the triggers that drive them to binge, but some male binge eaters find that they have a more difficult time than their female counterparts when it comes to understanding the relationship between food and feelings. That's because

- ✔ Men tend to be less connected with the emotions driving a binge and more focused on the food itself.

- ✔ In general, men may have a harder time acknowledging emotional or psychological problems, although this is certainly not true for all.

The unfortunate result is that men are far less likely than women to seek treatment for binge eating. And what's even worse is that by being out of the treatment loop, men may be missing out on participating in the studies that may help researchers figure out how to treat them in the most helpful and effective ways.

Whether you're in treatment now or just thinking about it, some of the battles you'll face will be different, but the techniques and coping skills you'll learn either in support groups or in direct treatment are universal to both men and women. The work you do in therapy and/or with a dietitian and/or support group is personalized and tailored to your situation and your challenges.

Understanding the Reasons Men Binge

The reasons that men binge are as varied and complex as men themselves. Just as there's no one reason or set of reasons that women binge, no one set of circumstances bring on binge eating for men.

What experts know is that although binge eating generally begins for women in their teens and twenties, for men, bingeing typically begins almost a decade later although certainly many men began bingeing as children. For many reasons, anxiety and stress tend to build for a longer time in some men, but the result is pretty much the same for men and women who don't have adequate coping skills in place. When the going gets tough, some turn to alcohol and drugs, some to work, and some turn to eating as a way to numb the pressure they feel.

One of the other theories you may hear is that men have begun to feel the kind of inadequacy about their bodies that women have been dealing with for years. Depending on how old you are, you may not feel as if you need to conform to unattainable ideals about the male body. But if you're in your 20s or 30s or perhaps even younger, you may feel more pressure than your father and grandfather did to have a perfect body. Although it's difficult to know for sure, the increased focus on body shape, size, and physical appearance may have contributed to the rise of eating disorders in men.

Fortunately, if you're interested in seeking help, the actual experience of binge eating is pretty similar in both men and women, which means that the same treatments that work for women can work for you.

In Chapter 3 and throughout this book, we discuss some of the reasons anyone might binge, but in the following list, we talk about those reasons as well as causes specific to men:

- **Biological reasons due to aging:** After age 30, men begin to experience a gradual decline in testosterone and other hormones, leaving some not only with a decrease in sex drive but also with less energy and reduced muscle tone along with the threat of more serious conditions such as heart disease, high blood pressure, diabetes, and depression among others. Although the change is gradual for most men, you may notice a dip over time, and that dip could lead you to overeat for more energy and to try to feel better.

- **Boredom:** Maybe you binge because there's nothing better to do. In many cases, overeating because you're bored slowly grows and morphs into bingeing. Eating is a visceral, sensory activity that charges up the senses, which is why it can sometimes be seen as a form of entertainment and activity in and of itself. It's also a favorite pastime when watching sporting events. Again, this is not exclusive to men, just more frequent.

- **Numbing feelings:** Whether you're a man or a woman, everyone faces negative emotions such as sadness, anger, and frustration, among others. If you don't know what to do with those feelings or how to channel them into healthy, constructive behaviors, you can very easily end up bingeing as a way to avoid dealing with discomfort.

✔ **Quitting another addiction:** If you're trying to give up another addiction, you may very easily find yourself turning to food for comfort and as a substitute for smoking, gambling, alcohol, or other addictive substances or behaviors. Many people battling addiction feel the need to keep their hands and mouths busy, so at first, eating may seem like an easy and harmless way to keep yourself distracted from whatever you're trying to quit. Unfortunately, in the long run, binge eating may become its own addiction and something you'll have to work just as hard to overcome.

✔ **Abuse in many forms:** Although the number of men with eating disorders who have suffered some form of abuse isn't often reported, studies show that up to 40 percent of women with eating disorders report having suffered some sort of abuse, be it physical, verbal, emotional, and/or sexual. Some studies put the number as high as 50 percent. It makes sense that if you were harmed in some way, you may have turned to food to dull the pain and shame of that abuse and/or to regain a sense of control.

✔ **Sleep issues:** Increasing occupational responsibilities or financial worries and their accompanying stress may keep you from sleeping well. Additionally, biological conditions such as sleep apnea can interfere with quality sleep As we discuss in Chapter 15 and throughout the book, sleep is critical for physical and emotional health. Being chronically sleep deprived not only puts you at risk for heart disease and high blood pressure among other serious conditions, it's also a significant risk factor for obesity. Whatever the reason you suffer from insomnia, getting a handle on your sleep issues is a key part of your recovery.

✔ **Stress and anxiety:** Whether it's due to stress such as a demanding boss or anxiety over a relationship, when life becomes stressful, both men and women eat to calm their frustration. Eating may give you a sense of control and power when the rest of your life seems out of your hands. In addition, the sensory experience of tasting food and the comfort of a full stomach may distract you from the problems facing you.

✔ **Life trauma:** It's difficult, if not impossible, to find a blanket definition for trauma, but any event in your life that produces upheaval, sadness, depression, or feelings of despair can qualify as one. Some examples include the death of a loved one, a move, a job loss, a change of school, abuse, divorce, and many, many other potentially traumatic incidents.

This is just a small sample of some of the triggers, both emotional and physical, that may contribute to binge eating. Your triggers may be some combination of these factors plus others. Every binge eater is a little different, and as you move forward in your journey, you can discover more about why you began bingeing in the first place and what you can do to slow and eventually stop the binges.

Getting Help That's the Right Fit

If you're thinking about getting help for binge eating or you're already in treatment, you may have a pretty clear idea of what you want and what you think might work best for you. Many men prefer a time-limited, task-oriented, and solutions-based approach to slowing down and eventually stopping their binges. You can create a program that takes a behavioral approach and gives you concrete strategies for changing your habits and your nutrition. While knowing that such strategies exist is useful and true for women as well, the statistics tend to show that many men prefer this approach to something more process-oriented or, shall we say, "touchy-feely" in nature.

Unfortunately, looking only at the behaviors themselves and ignoring the underlying causes of binge eating often does not work well over time. Most binge eating comes about for complicated, deep-seated emotional reasons, and without addressing those causes, you may find your results more short-lived or harder to achieve. Although you may not feel comfortable at the start talking about your feelings and the experiences that led you to seek help, hopefully you can find a way to include the psychotherapy you need in your game plan.

Finding the right psychological support

Ultimately, the most effective therapeutic experience for men and women may be very similar. As we discuss in Chapter 10, it takes time and patience to find the right therapist, but doing your homework at the beginning and finding someone who's a good fit saves you time and money over the course of your treatment and can be one way to improve your experience in therapy.

One thing we hear again and again is that some men say that they prefer a male psychotherapist, but that in and of itself may be an idea you should examine. If your preference is that strong, the reason is probably worth bringing up in therapy.

Find a therapist that's a good fit regardless of gender, but when it comes time to find a support group, it may be a good idea to look for one that has other men or is focused exclusively on supporting men recovering from disordered eating.

Establishing appropriate nutritional support

You may not have ever considered going to a dietitian before starting treatment for binge eating, but learning about nutrition and collaborating on a solid food plan is an important part of your recovery.

In general, meal planning and nutrition counseling for men tends to be more structured than for women. Men typically do better with more guidelines, specific foods, and a tightly organized plan for what they're going to eat. However, as we've said many times, everyone is different, and for some people, highly structured meal planning feels confining and controlling, two emotions that you may want to avoid if you're trying to break out of the dieting-losing weight-bingeing cycle so common for binge eaters.

In Chapter 12, we provide a sample meal plan geared toward women, and in Table 16-1 we provide an example for an average man based on typically greater caloric requirements, larger body size, and overall metabolism.

Table 16-1	Sample Meal Plan for Men	
Meal & Time	*Meal Plan & Ingredients*	*Preparation*
Breakfast 7:30 a.m.	Breakfast sandwich 2 slices whole-wheat bread 1 egg and 2 egg whites Cheese stick Pear	Scramble one egg and two egg whites in a non-stick skillet. Shred the cheese stick and let it melt on the toasted bread. Add the eggs and assemble the sandwich. Eat the pear on the side.
Lunch 1 p.m.	Turkey chili over baked potato Side salad with low-fat balsamic dressing served on the side.	Order from the diner at noon for 1 p.m. delivery.
Snack 3:00 p.m.	Yogurt, banana, and nuts	Slice or dip the banana in the yogurt. Eat the nuts on the side.
Dinner 7 p.m.	8-ounce chicken breast ½ cup couscous 2 cups broccoli Ear of corn	Preheat the over to 325 degrees. Season the chicken with 1 teaspoon olive oil and the seasonings of your choice. Bake the chicken for 20 to 30 minutes, turning once. Cook the couscous per package directions. Husk the corn and place it in a pot of boiling water for 5 to 7 minutes. Steam the broccoli for 4 to 6 minutes.

Other things to think about include

- Men, even men who are severe bingers and need to lose weight, still need to eat more than women. This is based on muscle mass, bone structure, and overall metabolism. You and your dietitian can work together to make sure your meal plan has enough food so as not to trigger a binge because of hunger.

- Nutrition is action-oriented, and meal planning supplies a great deal of structure, which typically appeals to men and tends to work faster for men than for women. If structure appeals to you, consider working on this sooner rather than later to jump-start your success.

- Whether or not you've been diagnosed with binge eating disorder, if you struggle with binge eating or emotional eating, you can benefit from treatment and from the ideas and techniques in this book.

- Concrete strategies can work well if you're working from a clear overall plan that takes preferences and cooking abilities into account. Men tend to be less open with their feelings than women are, but recording feelings and logging emotions is a critical strategy for binge eaters of both genders.

- Feelings and emotions can be logged (or even just noted) in another journal or later in the process of meal planning. Men tend to be more comfortable with a meal plan and food journal that doesn't include feelings and emotions at first. After you master your meal plan, logging your feelings may be easier to accomplish.

Chapter 17

Children and Bingeing

Canada, the United States, and the United Kingdom are currently suffering from an epidemic of childhood obesity that seems to be getting worse each year. According to the U. S. Centers for Disease Control and Prevention, childhood obesity has more than tripled during the past 30 years. In 1980, 7 percent of children 6 to 11 years old and 5 percent of adolescents 12 to 19 years old were considered obese. In 2008, those numbers had ballooned to 20 percent and 18 percent, respectively. Canadian and UK statistics are similar. In 2007, the Canadian Community Health Survey found that 29 percent of adolescents had unhealthy weights and reported that if current childhood obesity trends continue, by 2040 up to 70 percent of adults aged 40 years will be either overweight or obese. Statistics from a large-scale survey in the United Kingdom shockingly reveal that 25 percent of boys, and 33 percent of girls between 2 and 19 years old are overweight or obese — and there's little sign the incidence is slowing.

Whether childhood obesity can be attributed to actual binge eating is highly debatable. Children overeat for many reasons, and most don't have the means or the access to food to take in the excessive calories that would qualify as a binge. However, childhood obesity definitely can be considered a gateway to binge eating disorder in adulthood, and the earlier you intervene, the better the chance a child has to diminish the behaviors and negative emotions that might result in an eating disorder later in life.

The role of family and support networks in addressing childhood obesity and binge eating is critical. Because children are raised in a family setting, however family is defined, no treatment for a child can be effective without treating the whole family. Helping a child can be an opportunity, however challenging, to make changes that result in significant, long-lasting improvement for children and adults alike within the family.

In this chapter, we talk about the relationship between obesity and overeating in children. We also discuss the complex interplay between nature and nurture when it comes to overeating. Finally, we take a hard look at the teen years, when young people's bodies and emotions are constantly shifting and they become more vulnerable to eating disorders.

A Rising Tide: Kids and Binge Eating

For many reasons, more children across the developed world over the past 20 to 30 years have become overweight or obese. The constant availability and strategic marketing of processed, high-calorie foods make it desirable, easy, and convenient to overeat, often without even realizing it. For children growing up in a world with abundant and available junk food, it can be second nature to eat too much, and as they mature, these habits become more and more difficult to break.

For obese children, genetic factors and little-to-no physical activity can make the problems of poor nutrition worse. Imagine a kid who eats high-calorie, high-sugar, high-fat foods all day long and then spends hours watching television, playing video games, and/or on the computer instead of going out to play as kids did more regularly just a generation ago. Even if a child were extremely active, offsetting the effects of an unhealthy diet is difficult, but inactivity makes it much more likely that a child becomes overweight or obese.

Because obesity and overeating are intimately related, it's likely that overweight children are also bingeing even if they are doing so in a limited way. Although current research shows that the percentage of children and adolescents who meet criteria for full BED is very low, studies show that up to 40 percent of overweight children exhibit some BED symptoms. Also, many binge eaters of all ages report that their condition started in childhood.

Beyond the long-term risk of becoming a binge eater later in life, childhood obesity poses immediate risks for most kids. The most common problems are type 2 diabetes and heart disease, both of which are being diagnosed at younger and younger ages. Common health effects of obesity in children include

- ✔ **Heart disease:** Even though cardiovascular or heart disease has always been thought of as an adult problem, in a study of obese 5- to 17-year-olds, 70 percent suffered from at least one risk factor for heart disease such as high cholesterol or high blood pressure.

- ✔ **Diabetes:** Before a diagnosis of type 2 diabetes comes pre-diabetes, which is of great concern because blood glucose levels are higher than normal but not quite high enough to be full-blown diabetes. Nearly one in four obese adolescents has pre-diabetes or diabetes itself.

- ✔ **Joint problems:** Obesity puts great strain on a growing body, and overweight and obese children and adolescents often face bone and joint problems earlier than their peers. This also sets them up for early onset arthritis.

- ✔ **Sleep problems:** Like their adult counterparts, obese children can suffer from sleep problems including sleep apnea, a disorder in which pauses in breathing and shallow breaths can cause sleep disruptions. Not sleeping well then sets off a cascade of other problems including inability to focus, poor memory, little to no motivation for physical activity, and excessive fatigue to name a few.

- ✔ **Psychological problems:** Other children, and unfortunately some adults, can be cruel, and obese children suffer from significant social and psychological problems due to teasing, bullying, and low self-esteem.

In the long run, obesity affects a child's health in other devastating ways:

- ✔ If you're obese as a child, you're likely to become an obese adult with all the health concerns that brings. Even before adulthood, an obese child is at risk for heart disease, diabetes, stroke, several types of cancer, and osteoarthritis.

- ✔ Overweight and obesity are associated with increased risk for many types of cancer, including cancer of the breast, colon, endometrium, esophagus, kidney, pancreas, gall bladder, thyroid, ovary, cervix, and prostate, as well as multiple myeloma and Hodgkin's lymphoma.

Looking at communities at risk

Statistics show stark differences in obesity rates among medium-to-high-income communities and low-income ones. Although studies are still ongoing, early data suggests that the obesity rate in children living below the poverty line may be almost double that of those living in middle-class communities.

Although the exact reasons for financial instability vary from family to family and are incredibly complex, children in these families face food insecurity on a daily basis, which may be one reason among many that parents with fewer resources choose high-calorie, low-nutrient foods for their kids. In general, highly processed foods that are high in calories and fat are cheaper than fresh foods and require less preparation. Both cost and preparation are often major obstacles for families with limited financial resources. The time required to prepare food may also be limited because of the need for parents to spend more time outside the home working.

Another consideration is that low-income families often have less access to fresher, more nutritious foods depending on the availability of public transportation and whether or not a neighborhood has a full-service supermarket. For example, a large bowl of pasta is a very cost-effective and filling meal for a financially struggling family whereas meat, potato, and fresh vegetables is a more well balanced, but more expensive and difficult to prepare, dinner.

Because poorer children typically become obese at higher rates than kids of greater means, some government initiatives have been put in place to attempt to address the problem. Many school districts have stepped in to provide healthier meals for children who may not be eating well or at all at home. Legislators and school boards have also begun eliminating vending machines in schools and have put nutritional standards in place with an eye toward instilling healthier eating habits in students. Some communities also make efforts to offer nutritious versions of the local culture's most common foods so that these foods may be sought out and obtained outside of school when possible. These initiatives are ongoing and represent one approach to closing the nutritional gap that exists within the income gap.

Examining the role of dieting

Ironically, one of the factors at play in the development of eating disorders in children is early dieting. One of the most common behaviors leading to eating disorders is dieting, so it's alarming that, according to *Time* magazine, almost 80 percent of children in the United States have been on a diet by the time they've reached the fourth grade — whether they want to be or not.

A sense of deprivation, both emotionally and physically, is one of the main risk factors for binge eating and can be a significant trigger for binges. A child who gets on the dieting-bingeing-weight gain cycle early in life will have greater difficulty transitioning to healthier eating habits and use of consistent and appropriate coping skills to deal with negative emotions or situations as she gets older.

Dieting as a way of life takes an unfair toll on children as they grow up, both physically, due to inadequate nutrition, and emotionally because of the sadness of not being good enough just as they are. Rather than figuring out how to deal with the expected fluctuations in their sizes and shapes during childhood, adolescence, and adulthood, they instead assimilate persistent and unrealistic messages about the way they look and what it means about who they are.

Consider the following statistics based on surveys of adolescent and pre-adolescent children:

- 81 percent of 10-year-olds report that they're afraid of being fat. Fifty-one percent of 9- and 10-year-old girls feel better about themselves if they're on a diet.

- 42 percent of girls in first, second, and third grade say they want to be thinner.

- 46 percent of 9- to 11-year-olds are "sometimes" or "very often" on diets, and 82 percent of their families are "sometimes" or "very often" on diets.

Although it's not accurate to blame dieting for all eating disorders, you don't do your children any favors by creating or tolerating an environment in which dieting and weight loss is a preoccupation from early childhood. If you're an adult reading this book, you know that people come in all shapes and sizes, and that it can be difficult to be kind to yourself if your body changes in ways you don't like with age and life experience.

You can't shield your child forever from the world as it is with its obsession with youth and beauty, but you can do yourself and your children a great service building their self-esteem, teaching them to make healthy choices, and showing them how to accept themselves and to be gentle with themselves and their own physical and emotional health from a young age.

Supporting your child's appetite for self-esteem

As children grow up, they mimic what they perceive to be their parents' positive and negative self-perceptions. Although self-esteem is far more than just your attitude toward food and body, parents' attitudes toward their own bodies and eating habits, as well as those of their children, can have an impact on how a child feels about herself. If you're a parent, you can do a lot to foster and encourage a healthy attitude about health and self-worth in your children:

✔ Avoid negative and judgmental comments about the appearance of others.

✔ Don't compare your child to anyone else, especially siblings.

✔ Encourage your child to make his own healthy food choices. Don't force him to eat or not eat something.

✔ No one needs to be a member of the clean plate club. Its alumnae are miserable.

✔ Avoid negative comments about your own body or frequent mention of needing to go on a diet yourself.

Uncovering Genetic Risk Factors

If you're a binge eater yourself, you may already suspect that heredity plays a role in your eating disorder. Notice we didn't say it is a cause, but rather a possible contributing factor. Studies currently underway, along with conventional wisdom, suggest that both obesity and binge eating may come about due to a complex mix of genetic vulnerabilities and environmental factors that's not yet fully understood.

Even though new studies are ongoing, there's already convincing evidence that binge eating often includes a significant genetic component. One popular theory is that evolution is working against us now that we live in a world with plentiful and available food. The genes that helped us to survive during times when food was scarce now work against us when it comes to storing and using fat and calories. Think of it this way: The human body is designed for survival, meaning our genes are really good at conserving fat cells, not burning them. When food was not readily available this function was an evolutionary advantage that helped humans survive. However, in our current food climate, the body's ability to easily conserve fat is no longer an advantage.

Other studies seek to understand the links between inherited traits and specific physiological issues related to obesity and binge eating. Some of the current research focuses on

- ✔ The drive to overeat for both physical and emotional reasons
- ✔ The human body's diminished ability to use fat as fuel
- ✔ The body's ability to easily store increasing amounts of body fat
- ✔ The possibility of turning white fat into energy-burning brown fat. White fat is the less metabolically active of the two.

On the one hand, you may feel relieved knowing that something you have no control over is at work behind the scenes. But you may also feel discouraged if you've been trying to help yourself or your child overcome obesity.

Keep in mind that genetics is not destiny. As many scientists and therapists observe, "Genetics loads the gun, but environment pulls the trigger." Your family history means only that you have a greater chance of being affected. No matter what your genetic background, you and your children can still change some of the environmental factors and certainly affect the learned behaviors that play a major role in binge eating.

Looking for signs of binge eating

The relationship between obesity and binge eating takes on even more complexity when you talk about it in connection to children. Not all obese children binge nor do all children who binge become obese.

Although it's rare for children to receive a diagnosis of binge eating disorder, that may not mean that your child isn't bingeing at all.

Binge eating in children generally resembles binge eating in adults in the most important ways. However, because children rarely have the time, money, or access to food that would allow them to binge like adults, one of the most important qualities of childhood binge eating is a sense of loss of control regardless of exactly how much food is eaten.

Even though binge eating in children is different, *bingeing* is defined as eating much larger amounts of food than would normally be consumed within a distinct period of time (usually less than two hours). Eating binges occur at least twice a week for at least several months and may occur as often as several times a day.

If you're reading this chapter, you may be asking yourself, "How can I tell whether **my child is bingeing?**" Some of the signs and symptoms you may notice include

- Fast eating of excessive amounts of food in a short period of time. If you're not sure what's excessive, it's a good idea to check in with your child's pediatrician so as not to jump to conclusions.

- Secretive eating.

- Hiding or hoarding food. Food frequently disappearing from the kitchen or food hidden in another room such as a bedroom. This one gets complicated when multiple people live under the same roof.

- Eating a lot even when not hungry.

- Peculiar eating habits or food rituals.

- Anxiety when not eating, which is calmed when given food.

- Feelings of dissatisfaction with themselves and their bodies.

- Depression and/or sadness, especially when in combination with other symptoms or behaviors.

- Preoccupation with food, weight, and body shape — always asking about the next meal or what there is to eat. Constantly expressing the desire to lose weight, or being hypercritical of both her shape and of others' bodies.

- Significant weight gain in a short period of time not related to a growth spurt. Once again, it's a good idea to check in with your pediatrician to evaluate this.

If your child is overweight, obese, and/or bingeing, your first priority is a trip to the pediatrician. A good physician can put any problems in context and educate you and your family about what's normal and developmentally appropriate for your child and which concerns may need to be addressed immediately.

Bingeing by Example

You teach what you know, and even parents with the best intentions can unwittingly pass on negative perceptions and behaviors regarding food to their children. The good news is that by learning about and recognizing the habits and beliefs you hope to change in yourself, you can make an enormous difference in the life of your child.

The family that binges together

You may never have considered that anything out of the ordinary is going on in your family especially if overweight is the norm, but perhaps something or someone called attention to the fact that your son or daughter has been having trouble, and you can't help but wonder whether it has something to do with overeating and the effects of doing so.

Often a family's idea of what's a normal amount of food is skewed. This makes it even harder to break the bingeing cycle for a child because the entire family has no clue that they're all bingeing.

If Mom and Dad are bingers or simply have big appetites and aren't aware of how much food is appropriate for a child, they may serve their children adult-size portions. It's not unusual for a parent to serve the same amount of food to her 8-year-old, her 12-year-old, and to herself.

Just remember these food facts:

✔ Kids aged 5 to 12 need an appropriate amount of food and calories based on their body weight, but the amount rarely totals more (or even the same) amount that an adult needs.

✔ If you're serving your young child the amount that you eat as an adult, you may be unintentionally teaching him how to binge by setting him up to think he needs much more food than he actually does. Instead, teach him to recognize and follow appropriate hunger and satiety cues. (We talk about recognizing these cues in Chapter 12.)

Breaking the cycle

There's nothing more difficult than seeing your child struggle, especially if you know the pain and suffering she's dealing with firsthand. You may be scared by the possibility that your child's overeating could spiral out of control. You may be angry at your child or at yourself. You may be ashamed because you think your own habits played a role in what's happening with your child.

Even if you've never had a diagnosed eating disorder yourself and are perplexed by what's happening with your child's eating patterns, how you talk about food and the food you make available in your home are key factors to breaking this cycle.

No matter where you, your children, and your entire family are in this process, you can find ways to break the patterns of behavior that may have contributed to either obesity, binge eating, or both.

Ways to promote some healthier choices and eating habits include:

✔ **Eating dinner together as a family.** Studies show that families that eat dinner together are slimmer and healthier overall. In addition, children of families that eat together with regularity tend to be much less engaged in addictive, rebellious, or harmful behaviors. Even if you can't eat dinner together every night, just a few days per week can make a difference.

✔ **Serving meals buffet style, not family style.** Leave food on the stove, and if someone wants more, have them go get it. Bringing all the food to the table makes it too easy to eat seconds or thirds and harder to pause properly to assess your fullness or hunger cues. If you portion meals in the kitchen and allow time for the meal to settle after you and your child have finished eating, you'll both eat a lot less than if the bowl is six inches in front of you on the dinner table.

✔ **Prohibiting eating in front of the television.** Eating in front of any electronic media promotes mindless eating. It's a surefire path to overeating and to losing touch with fullness cues. A Friday dinner-with-a-movie night is fine as long as you do it infrequently.

✔ **Shopping and preparing meals together.** Even if you can't make a full homemade dinner, the more the entire family is involved in the meal process, the better. Set the table together, create a grocery list, ask your child to choose or even make certain parts of the meal. For example, ask, "Would you rather have chicken or fish? Broccoli or cauliflower?" Including your child in these basic aspects of meal planning and preparation gives her control and teaches her to make healthy choices. Because bingeing often serves as a way to cope with feeling out of control, having the final say or a sense of control over food choices can translate into more positive coping mechanisms overall.

✔ **Not buying junk food.** Everyone enjoys snack foods now and then, and eating them occasionally is fine. However, convenience foods shouldn't be a daily routine for anyone, especially for a child who struggles with overeating. Having junk food in the house is a set-up. Better to not purchase the food and to plan ahead for special times when a dessert is appropriate.

You don't have to make all your changes right away. Try picking two and really stick with them for the next couple of weeks.

Facing Adolescence and the Teenage Years

It's not easy growing up, but for adolescents and teens struggling with binge eating, overweight, and obesity, life can be particularly tough. Relentless teasing and feelings of isolation often drive the stress, anxiety, depression, and other negative emotions that may lead to emotional or binge eating.

Binge eating is a mixed-up way of dealing with or avoiding difficult emotions. Teens who binge eat aren't necessarily aware of what's driving them to overeat. This is especially true for adolescents and teens who are already struggling to get to know themselves and who generally lack the insight and maturity level needed to understand such a complicated process.

On top of their own complex, but developmentally appropriate emotions, adolescent and teenage girls are especially susceptible to the media's non-stop emphasis on body image and dieting. Studies show that at least half or more of teenage girls are on or have been on more than one diet. Often these diets are extreme in nature or set up unrealistic expectations. And at their worst, restrictive diets can be a significant trigger for all forms of serious eating disorders.

Dealing with shifting hormones

As every adult knows, the teenage years can be a rather stressful time. No matter how much their parents have told them or how many books they've read, many teens don't really understand or aren't comfortable with the changes happening to their bodies and in their lives. The feeling of being out of control coupled with low self-esteem and isolation can lead to all sorts of negative behaviors, including binge eating.

The hormonal changes that happen during puberty are one of the greatest biological shifts in the human life cycle. Hormones change a teenager's appearance and behavior while also adding intensity to physical and sexual desires. Although they may have more drive to experience sex, many teens still have one foot in the world of childhood feelings and behaviors. In general, teens are self-conscious, vulnerable to comments from others, and desperate to be different and individual — since everyone else is too! They're prone to anxiety and fear about themselves and their futures. Their emotions can swing unpredictably from one extreme to another.

Unfortunately, the hormonal imbalance that occurs as teens mature can lead to depression, anxiety, headaches, and other problems, all of which increase the urge to binge and decrease the emotional strength to reason and fight the urges. And new studies suggest that these changes occur much earlier than previously believed.

Another area of rising concern is diagnosable hormone imbalances in teens such as hypothyroidism, polycystic ovary syndrome (PCOS), and premenstrual syndrome (PMS), which are becoming increasingly common due to changes in diet and other environmental factors. Hormone imbalance has previously been thought of as something that usually affects older women in their forties and fifties. Today, more teenage girls show signs of these imbalances. Possible reasons for the increase include the fact that overall food intake can greatly affect hormone levels. Teens who eat a lot of processed foods with artificial flavors and colors are more at risk of hormonal imbalance and struggle less effectively with natural hormonal shifts. Factors affecting girls as they enter adolescence that can influence eating habits include:

✔ **Depression:** Recent studies show that girls between the ages of 12 and 15 are more than three times as likely to suffer from depression than boys are. Some studies show that depression itself can actually impact hormone levels in teenage girls, leading to weight gain and obesity. A "chicken or egg" dilemma for sure.

✔ **Increased stress and cortisol levels:** The body generates higher levels of the hormone cortisol as a reaction to stress. Scientists know that depression and cortisol are linked to obesity, but they have not yet determined the exact biological mechanism. The latest findings indicate that the increased levels of cortisol in young girls can affect their metabolism and lead to weight gain.

✔ **Hormonal surges:** When a girl enters puberty, hormones stimulate the production of estrogen in the ovaries, resulting in breast growth and the beginning of menstruation. Estrogen surges naturally cause teenage girls to focus on their looks — to serve the biological imperative to attract a mate. These same hormones may drive girls' concerns about looking, dressing, and acting out.

For overweight or obese teens, it's normal to strive for attention and affection even though their perceived rate of rejection seems high. That rejection can set in motion a vicious cycle for teens with vulnerability toward bingeing and who may use eating as a coping mechanism.

Coping with changing expectations and societal triggers

Teenagers aren't children, but they're definitely not yet adults either. The struggle to find their way and to figure out their place in the world can be a stressful, lonely experience even if many of their friends experience the same things at the same time. At the same time that they want more independence and privileges, they may not actually be ready for increased responsibilities and for dealing with the consequences of their actions. Living for years in this strange middle ground can take a toll on them and their families. When you think about it, the emotions and day-to-day struggles every teen experiences at some point are also triggers for seeking out the ability to numb or self-soothe emotional discomfort, including binge eating, and other forms of disordered eating or addictive behaviors.

Many adults who binge eat or overeat in any way report that they began to turn to food for comfort as teenagers. For a complicated series of reasons that we discuss in Chapter 3 and throughout the book, some individuals, particularly children with the genetic and environmental vulnerabilities, are susceptible to unhealthy coping strategies such as binge eating that provide a quick fix for negative emotions but which can cause far more serious problems down the line.

In addition to the eating- and weight-specific strategies we outline in the next section, one of the best ways to help kids who may turn to disordered eating of any kind during the teenage years is to help them find healthier, more productive ways to deal with their confusion, sadness, anger, depression, boredom, or other unpleasant emotions. We talk about alternate coping strategies in Chapter 11, and there are a multitude of books and websites that can help you learn more in addition to working on this skill with your psychotherapist, dietitian, or any group you or your kids may be in to work on changing negative behaviors.

Having healthy coping skills and knowing how to adapt them to many different situations or feelings is something that serves kids (and adults!) well for a lifetime.

Helping Kids Deal with Binge Eating and Emotional Eating

How you deal with your kids and their tendencies to look toward food for comfort can shape much of their future relationship with food and how they use it to deal with their feelings.

In other parts of this book, we talk about being compassionate toward yourself if you're a binge or emotional eater. That goes double if you're trying to help your child to deal with obesity and the prospect of binge eating now or in the future. Although you may get frustrated or scared, remember that your role is to support your child and help him develop the coping skills and habits that will serve him well for the rest of his life.

The most important thing you can do for your child is to love and accept her for who she is. By being kind and gentle to her and to yourself, you model the way she should treat herself now and in the future. Life is full of ups and downs, some having to do with weight and body image, some not, but if you can teach your children to accept themselves and others, you go a long way toward helping them learn to deal with unpredictability and setbacks.

Tips for helping an obese or bingeing child in your life include:

- ✔ **Don't single out overweight or obese kids with information about healthy eating and lifestyle habits.** Empower kids of all shapes and sizes to make healthy choices by teaching them about eating right and exercising from an early age. Childhood and adolescence are times of great change and growth. A kid who's overweight now may grow out of it in several years, and one that never seemed to have trouble in middle childhood may develop an eating disorder as a teenager.

- ✔ **Don't focus on weight loss.** It's tempting to use weight as a measure of progress, but the solution to dealing with obesity or bingeing doesn't have as much to do with the number on the scale as you might think. Eating better and exercising more can be its own reward for your children and your family.

- ✔ **Find a balance between concerns about health and concerns about emotional well-being.** It's easy to feel like being fat means you're bad or worthless, but as best you can, try to separate weight and eating from who a child is at the core. Everyone's body is different, and size and shape doesn't determine character or worth.

Chapter 18

The Endocrine System and Binge Eating

*O*ver the course of this book, we talk a great deal about the complex interactions of heredity, environment, neurobiology, and emotional states that trigger binge eating and compulsive or emotional overeating. However, these behaviors sometimes also come about for other reasons, for example, as a result of medical or physical conditions that upset the body's hormonal balance.

One medical reason women may be more vulnerable to overeating and binge eating is due in part to polycystic ovary syndrome or PCOS, which is typically diagnosed in a woman's 20s or 30s. Another common syndrome is hypothyroidism, which can be present at any age but tends to be most commonly found in women 50 and older. While these illnesses affect the hormonal system in different ways, both create a physical vulnerability to overeating that can make sufferers more susceptible to overweight, obesity, and the health problems they bring about.

In this chapter, we talk about the endocrine system and how it works as well as take a closer look at hypothyroidism and PCOS. We examine the way each of these conditions may make you susceptible to overeating or bingeing, and discuss how each one is treated with respect to diet and exercise. Finally, we discuss hormonal shifts or cascades and explain that sometimes people over-eat or binge to offset the fatigue and depression that can come along with these changes.

Understanding the Endocrine System

Eleven interconnected systems regulate and support the function of the human body. Each one is essential to an individual's health and survival, and when they work well and work together, they make it possible for you to breathe and move and eat and feel and think among thousands of other essential functions, both voluntary and involuntary, each and every day.

The endocrine or hormonal system is one of several systems that influence all cellular functions within your body. *Hormones* are chemical messengers that move through the bloodstream, signaling the processes that keep your body functioning optimally. Most hormones have a single job and perform just one function although each function forms one tiny part of the intricate and multifaceted framework that makes up the endocrine network. Some of the most important hormonal functions include the regulation of metabolism, growth and development, mood, and reproduction.

The endocrine system, shown in Figure 18-1, is made up of a series of glands located throughout the body. A *gland* is a group of cells that produces and secretes hormones. The endocrine system is unique in that it simultaneously uses glands and cells within multiple organs that are all closely related to other body systems. The pancreas, for example, is part of both the endocrine and digestive systems. Some of the major glands of the endocrine system are the hypothalamus, pituitary gland, and pancreas.

n general, the endocrine system is in charge of bodily processes that happen relatively slowly, such as cell growth. Faster and more immediate processes such as breathing and body movement are controlled by the nervous system. The endocrine and central nervous systems are separate, but they work closely together to regulate every body function properly through what's called the neuroendocrine pathway.

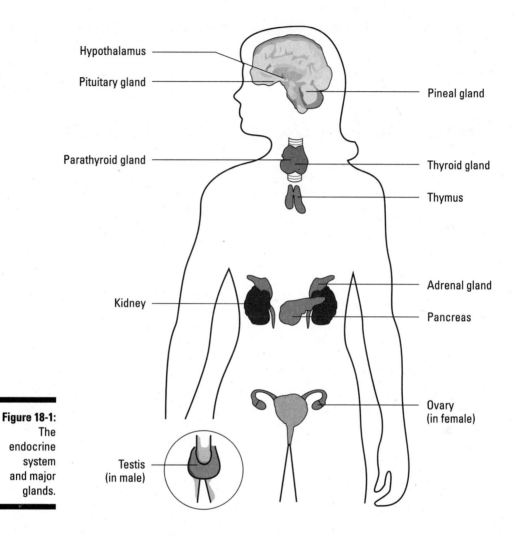

Hypothalamus

Pituitary gland

Pineal gland

Parathyroid gland

Thyroid gland

Thymus

Kidney

Adrenal gland

Pancreas

Ovary
(in female)

Figure 18-1:
The
endocrine
system
and major
glands.

Testis
(in male)

Connecting Hypothyroidism and Binge Eating

Everyone goes through periods of feeling tired or weak. A few weeks of low energy here and there are probably the byproduct of the ups and downs of everyday life, such as a schedule change that forces you to get up earlier or a stressful new project at work. Perhaps one day you notice you aren't feeling well, so you get into bed earlier or take more time for yourself in the form of exercise, meditation, reading, or any other activity you enjoy. You may cut down on sweets after eating too many at the holidays. However you felt and whatever your own remedies, time passed, and one morning you woke up feeling more energetic, refreshed, and alert again.

Imagine that your feelings of fatigue and weakness have been going on for two or more weeks without a logical reason, and no matter what you do, you still feel tired and are getting worse. You notice joint and muscle pain from the moment you wake up, and your skin and hair have gotten dull and brittle. Even though you're doing your best to rest and recover, you can't, and you've started to suspect that something more serious may be wrong.

If this describes how you feel day in and day out, it may be time to get tested to see whether you have hypothyroidism, a treatable condition that affects mostly women aged 50 and older.

Explaining hypothyroidism

Hypothyroidism, or underactive thyroid, is a disorder of the thyroid gland, located in the front of the neck just below the hollow of your throat. If you have hypothyroidism, your thyroid doesn't produce enough of the hormone needed to regulate your metabolism. Hypothyroidism upsets the normal balance of chemical reactions in your body, but it rarely causes symptoms in the early stages. Most people are unaware they have hypothyroidism for years, but if not treated, it eventually causes a number of health problems including obesity, joint pain, infertility, and heart disease — to name just a few.

Metabolism is the process that allows your cells to grow, to reproduce, to maintain themselves, and to react to changes in their environments. Many people refer to metabolism as the way the body absorbs and uses nutrients and food to fuel itself, but metabolism actually refers to all the chemical processes going on in your body during which energy is processed and utilized.

Anyone can develop hypothyroidism, but women 50 and older are most likely to suffer from it. In the United States and most of the developed world, the most common cause is *Hashimoto's thyroiditis,* an autoimmune disease that leads to an inadequate production of thyroid hormone. Another common cause of hypothyroidism is swelling and inflammation due to some of the following:

✔ An attack of the thyroid gland by the immune system

✔ A cold or other respiratory infection

✔ *Postpartum thyroiditis,* a condition that affects about five percent of new mothers within a year of giving birth

Other causes include

- ✔ The use of certain drugs, such as lithium-based mood stabilizers and *amiodarone,* a medication used for cardiac rhythm irregularities
- ✔ Congenital birth defects
- ✔ Cancer of the thyroid gland
- ✔ Radiation treatments to the neck or brain to treat different cancers
- ✔ Radioactive iodine used to treat an overactive thyroid gland
- ✔ Surgical removal of part or all of the thyroid gland
- ✔ *Sheehan syndrome,* a condition that may occur in a woman who bleeds severely during pregnancy or childbirth and causes the destruction of the pituitary gland

Even though hypothyroidism is most common in adults, it also occurs in newborn infants. Congenital hypothyroidism (CH) can be mild, moderate, or severe, with approximately 1 in 4,000 newborn infants suffering from a significant deficiency of thyroid function. If left untreated, severe CH can lead to growth failure and permanent mental retardation. Treatment consists of a daily dose of thyroid hormone (thyroxine) by mouth. Because the treatment is simple, effective, and inexpensive, nearly the entire developed world practices newborn screening to detect and treat congenital hypothyroidism in the first weeks of life.

Hypothyroidism in real life

For months, Delores, a 55-year-old real estate agent, felt tired and didn't have the energy to exercise or to go to weekly salsa class with her husband. The real estate market's been difficult and her job's been stressful, so she assumed that when she sells a house or two and her work life gets back to normal, she will too.

One Saturday, after showing several houses to potential buyers, Delores fell down the stairs as she finished with her clients. Although she bruised her hip and shoulder, her doctor said she didn't have any head injuries, so she went back to work the following week. During the next two months, her body started to ache more

regularly, and she started to be more forgetful. She also felt so tired some mornings that she couldn't get out of bed and called in sick.

Finally, Delores' husband insisted she go back to the doctor for a physical. During a routine examination, her doctor noticed her enlarged thyroid and sent her for a biopsy. The biopsy revealed a growth on her thyroid, which she had surgically removed along with a piece of her thyroid. Now she's taking thyroid hormone and starting to feel like herself again even though her medication still needs to be adjusted depending on how she responds to treatment.

Symptoms and diagnosis

Hypothyroidism comes on slowly, and you may not notice the symptoms for months or even years, especially because it's easy in the midst of a busy life to attribute general symptoms such as fatigue or constipation to working too late or not eating well.

But at a certain point, if you actually have hypothyroidism, your symptoms will become more serious and hard to avoid. Some of the things to look for may be

- Fatigue, even after more and more rest or sleep
- Increased sensitivity to cold
- Unexplained weight gain
- Brittle nails and/or thin or brittle hair
- Muscle weakness and/or muscle aches, tenderness, or stiffness
- Pale or dry skin, which may be cool to the touch
- Swelling of the arms and legs

Diagnosis of any thyroid abnormality generally begins with a physical examination by your doctor to look for an enlarged thyroid, which may indicate a growth. She'll also look for any signs or symptoms you may not have noticed or reported, and you'll give blood for lab tests to determine thyroid function as well as

- **TSH levels:** The thyroid-stimulating hormone (TSH) test is the most accurate measure of thyroid activity. The pituitary gland, located at the base of the brain, secretes TSH when it senses the thyroid gland becoming too sluggish to produce T4, one of the thyroid hormones. The pituitary gland works hard to keep T4 in the normal range, so it will be elevated long before T4 actually drops enough to produce low thyroid function. Because this test is extremely sensitive, abnormal thyroid function can be determined before a patient complains of symptoms.

- **T3/T4 and Free T3/T4:** T3 is the most active thyroid hormone, and the body converts it as needed from T4, which is more plentiful. The absence of certain vitamins and minerals and/or stress can interfere with this conversion.

- **Blood cholesterol levels:** High cholesterol is often associated with hypothyroidism because when the thyroid function slows it slows the body's ability to process cholesterol.

> ✔ **Complete blood count (CBC):** CBC measures red and white cells in the blood and can offer clues or confirm diagnoses of other conditions.
>
> ✔ **Liver enzymes:** Thyroxine-binding globulin (TBG) is an enzyme manufactured in the liver. TBG binds to T3 and T4, and is an indicator of irregular T3 and T4 levels.

Some patients who do not experience symptoms may still have a mild form of hypothyroidism and need to be screened periodically to monitor any changes.

In addition, doctors generally recommend that pregnant women be tested for hypothyroidism so that if they do have it, they can take iron supplements to prevent the baby from being born with the same condition. Older women are also encouraged to be screened for the disorder annually.

Linking thyroid irregularities and bingeing or overeating

The primary effects of hypothyroidism mimic the very same triggers that overeaters and binge eaters deal with on a daily basis. If you have hypothyroidism, you may face depression, fatigue, weight gain, and an overall sense of weakness among other symptoms; and if you're not feeling your best, you can be vulnerable to using food to soothe yourself.

If you were already prone to overeating and bingeing, the symptoms of hypothyroidism may be the last straw in your efforts to avoid using food as a coping mechanism. But even if you've never had problems with food and eating, there's a first time for everything, and hypothyroidism may be the reason you binged in the first place. This may be especially true if you've not yet been diagnosed and can't quite figure out the reason for the changes in your body.

A word of caution: It would be easy to look to thyroid dysfunction or any other physical or medical condition as the magic bullet for why bingeing or overeating takes place. If only. It may certainly be a factor, and it's worth checking out, but in the final analysis, the work to be done to deal with the consequences still need to focus on your reactions to potent emotional triggers, developing new strategies to calm your body, and adapting new coping behaviors that can replace entrenched and, dare we say, comfortably uncomfortable habits.

Dealing with the whole picture

The standard treatment for hypothyroidism is generally straightforward and effective. Most patients respond well to a daily dose of thyroid hormone, and typically begin to feel better within a short period of time after refining the dosage. Over time, depending on how you feel and after evaluating regular testing to determine levels of thyroid hormone in your blood, together you and your doctor can manage your hypothyroidism, and you can live a more healthy life.

Generally, there's no hypothyroidism diet. Although claims about such diet plans abound, there's no evidence that eating or avoiding certain foods improves thyroid function in people with hypothyroidism. If you have hypothyroidism, take thyroid hormone replacement as directed by your doctor — generally on an empty stomach. It's also important to note that too much dietary fiber can impair the absorption of synthetic thyroid hormone. Certain foods, supplements and medications can have the same effect.

A variety of nutritional factors affect thyroid function. In order to make informed choices, it's important to work with a dietitian and/or a medical doctor who know your thyroid function blood results and your symptoms in order to establish the most appropriate diet and supplements for you. Thyroid hormone should be taken at the same time each morning half an hour to an hour before eating breakfast — follow your doctor's instructions.

Note that we're not saying not to have any fiber if you take synthetic thyroid hormone, as fiber is a very important part of your food intake. However, follow your doctor's advice about how much fiber to include in your diet.

According to the Mayo Clinic, you should avoid taking your thyroid hormone at the same time as these foods and medications:

- Walnuts.
- Soybeans: Soy-based foods reduce absorption of medication, so if you eat soy products, don't have them within three hours of taking your medication.
- Cottonseed meal.

To avoid potential interactions, eat these foods or use these products several hours before or after you take your thyroid medication.

Some supplements and medications interfere with your body's ability to absorb thyroid hormone medication if they're taken too closely together — or at all. They include

- ✔ **Aluminum and magnesium:** Antacids may contain these minerals, which can interfere with thyroid hormone absorption.

- ✔ **Calcium:** Don't take calcium supplements or calcium-fortified foods within three hours of taking your thyroid medication.

- ✔ **Cholesterol-lowering drugs:** Cholestyramine (Questran) and colestipol (Colestid) are two. Your doctor can advise you on how to take these medications when on thyroid hormone.

- ✔ **Iron:** Don't take iron supplements or multivitamins that contain iron within three hours of taking your thyroid medication as iron may compete for absorption.

- ✔ **Lemon balm:** This herb may interfere with medication absorption and should be avoided while you're on thyroid medication. Check any herbal teas you drink regularly to see whether lemon balm is an ingredient.

- ✔ **Ulcer medications:** Sucralfate (Carafate) can interfere with absorption, so check with your doctor about any ulcer medications.

Coping with Polycystic Ovary Syndrome

Another hormonal disorder that may trigger overeating or bingeing is polycystic ovary syndrome (PCOS), a condition in which a girl or woman has an imbalance of female sex hormones. Although PCOS notably causes problems with a woman's reproductive system, the hormonal imbalance that results can also lead to high insulin levels, which can produce unexplained weight gain and low blood sugar, leaving PCOS sufferers hungry and craving carbohydrates.

If you think you may have PCOS or if you've already been diagnosed, the struggle with weight and body image can leave you feeling exhausted, depressed, anxious, or sad. Unfortunately, the psychological impact of PCOS presents another challenge because negative feelings and a sense of being out of control can also lead to emotional eating or bingeing. Although it may sometimes be difficult both physically and psychologically, it's possible to manage your PCOS and find ways to manage some of its challenges.

Defining polycystic ovary syndrome

Polycystic ovary syndrome (PCOS) is a condition in which a woman has an imbalance of female sex hormones. As girls reach puberty and begin to menstruate, the ovaries release a single egg every month in addition to producing the female sex hormones estrogen and progesterone. The ovaries are also meant to produce a tiny amount of *androgens,* or male sex hormones. Women suffering from PCOS produce a greater than normal amount of androgens, and as a result, many do not get their periods or have irregular periods. Along with changes in menstrual cycles, PCOS typically causes cysts in the ovaries and difficulty getting pregnant.

In addition to affecting the reproductive system, the hormonal imbalance triggered by PCOS tends to lead to overweight, obesity, and insulin resistance due to changes in metabolism. Unfortunately, insulin resistance often causes unexplained weight gain and can lead to irregular blood sugar levels, which can trigger overeating or bingeing. PCOS sufferers also may experience

- ✔ Increased abdominal weight
- ✔ High levels of triglycerides, a specific form of blood fats
- ✔ Low levels of good cholesterol or HDL, another form of blood fats
- ✔ High blood pressure
- ✔ High fasting blood sugar

The result is that PCOS sufferers have a higher risk of developing the most common obesity-related conditions including type 2 diabetes, high blood pressure, high cholesterol, and heart disease. And though weight loss is one of the most effective treatments for PCOS, it's also a challenge because of the hormonal swings that leave women with PCOS hungry and gaining weight. Studies show that

- ✔ PCOS is associated with a higher amount of abdominal fat, and it's common to find an overlap between obesity and PCOS. Patients with PCOS also show greater cravings for sweets.

- ✔ Patients with PCOS may have difficulty regulating their appetites due to insufficient production of the hormone cholecystokinin (CCK), which signals fullness. Therefore, the rates of bingeing among PCOS sufferers tend to be higher.

On top of the physical symptoms, it's no surprise to discover that some evidence links PCOS to feelings of anxiety and depression. Whether these are due to hormonal fluctuations or to the sense of feeling out of control of your body, the resulting negative feelings may trigger emotional eating or binge eating no matter what their origin.

Managing PCOS through nutrition

There's no cure for PCOS, but committing to regular exercise, eating a nutritious, balanced diet, and maintaining a healthy weight can go a long way toward managing the condition. Doctors usually first attempt to treat PCOS with an anti-diabetic drug called metformin, which can help reduce insulin sensitivity, lower cholesterol and triglyceride levels, and reduce cardiovascular risks. By lowering insulin sensitivity, metformin can assist in decreasing cravings and urges to binge and also lead to some weight loss. Some doctors may also prescribe hormone therapy, particularly if you're trying to get pregnant, but unfortunately, taking hormones regularly cannot control the risk factors that may lead to a higher risk of heart disease, high blood pressure, diabetes, and high cholesterol.

Because insulin resistance causes most PCOS symptoms, the changes you may make to your nutrition and lifestyle mainly focus on treating insulin resistance and its long-term health effects. In general, a PCOS food plan is just like any other healthy, low-fat, high-fiber diet. The following recommendations have proven successful in treatment.

- ✔ **Begin with a manageable amount of weight loss.** Even a ten percent reduction in body weight decreases insulin resistance.

- ✔ **Don't skip meals.** Aim to eat every three to four hours, so that you can maintain stable blood sugars and diminish extreme hunger, which frequently leads to bingeing.

- ✔ **Balance your carbohydrate intake throughout the day.** Meals and snacks throughout the day should have a consistent amount of carbohydrate to keep your blood sugar stable. When you eat too many or too few carbohydrates at any one time, you're more likely to have unstable blood sugar and experience food cravings.

- ✔ **Increase your fiber intake.** This may need to happen gradually, but over time, you should aim for 30 to 40 grams of fiber per day. A higher fiber diet can help keep your weight stable, digestion optimal, and is associated with reduced rates of several cancers. Choose high fiber carbohydrates such as

  - • Whole grain breads, rolls, and bagels

  - • Whole-wheat pasta

  - • Brown and wild rice

  - • High-fiber cereals including oat and barley cereals

  - • Legumes (peas, beans, and lentils), corn, bran, seeds, nuts

  - • Fresh and dried fruit and most vegetables

✔ **Focus on lean protein foods.** You can do this by including protein with most meals and snacks. Lean protein helps maintain healthy blood sugar.

✔ **Moderate fat to about 25 percent to 30 percent of your total intake.** Aim to eat mostly low-saturated fats and avoid foods containing trans fats. Increase your intake of monounsaturated and omega-3 fatty acid food choices such as avocado, canola, olive, and peanut oils; olives; nuts such as almonds, cashews, peanuts, and pecans; peanut butter and nut butters; and sesame oil, seeds, and paste.

✔ **Include two to three servings of low-fat dairy foods per day.** These foods include skim milk, fat-free yogurt, lite cheese, cottage cheese, and so on.

✔ **Eat foods high in phyto-nutrients, which improve insulin resistance.** Foods high in insulin-improving phytochemicals are low-fat dairy foods; nuts, especially walnuts; orange and leafy green vegetables such as spinach and kale; carrots; yams; and sweet potatoes.

✔ **Control portions.** Keep a close eye on how much you're eating, especially from restaurants or fast food places. Most restaurant portions are 50 percent more than your body needs. Ask for the to go container when the meal arrives and put aside part of the meal.

PCOS in real life

Teresa's always been overweight, and in her teens, the hair on her upper lip and sideburns turned so dark and coarse that she was embarrassed to go to school. Luckily, her mother noticed and made appointments for electrolysis, which removed much of the hair and helped her cope with the humiliation she felt. In her 20s, Teresa has tried constantly to lose weight without success, and several times a year, she finds herself bingeing out of frustration and anger.

Now in her 30s, Teresa and her husband would like to have a baby, but after a year of trying, her doctor ran routine tests and has diagnosed her with polycystic ovary syndrome. The first couple weeks were difficult for her because she knows there's no easy solution, but after meeting with a nutritionist, she feels ready to start the PCOS diet so that she can get healthier. Although the prescribed meal plan is no picnic in any sense of the word, with the support of her husband and the goal of pregnancy to motivate her, Teresa is losing weight and hopeful of becoming pregnant in the coming year.

Chapter 19

Menopause and Bingeing

· ·

In This Chapter

▶ Experiencing the cycle of menopause

▶ Making the connection between menopause and bingeing

▶ Taking a multi-pronged view of treatment

· ·

*1*n recent years, women, their doctors, their partners, and the larger medical community have begun to turn their attention and energy to understanding and treating some of the issues that arise during the stages of menopause. *Menopause* literally means "end of monthly cycles." It's the gradual process in which a woman's period ceases and she's no longer able to have children. Menopause is the result of a reduction in the production of female hormones by the ovaries.

Although sometimes defined as distinct stages, *perimenopause,* the transition toward menopause, and menopause itself form part of a progressive and continuous hormonal and metabolic shift that occurs as a woman ages. Just as the hormonal shifts of adolescence are a normal part of life, perimenopause and menopause are also part of the cycle of every adult woman. The final phase is *postmenopause,* which occurs after a woman has not had her period for an entire year.

In some cases, menopause brings about hormonal imbalances that trigger overeating, binge eating, or other types of excessive eating unrelated to actual physical hunger. Some of these triggers include unpredictable mood and energy shifts due to changing hormones; an unusually high level of angst, anxiety, and/or depression; and perhaps most frustratingly, weight gain for what seems like no apparent reason. Any one of these triggers or a combination can contribute to the impulse to use food as a way to self-soothe.

In this chapter, we talk about the realities of menopause and why you may binge or overeat at various points before, during, and after this stage of life. We also discuss the nuances of seeking treatment during this time and give you information about finding equilibrium in the face of significant physical changes.

Shifting Hormonal Seas of Menopause

The onset of perimenopause and eventually menopause itself signals great change in your physical and emotional life. Incremental shifts come on for months and years before menopause sets in, although some women experience few symptoms. These physical changes are often accompanied by psychological ones as you confront the realities of aging and try to deal with the mood shifts that often come along with hormonal change and hormonal imbalance.

Because your hormones are off-kilter, you may be more susceptible to depression, fatigue, moodiness, and food cravings. Unfortunately, these side effects are some of the more potent triggers for binge eating and/or other types of emotional or compulsive eating. Even if you've never had a troublesome relationship with food before or you've successfully managed any eating issues for years, you may find yourself turning to food if you feel tired, depressed, frustrated, or angry about the changes in your body.

If you've rarely eaten out of anything other than physical hunger, you may be shocked to find yourself now eating compulsively or bingeing. The shift in your eating habits doesn't necessarily mean you're a binge eater, but it does mean that something in your life and/or in your body is shifting. A thorough work-up including visits to your doctor, gynecologist, a psychotherapist, and/or dietitian can help you get a better picture of what's going on and begin to give you the coping skills you'll need to face menopause with a healthy, optimistic outlook.

Understanding perimenopause

If you've heard your girlfriends complaining about menopause, they're likely talking about the ups and downs of perimenopause, the months and years that typically precede menopause, when your hormones fluctuate in a way that may make you feel like a moody teenager all over again.

The changes in your body and your mind are largely caused by natural changes in your body's hormone production. during perimenopause, your body starts decreasing production of the female sexual hormones — estrogen and progesterone — and other hormones as well. Like many changes that happen during perimenopause, these may have been gradual but then ramp up in ways that are impossible not to notice.

Although perimenopause typically begins in a woman's 40s, some women may notice the signs as early as their 30s. These signs and symptoms include hot flashes, night sweats, insomnia, irregular periods, vaginal dryness, and/or changes in your sex drive. Other changes include

- ✔ **Irregular periods and/or a change in your menstrual cycle:** No matter what your periods have been like before and how often they've come, everything's starting to change now. Your period may come more or less often, and be heavier or lighter than it's been before for more or less days per cycle. You may even skip periods when you never have before. Whatever the differences, you know your body's changing.

- ✔ **Hot flashes:** You've heard women complaining about hot flashes, but you never understood what the big deal is — until now. About 65 to 75 percent of women experience hot flashes. A hot flash comes on quickly and can feel like a surge of warmth or like burning up from the inside out, leaving you flushed, sweaty, and confused. They don't last long but are hard to miss. In "Treating the symptoms of menopause" later in this chapter, we talk more about the clever ways women come up to deal with hot flashes. When a hot flash occurs while you're sleeping, it can cause disrupted sleep and night sweats.

- ✔ **Insomnia and night sweats:** A balanced hormonal cycle is one part of what made sleeping easier when you were younger. But now that your hormones have begun to shift, drifting off to sleep and staying asleep isn't as easy as it once was. You may find yourself restless and wide awake in the middle of the night, and if you're having night sweats, a close relative of hot flashes, even if you do get to sleep, you can wake up so clammy and chilled that you need to get out of bed to change your nightclothes, and maybe even your sheets.

- ✔ **Vaginal and bladder problems:** Over time, lower estrogen levels lead to less elasticity and lubrication in the vagina, and you may find sexual intercourse uncomfortable as a result. Less estrogen also may mean more vaginal or urinary infections for some women. During perimenopause, some women also experience a degree of urinary incontinence.

- ✔ **Decreased interest in sex:** If you're less interested in sex these days, it may be because it's physically uncomfortable or because you have less sex drive and desire than you did in your 20s and 30s, or a combination of factors. The combination of physical and emotional changes can make sex less appealing for many women during perimenopause.

✔ **Bone loss:** *Osteoporosis* is a disease of the bone that occurs when you lose bone and/or make too little bone. The result is that bones become weak and can break from a minor injury. Osteoporosis risk rises during menopause because with less estrogen, you begin to lose bone faster than you replace it. The risk of osteoporosis is greater for Caucasian and Asian women, and some studies suggest that this difference can be attributed greater numbers of protective melanin receptors in darker skin pigment.

✔ **Rising cholesterol levels:** Your blood cholesterol levels may have always been within normal ranges, but perimenopause and menopause can cause shifts that affect those levels and put you at greater risk for heart disease. In some cases, your bad cholesterol (LDL) can increase just as the good cholesterol (HDL) starts to drop. The double whammy can leave you vulnerable to diseases of aging.

For many women, the signs and symptoms of perimenopause are no more than an inconvenience, but if you find that you're unable to go about your daily life, make sure to see your doctor to discuss alleviating your symptoms.

Detecting menopausal hormone shifts

If you've noticed symptoms of perimenopause, or are approaching your menopausal years, you may want to consider seeing your doctor. Simple tests can confirm if you are in or entering menopause, and regular blood testing can establish a baseline so you can understand how your hormone levels shift over time.

Both blood and urine tests can be used to look for changes in hormone levels. Test results can help your doctor advise you on treatment options, whatever stage of menopause you're in.

Your blood may be tested for

✔ **Estrogen levels:** Estrogen levels drop during menopause

✔ **FSH (follicle-stimulating hormone):** FSH levels rise during menopause.

✔ **LH: (luteinizing hormone):** LH stimulates ovulation.

Your doctor will also perform a pelvic exam to check for signs of changes in the lining of the vagina.

Because bone loss slowly increases during the first few years after your last period, your doctor may also do a bone density test to look for bone loss related to osteoporosis.

Completing the cycle

Perimenopause can go on for several years, but menopause is considered complete when you've had 12 consecutive months without a period. For most women, this happens some time between the ages of 45 and 55. Although the change is gradual, the transition from perimenopause, through menopause, and eventually post-menopause, which you enter 24 to 36 months after your last period, slowly bring about less intense symptoms of hormonal imbalance.

If you gained weight or were depressed during perimenopause, you may continue to be vulnerable to certain binge-eating triggers during menopause and beyond. You may be more prone to weight gain now than you were when you were younger, and that may frustrate and depress you. In addition, as your ovaries completely stop producing estrogen and progesterone, hormonal equilibrium may still seem out of reach.

Surgical menopause

Although most women experience the gradual changes associated with natural menopause, a small group find themselves menopausal due to medical or surgical causes. *Surgical menopause* is the result of having to remove both ovaries or what's called a bilateral oophorectomy. A woman's ovaries produce female sex hormones estrogen and progesterone, and after surgery, the sudden drop in these hormones can produce menopausal symptoms that can be more severe than they might be during natural menopause.

The most common reasons a woman may have her ovaries removed include

- ✔ Cancer (including endometrial or ovarian cancer)

- ✔ Hysterectomy (although not all hysterectomies result in oophorectomy)

- ✔ Endometriosis, a condition when cells from the womb lining grow outside the uterus causing pain at many points during a woman's cycle

- ✔ Myomectomy, the removal of uterine fibroids, non-cancerous tumors that grow into the uterine wall and may cause excessive bleeding, pain, or infertility

- ✔ Treatment for other infections or conditions

As a result of surgical menopause, the signs and symptoms of menopause are likely to come on quickly and powerfully. Although some doctors still prescribe estrogen to prevent or control these intense changes, the use of synthetic hormones has become controversial during the past decade after studies showed that hormone replacement causes an increased risk of heart disease and some cancers.

Hopefully, if you've had a hysterectomy due to intense pain or bleeding or an oophorectomy due to the presence of ovarian cancer or because of an increased risk of ovarian cancer, you're now free from the intense symptoms that led to the need for the surgery in the first place. As with all things related to menopause, educating yourself and adopting as positive an attitude as you can goes a long way toward living healthily and living well during this transition.

Seeking Treatment and Finding Balance

The relationship between menopause and bingeing is a complex one because menopause brings about both physical and emotional changes that are often difficult, if not impossible, to untangle.

Getting treatment for compulsive eating, emotional eating, or binge eating during menopause is best undertaken with a complete medical and psychological evaluation that can allow you to address each of the complex issues that triggered your eating issues. At first, it can be difficult to determine whether the undesirable behaviors you're trying to change have come about because of hormonal shifts or emotional shifts, but no matter what the origin of the shift, it's important to develop a multipronged approach to slowing and eventually stopping your use of food as self-soothing technique.

Accepting change and yourself

What does it mean to age? On a good day, you can look in the mirror and see the scope of your life experience, wisdom and all that you know and have to offer to the world. You may not look 20 years old anymore, but you look good, feel confident, and are looking forward to what life has in store for you.

On a bad day though, if you're going through menopause, you may beat yourself up for changes that are completely natural. Gravity is having an all-out war with various muscle groups in your body and, much to your surprise, you look in the mirror and often see none other than your own mother looking back at you! Perhaps there's a bit more facial hair than you've ever had before. You have more belly fat, you have to exercise twice as hard and twice as long to keep your body as it is, and you're facing an inevitable, but perhaps not entirely welcome, phase of life. It's no surprise that you may be feeling anxious, depressed, angry, afraid, frustrated, or even victimized by these changes.

If you've ever had trouble with eating before, it can easily resurface or get worse during perimenopause and menopause. Both your physical and psychological foundations may be shifting, and initially it can be easy and appealing to turn to food for comfort. If you find yourself binge eating, it may be time to ask for help. You may also consider seeing a psychotherapist specializing in eating disorders or in treating anxiety states if you find yourself compulsively overeating in ways you cannot seem to control. Any kind of eating disorder can compromise your health just as it becomes more important than ever to take care of your body and mind.

The truth about weight gain and menopause

Losing weight is difficult for most women especially when they're menopausal. Add binge eating disorder into the mix, and losing weight may seem impossible. During perimenopause, estrogen production diminishes. Simultaneously, levels of the male hormone androgen increase, causing a redistribution of weight to the belly, an area where men typically store fat. However, your body still needs estrogen. Because the fat cells in your body are able to produce estrogen, the brain sends a message to preserve fat stores at all costs and convert excess calories to fat, especially in the belly.

Unfortunately, when the body's stressed, as it typically is during menopause, hormones block weight loss, and even more weight accumulates around the waist and hips. Despite adequate food, the body acts as if it's in a famine state and stores all spare calories as fat.

Women struggling with binge eating tend to eat high-carbohydrate and higher-fat diets with a lot of processed foods. Eventually this kind of diet causes obesity and promotes insulin resistance. Also, when a woman is bingeing on a high-carb diet she is often barraged with a craving for sweets because when the body can't maintain optimal blood sugar and serotonin levels, high-carb/high-fat snacks and caffeine tend to make you feel better. That makes insulin resistance worse and accelerates the vicious cycle of dieting, bingeing, gaining weight..

Even though you may feel as if no matter what you do, nothing will change, it's important to follow a healthy diet and exercise routine no matter what your age. Even if you're frustrated by menopausal weight gain, remember that your overall health is more important than what the scale says.

As you begin to find your way through perimenopause and menopause and try to tackle why you might be binge eating, remember

✔ Be kind to yourself.

✔ Stay connected to friends and family even when you feel old, ugly, and fat.

✔ Develop new coping mechanisms that speak to your current interests and abilities.

✔ Knowledge is power. Read as much as you can on the subject of perimenopause and menopause because there are several different treatment approaches for the hormonal shifts — synthetic estrogen replacement therapy, bioidentical hormones, or, in some cases, doing nothing and letting things take their course — and you must make your own based on your family history, philosophical beliefs, and health history and risk factors

Reframing your self-defeating thoughts

Reframing is a common technique that simply means taking the same information, facts, or events and reinterpreting them in a different way.

For example, you may wake up one day and think, " I'm aging faster than ever. Soon I'll be completely undesirable, and no one will notice me. I'm now officially old. But with any luck, my newly fuzzy brain will help me not remember how bad I feel!" None of these thoughts is particularly accurate or empowering.

Try this reframe: "Well, it's a privilege to wake up each new day and to be slowly and gently growing older. Some never get to do so. I am like a fine wine. Every day I get wiser and more robust with much more depth and refinement. And isn't it great that I really no longer have to worry about what others think of me to nearly the same degree I used to? I am my own person. Full speed ahead!"

Treating the symptoms of menopause

After you visit your doctor and know more about the scope of your peri-menopausal or menopausal symptoms, you can decide together which treatment is right for you — if you need any treatment at all. Hormone replacement therapy (HRT) used to be standard treatment for many women, but it's no longer routine due to several important studies that suggested that HRT can increase a woman's risk for heart disease and breast cancer.

Most treatment options really depend on how bad your symptoms are. With your doctor's recommendations and guidance, you can decide if medication, lifestyle changes, vitamin/mineral/herbal supplements, or a combination is best for your situation.

Trying hormone replacement therapy

Hormone replacement therapy (HRT) or treatment with estrogen and/or pro-gesterone, may help if you have severe hot flashes, night sweats, or mood swings. Current guidelines support the use of HRT for the treatment of hot flashes; however, several major studies have questioned the health benefits and risks of hormone therapy, including the risk of developing breast cancer, heart attacks, strokes, and blood clots. Your family history is an important deciding factor as well.

Talk to your doctor about the benefits and risks of hormone replacement therapy. Your doctor should be aware of your entire medical history before prescribing HRT. You should also learn about options that do not involve taking hormones.

Specific recommendations for HRT include

- ✔ HRT may be started in women who have recently entered menopause.

- ✔ HRT should start as soon as possible when symptoms begin and should not be used in women who started menopause years ago.

- ✔ HRT should not be used for longer than five years.

- ✔ Women taking HRT should have a low risk for stroke, heart disease, blood clots, or breast cancer.

To further reduce the risks of estrogen therapy, your doctor may recommend:

- ✔ A low dose of estrogen or a different estrogen preparation, for example, a vaginal cream or skin patch rather than a pill

- ✔ Frequent and regular pelvic exams and pap smears to detect any problems as early as possible

- ✔ Frequent and regular physical exams, including breast exams, mammograms, and other more sensitive breast ultrasound or thermograph tests if needed

Going with alternative medications

If hormone replacement therapy isn't a good option for you, there are alternatives. Your doctor may recommend individually formulated *bioidentical hormones,* which are compounded specific to your needs and derived from natural plant compounds meant to duplicate the exact structure and function of the body's hormones (soy is often used). Besides hormones, other medications can help with mood swings, hot flashes, and other symptoms. These include

- ✔ Antidepressants such as paroxetine (Paxil), venlafaxine (Effexor), bupropion (Wellbutrin), and fluoxetine (Prozac)

- ✔ A blood pressure medication called clonidine

- ✔ Gabapentin, an anti-seizure drug that also helps reduce hot flashes

Taking supplements

The symptoms of menopause can be unpleasant and hard to manage.

Some women opt for dietary supplements and/or herbs, but the research on their effectiveness is often inconclusive. In the U. S. market, dietary supplements and herbs are rarely tested thoroughly, and their manufacturers make health claims that aren't always backed up by reputable scientific studies. According to the FDA, a supplement label cannot say it treats a specific disease, but it can claim to benefit a disease or support general well-being. For example, a supplement cannot say it "aids joint health to treat arthritis," but it can say it "promotes healthy, flexible joints." In 2012, the Department of Health and Human Services (DHHS) released a report stating that many products on the supplement market are illegally labeled, and even more lack the scientific evidence to support their purported health claims. This means that women in the United States must use extra caution when choosing a supplement or herb. Always consult with a dietitian or medical doctor first.

Unlike in the United States, where dietary supplements are monitored only after being put on the market, Canada requires products to be licensed by the Natural Health Products Directorate (NHPD), a branch of Health Canada, prior to market entry. Regulatory requirements are much more rigorous than in the United States, and many supplement companies are having difficulties meeting them. In fact, since 2004 the NHPD has completed reviews of about 33,000 of 43,000 applications submitted. Out of these, 48 percent have either been withdrawn or refused.

If you're considering taking a supplement or herb, be sure to check with your doctor first.

Some research indicates that 400 to 800 IU (international units) of vitamin E taken at night may have an impact on reducing night sweats. However, it's critical that you check with your dietitian or physician first, especially if you're taking any blood-thinning medications. Because there's a direct relationship between the lack of estrogen after menopause and the development of osteoporosis, the following supplements, combined with a healthy diet, may help prevent the onset of this condition:

- **Calcium:** If you think you need to take a supplement to get enough calcium, check with your doctor first. A study published in June 2012 in the journal *Heart* suggests that taking calcium supplements may increase risk for heart attacks in some people; however, the study showed that increasing calcium in the diet through food sources did not seem to increase the risk.

- **Vitamin D3:** Your body uses vitamin D3 to absorb calcium. Treatment regimens vary widely, ranging from 600,000 IU of vitamin D2 or D3 as a single dose every three months. In general, 2,000 to 4,000 IU daily is considered enough to prevent deficiency and maintain healthy vitamin D stores. Again, check with your medical advisor.

Changing your diet and lifestyle

Even though hormones were used for many years to control or reduce the symptoms of menopause, if you're not a good candidate for HRT or you'd prefer to try something else first, making changes to your lifestyle and nutrition can go a long way toward making your symptoms more manageable.

If you can, make changes when you first begin to notice the symptoms of perimenopause rather than waiting until you feel really low, either physically or psychologically. Not only can you moderate some of the signs of hormonal change going on in your body, but you also jump-start good habits that can help you live longer and feel better.

Working with your diet

Everyone would do well to eat a variety of foods to get a proper balance of vitamins and minerals, but it's particularly important as you get older to make time and space in your life for taking care of your nutritional needs. If you haven't paid much attention to what you're eating before now, menopause may be the first step toward sitting up and taking notice of your diet. Because of a slowing metabolism and health risks that rise with age, it's clear how important it is to make everything you eat truly count.

How do you set nutritional priorities in the face of an urge to binge and/or other medical needs? If you want to stay healthy and yet not overdo the diet mentality which so often leads right into a binge, follow these guidelines when making your daily choices:

- ✔ **Get enough calcium to reduce the risk of osteoporosis:** Eating and drinking two-to-four servings of low-fat or non-fat dairy products and calcium-rich foods a day helps ensure that you get enough calcium in your daily diet. Calcium is found in dairy products, fish with bones (such as sardines and canned salmon), broccoli, and legumes. An adequate intake of calcium for women aged 51 and older is 1,200 milligrams per day.

- ✔ **Pump up your iron intake to improve energy:** Eating at least three servings of iron-rich foods a day helps you meet your recommended daily allowance for iron — 8 milligrams a day in women over 50. Iron is found in lean red meat, poultry, fish, eggs, leafy green vegetables, nuts, and enriched grain products.

- ✔ **Get enough fiber to keep your digestion working smoothly:** Help yourself to foods high in fiber such as whole-grain breads, cereals, pasta, rice, fresh fruits, and vegetables. Most adult women should get about 21 grams of fiber a day.

- ✔ **Eat fruits and vegetables to get essential vitamins and minerals and to fill you up:** Include at least one-and-a-half cups of fruit and two cups of vegetables each day.

- ✔ **Experiment with adding soy to your diet to balance your hormones:** Plant-based foods that contain *isoflavones* (plant estrogens) work in the body like a weak form of estrogen. For this reason, soy may help relieve menopause symptoms, although research results are contradictory. Some studies suggest that eating soy may help lower cholesterol levels and relieve hot flashes and night sweats. Isoflavones are found in foods such as tofu and soy milk.

- ✔ **Avoid trigger foods and beverages to ward off menopause symptoms:** If you're having hot flashes, avoiding spicy foods, chocolate, caffeine, and alcohol may lessen their severity and frequency.

✔ **Read labels to understand what you're eating:** Use the package label information to help you to make the best selections for a healthy lifestyle. Pay close attention to the ingredients list. If you see high fructose corn syrup or hydrogenated oils, choose something else. Overly processed foods can add fuel to your worst menopause symptoms and cause weight gain.

✔ **Drink plenty of water to stay hydrated:** It's impossible to determine how much water you need because the amount depends on many factors: how much you eat, the climate you live in, and how active you are. As a general rule, drinking eight, eight-ounce glasses of water every day fulfills the daily requirement for most healthy adults.

✔ **Maintain a healthy weight to optimize your health and feel your best:** Lose weight if you are overweight by cutting down on portion sizes and reducing foods high in fat, not by skipping meals. A registered dietitian or your doctor can help you determine your ideal body weight.

✔ **Reduce foods high in fat:** Fat should provide 25 percent to 35 percent or less of your total daily calories. Also, limit saturated fat to less than 7 percent of your total daily calories. Saturated fat raises cholesterol and increases your risk for heart disease. You can limit saturated fat by limiting fatty meats, whole milk, ice cream, and cheese in your diet. Also try to minimize your intake of trans fats or hydrogenated oils, found in vegetable oils, many baked goods, convenience and pre-packaged foods, and some margarines. Trans fat raises cholesterol and increases your risk for heart disease.

✔ **Use sugar and salt in moderation:** Too much sodium in the diet is linked to high blood pressure. Also, go easy on smoked, salt-cured, and charbroiled foods — these foods contain high levels of nitrates, which have been linked to cancer.

✔ **Limit alcohol and caffeine intake:** Women should limit their consumption of alcohol to one or fewer drinks a day, and caffeine to two cups per day.

Including exercise and relaxation

At all stages of life, exercise is one component of living well. The physical and emotional benefits of exercise are well documented, and even though it can sometimes be tempting to skip your workout, menopause is no time to give up regular exercise. In addition to your physical fitness, breathing exercises and meditation are two tools you can use to create and maintain balance and stability as you enter this new phase of life.

✔ Get plenty of exercise.

✔ Practice slow, deep breathing whenever a hot flash starts to come on. Try taking six breaths a minute.

✔ Try yoga, tai chi, or meditation.

Chapter 20

Obesity and Bingeing

· ·

In This Chapter

▶ Defining what it means to be obese

▶ Examining the links between binge eating and obesity

▶ Finding a balanced treatment

· ·

*T*he link between obesity and binge eating is a complicated one. *Overweight* and *obese* are official labels for weight ranges that are both higher than what's healthy for a given height and that have been shown to increase the possibility of developing certain diseases and other health problems. Obesity can come about for any number of reasons; binge eating disorder is a psychological issue that may or may not result in obesity. Even though it's tempting to try to establish a direct cause-and-effect relationship between the two, as with many things related to bingeing, simple definitions and explanations don't really speak to the complex situations and circumstances that precede and contribute to binge eating in particular and/or obesity in general. What can be confusing is that not all emotional eaters, compulsive overeaters, and binge eaters who are obese can be diagnosed with binge eating disorder or any eating disorder.

As much as obesity has been studied, measured, and specified, the numbers don't tell the whole story about how people become obese and what can be done to help them.

Obesity isn't something that just happens from one day to the next. It often develops over a period of months and years for genetic, biological, behavioral, and/or environmental reasons. Chances are if you're obese, you already know that multiple factors got you here.

In this chapter, we'll review the medical definition of obesity and talk more about what it means socially, financially, and emotionally to be obese. Then we discuss how the obese population and binge eaters overlap, and finally we outline how to approach treatment and recovery if you're an obese binge eater.

Explaining What It Means to Be Obese

Obesity is a medical condition, yet the experience of being obese is one that encompasses far more than a person's physical experience. If you're obese, you know that it's more than excess fat that weighs you down. You may also face health problems, social stigma, discrimination at work, embarrassment, and depression to name just a few.

According to the U.S. Centers for Disease Control and Prevention (CDC), the rates of obesity in the United States have grown dramatically during the past 20 years, as shown in Figure 20-1. In the most recent studies, more than one third of adults and 17 percent of children and adolescents in the United States are obese. Although the problem varies from country to country, obesity is also a growing problem worldwide especially in wealthy, highly industrialized nations where food is abundant, and there's little to no physical labor.

Obesity Trends in the U.S.: 1985 – 2010

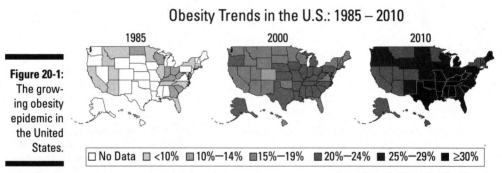

Figure 20-1: The growing obesity epidemic in the United States.

☐ No Data ☐ <10% ◻ 10%–14% ■ 15%–19% ■ 20%–24% ■ 25%–29% ■ ≥30%

Source: Centers for Disease Control and Prevention

Canada's published statistics for 2005 show the rate of obese Canadians (BMI higher than 30) almost doubled between 1978 and 2005, rising from 13.8 percent to 24.3 percent of the adult population or almost 1 in 4 individuals. Aside from the obese, in 2005, 36 percent of the adult Canadian population was considered overweight while only 39 percent had a healthy weight. And the United Kingdome isn't far behind. Data compiled by the Health and Social Care Information Centre reports there's been a marked increase in obesity rates over the past eight years: In 1993, 13 percent of men and 16 percent of women were obese; in 2011, this rose to 24 percent for men and 26 percent for women.

Explaining obesity medically

Most people don't go to the doctor to talk about their weight. More often they go to deal with some of the side effects of overweight and obesity. If your blood pressure is high, you've developed type 2 diabetes, or if you find yourself exhausted day in and day out from not sleeping well, whether or not you want to visit your physician, you may find yourself with no other choice. It may be difficult to treat any condition brought about by overweight or obesity without discussing the root cause.

If your doctor is doing a thorough work-up, one of the first things she may do after a physical exam is a quick calculation of your *BMI,* or *body mass index.*

For adults, scientists and doctors determine overweight and obesity ranges by using the ratio of weight to height to calculate BMI. Figure 20-2 shows the chart used.

Although these numbers provide a benchmark, if you're facing serious health risks that require weight loss, ultimately they're only numbers, and they can't measure healthfulness, which is your ultimate goal no matter what your weight.

Weight in Pounds

Height	100	110	120	130	140	150	160	170	180	190	200	210	220	230	240	250
4'	30.5	33.6	36.6	39.7	42.7	45.8	48.8	51.9	54.9	58.0	61.0	64.1	67.1	70.2	73.2	76.3
4'2"	28.1	30.9	33.7	36.6	39.4	42.2	45.0	47.8	50.6	53.4	56.2	59.1	61.9	64.7	67.5	70.3
4'4"	26.0	28.6	31.2	33.8	36.4	39.0	41.6	44.2	46.8	49.4	52.0	54.6	57.2	59.8	62.4	65.0
4'6"	24.1	26.5	28.9	31.3	33.8	36.2	38.6	41.0	43.4	45.8	48.2	50.6	53.0	55.4	57.9	60.3
4'8"	22.4	24.7	26.9	29.1	31.4	33.6	35.9	38.1	40.4	42.6	44.8	47.1	49.3	51.6	53.8	56.0
4'10"	20.9	23.0	25.1	27.2	29.3	31.3	33.4	35.5	37.6	39.7	41.8	43.9	46.0	48.1	50.2	52.2
5'	19.5	21.5	23.4	25.4	27.3	29.3	31.2	33.2	35.2	37.1	39.1	41.0	43.0	44.9	46.9	48.8
5'2"	18.3	20.1	21.9	23.8	25.6	27.4	29.3	31.1	32.9	34.7	36.6	38.4	40.2	42.1	43.9	45.7
5'4"	17.2	18.9	20.6	22.3	24.0	25.7	27.5	29.2	30.9	32.6	34.3	36.0	37.8	39.5	41.2	42.9
5'6"	16.1	17.8	19.4	21.0	22.6	24.2	25.8	27.4	29.0	30.7	32.3	33.9	35.5	37.1	38.7	40.3
5'8"	15.2	16.7	18.2	19.8	21.3	22.8	24.3	25.8	27.4	28.9	30.4	31.9	33.4	35.0	36.5	38.0
5'10"	14.3	15.8	17.2	18.7	20.1	21.5	23.0	24.4	25.8	27.3	28.7	30.1	31.6	33.0	34.4	35.9
6'	13.6	14.9	16.3	17.6	19.0	20.3	21.7	23.1	24.4	25.8	27.1	28.5	29.8	31.2	32.5	33.9
6'2"	12.8	14.1	15.4	16.7	18.0	19.3	20.5	21.8	23.1	24.4	25.7	27.0	28.2	29.5	30.8	32.1
6'4"	12.2	13.4	14.6	15.8	17.0	18.3	19.5	20.7	21.9	23.1	24.3	25.6	26.8	28.0	29.2	30.4
6'6"	11.6	12.7	13.9	15.0	16.2	17.3	18.5	19.6	20.8	22.0	23.1	24.3	25.4	26.6	27.7	28.9
6'8"	11.0	12.1	13.2	14.3	15.4	16.5	17.6	18.7	19.8	20.9	22.0	23.1	24.2	25.3	26.4	27.5
6'10"	10.5	11.5	12.5	13.6	14.6	15.7	16.7	17.8	18.8	19.9	20.9	22.0	23.0	24.0	25.1	26.1
7'	10.0	11.0	12.0	13.0	13.9	14.9	15.9	16.9	17.9	18.9	19.9	20.9	21.9	22.9	23.9	24.9

Height in Feet and Inches

☐ Underweight ■ Normal ☐ Overweight ■ Obese

Figure 20-2: A standard BMI chart.

Source: National Institutes of Health

Calculating your BMI

If you're overweight or obese, your body mass index, or BMI, is one of the first numbers your physician looks at. The formula is the same for adults and children and for all genders and ethnicities. BMI is an indirect measure of a person's body fat. However, the BMI formula does differ slightly depending on whether you're using the English or metric system.

With the English system:

1. Multiply your height in inches times your height in inches — height squared.

2. Divide your weight by the number you arrived at in Step 1.

3. Multiply the number you came up with in Step 2 by 703.

Weight in pounds (lbs) divided by height in inches (in) squared and multiplied by a conversion factor of 703 (weight (lbs) / [height (in)^2] × 703).

For example, for a person weighing 150 pounds who's 5'5" (65 inches) tall, the

BMI calculation is $[150 \div (65)^2] \times 703 = 24.96$

If you're using the metric system, you can calculate BMI by using a similar formula: Divide your weight in kilograms by your height in meters, squared. Because height is commonly measured in centimeters, divide your height in centimeters by 100 to obtain your height in meters.

So, the formula for a person 165 centimeters tall, or 1.65 meters, who weighs 68 kilograms looks like this: $68 \div 1.65^2 = 24.98$

You may already have a sense of where you may fall on the spectrum, but BMI can give you and your doctor a more concrete idea. An adult who has a BMI between 25 and 29.9 is considered overweight, and an adult who has a BMI of 30 or higher is considered obese. In unusual cases, such as those of athletes, BMI may identify someone as overweight or obese even though they do not have excess body fat, but for most people, BMI correctly correlates with the amount of body fat.

Some doctors use other methods of estimating body fat and body fat distribution including

- ✔ Measurements of skinfold thickness and waist circumference

- ✔ Calculation of waist-to-hip circumference ratios

- ✔ Techniques such as ultrasound, CT scan, and magnetic resonance imaging (MRI)

In recent years, the definitions of obesity have been expanded to account for an ever more complicated picture of who's at most risk of health problems and early death due to weight-related issues. According to the World Health Organization (WHO), obesity is classified as

- ✔ Class I for a BMI between 30 and 34.9 (moderate risk of mortality)

✔ Class II for a BMI between 35 and 39.9 (high risk of mortality)

 ✔ Class III for a BMI ≥ 40 (very high risk of mortality)

If you've recently seen your doctor, you may already know your BMI. But if you don't know it, take a moment to calculate it using the formulas in the sidebar.

One of the other parts of your exam may be to measure your waist circumference. Though it may seem unnecessary when you already know your BMI, the health risks of being overweight or obese are more serious for people with excess abdominal fat. If you store fat around your abdomen, you're at greater risk for disease no matter what your weight but especially if you're overweight or obese.

Excess abdominal fat is clinically defined as a waist circumference greater than 40 inches in men and greater than 35 inches in women.

Assessing your health risks

Altogether, obesity affects at least nine organ systems of the body. If you're overweight or obese, you may have heard your doctor talk about metabolic syndrome, a group of risk factors that raises your chances of developing heart disease or other chronic diseases. The metabolic risk factors include

 ✔ Large waistline, particularly with fat concentrated around your waist

 ✔ High cholesterol, meaning that you have high levels of triglycerides and low LDL or good cholesterol

 ✔ High blood pressure

 ✔ High blood sugar

Are you an apple or a pear?

Has anyone ever asked you if you're an apple or a pear? If you're a pear, you store weight in your hips, thighs, and buttocks, but if you're an apple, you store weight in your abdomen. Even though you may not think the shape of your body matters if you're overweight or obese, it may make all the difference as far as your risk of chronic diseases.

Though doctors don't know exactly why, chances are the distribution of excess fat tissue around the abdominal organs puts more stress on the heart and circulatory system thus increasing risk of heart disease and other related conditions.

The more of these risk factors you have, the higher your risk of heart disease, stroke, or diabetes to name a few. If you already know that you suffer from one of these risk factors, check with your doctor to see whether you're affected by others you don't know about especially because overweight and obesity increase your disease risk even further. In fact, if you have metabolic syndrome, you're twice as likely to develop heart disease and five times as likely to develop diabetes as someone who doesn't.

In addition, you may also be at risk for

- ✔ Gout, the build-up of uric acid in the joints is a very painful form of arthritis where the joints to become swollen, red, and hot. Overweight and obesity is a primary factor in the development of gout.
- ✔ Gallbladder disease and gallstones.
- ✔ Joint pain or osteoarthritis.
- ✔ Cancer.
- ✔ Early death.

Just as overweight or obesity comes on slowly, you may not experience the most dangerous effects of these diseases right away. But over time, they can worsen with continued weight gain, and some symptoms and risks may get harder to control with medication than they were when you were first diagnosed.

Good health is the goal. Over time, yo-yo dieting can be much more risky and harder on your body than obesity. Setting realistic, attainable goals is a better strategy than trying to make dramatic, unsustainable changes.

Unfortunately, you may have also noticed that depending on whether you're mildly, moderately, or severely obese, your worsening quality of life may be closely linked to increasing body weight and the many medical symptoms and conditions that may result. Though it may be difficult, some conditions only improve through weight loss.

Facing the social and emotional costs of obesity

If you're obese and facing difficulties, you already know that you can't pin all your troubles on just one trigger or situation. Looking at the bigger picture, it's probably a combination of social, psychological, and medical factors contributing to the decline in your general health and your quality of life.

The social and psychological complications of obesity can be as significant as the physical health concerns. If you're obese, and particularly if you fall into the category of extreme obesity, you may experience discrimination and other difficulties in the workplace or in personal relationships which often lead to poor self-esteem, social withdrawal, depression, and other mental health problems.

Interestingly enough, being overweight or obese doesn't put you in the minority in many countries, especially in the United States. In fact, if you live in the United States and are overweight, you're part of more than 60 percent of the population. But no matter what the statistics say, you may be extremely hard on yourself and on others for weight-related reasons. Whether you're more self-conscious or people around you are more judgmental or both, you may go through the world with the sense that

✔ Everyone is watching you when you eat with friends and family either at home or in a restaurant.

✔ Everyone thinks you just need more discipline and willpower.

✔ You never know where you stand at work. You wonder whether you're being passed over for a promotion because of how you look.

✔ You may be putting your relationships at risk. Very often obesity negatively affects your ability to be intimate. There may also be a strain on any close relationship if a loved one is often worried by the increasing overweight

Though there has been some progress in recent years toward removing some of the stigma around overweight and obesity, there's still a long way to go. Until then, you may find yourself in uncomfortable positions more often than you'd like, both literally and figuratively, and the feeling may take more of a toll than you'd like to admit.

Looking at the societal implications

Numbers don't lie, and one of the clearest and most unfortunate pieces of information to emerge from the studies on obesity is that obesity is not an equal opportunity condition.

In the United States, the overweight and obesity rates are increasing across all racial and ethnic groups. However, according to the CDC, compared with Whites, Blacks have 51 percent higher and Hispanics had 21 percent higher obesity rates, which means that in order to reduce racial and ethnic disparities in obesity rates, there must be more outreach and education in the communities that need it most. Figure 20-3 shows the survey results in graphic form.

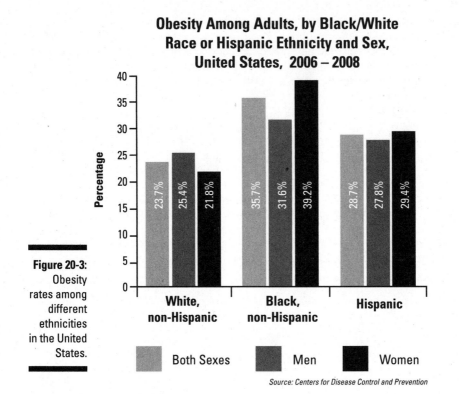

Figure 20-3:
Obesity
rates among
different
ethnicities
in the United
States.

According to data from the Canadian Community Health Survey, Aboriginal men and women had the highest prevalence of overweight and obesity; East/Southeast Asians, the lowest. Independent of age, household income, education, and physical activity, Aboriginal people had elevated odds of overweight and obesity compared with Whites; South Asians and East/Southeast Asians had significantly lower odds. Recent immigrants (then years or less) had significantly lower prevalence of overweight, compared with non-immigrants, but this difference tended to disappear over time.

At least three reasons may account for the racial and ethnic differences in obesity:

✔ **Diet and exercise opportunities:** Differences still exist in access to affordable, healthful foods and safe locations to be physically active. Limited access to both can negatively impact diet and physical activity levels. For example, some low-income neighborhoods don't have full-service grocery stores with fresh produce, and people living there may be dependent on convenience stores for food shopping.

✔ **Attitude about weight:** Individual attitudes and cultural norms related to body weight vary. For example, the traditional foods may not represent a balanced diet. In addition, some cultures put a high value on a curvaceous or plump body for women and see it as a sign of physical strength in men.

✔ **Income level:** Poverty rates among African-Americans and Hispanics, as well as other minority communities, are significantly higher than among Caucasians, and both physical and sexual abuse is reportedly more prevalent in lower income groups. There's a frequent and common link between shame and fear of abuse and the need to eat to self-soothe and numb those feelings.

To reduce racial and ethnic disparities in the prevalence of obesity, an effective public health response must include policies, programs, and supportive environments through the effort of government, communities, workplaces, schools, families, and individuals. These efforts can't come from outside the community. They're more effective if coming from leaders and organizers within the communities themselves.

Analyzing the economic costs

According to the CDC, in 2008, overall medical care costs related to obesity for adults in the United States were estimated to be as high as $147 billion. Medical costs for an obese person averages $1,429 higher per year than the cost for a person of normal body weight. Obesity also has been linked to reduced worker productivity and chronic absence from work.

The causes of obesity are complicated and numerous, and they occur at social, economic, environmental, family, and individual levels. Life in many first-world countries has become characterized by environments that promote physical inactivity and increased consumption of less healthy food, so it's no wonder disordered eating of all types is on the rise or that binge eating is now being recognized as a diagnosable eating disorder.

Public health approaches that can reach large numbers of people in multiple settings — such as in childcare facilities, workplaces, schools, community centers, and health care facilities — are needed to help people make healthier choices. As we establish throughout this book, the easier it is for someone to choose a healthier food option, the more likely he is not to fall into a binge. Policy makers are starting to recognize the power of how healthy easy, options can make a difference. Policy and lifestyle approaches that make healthy choices available, affordable, and easy can be used to raise awareness and support people who struggle with overeating and want to make healthy changes.

Understanding the Connection between Binge Eating and Obesity

Although the majority of people suffering from binge eating disorder are overweight or obese, the majority of people who are obese are not suffering from binge eating disorder. In fact, less than five percent of the obese population is diagnosed with BED.

People become obese for all sorts of reasons, but only a small group meet the diagnostic criteria for binge eating disorder. Within this group, some may maintain a weight within the normal or even overweight range, but for most, regular episodes of compulsive overeating or binge eating take an inevitable toll on the body in the form of weight gain.

Everyone is different, but if you're a binge eater, you can consume a very large amount of calories in a single episode of bingeing even if you don't know exactly how much you've eaten. Binge eaters typically turn to junk food or empty, carbohydrate-laden food (also known as _beige comfort foods_) during binges. Many of these foods are heavily processed and made almost exclusively from whole milk, white flour, and/or white sugar including ice cream, baked goods, and pasta. The average binge can consist of 2,000 to 5,000 calories or more. The frequent consumption of massive amounts of calories inevitably leads to weight gain.

It's important to note that even if you might not technically have binge eating disorder, you may still be eating far more than your body needs. Over time, repeatedly eating for reasons other than physical hunger results in weight gain unless you're offsetting your overeating with compensatory behaviors such as over-exercising or yo-yo dieting.

What that means is that whether or not you're a binge eater, the impact on your body may be the same. Although the psychological treatment may vary depending on what drives your overeating, the physical result — overweight and obesity — puts your health at risk no matter what the underlying motivation.

Seeking the Right Kind of Treatment

While obesity is often a result of BED and the two conditions need to be treated together, some aspects of treatment are distinct, especially when an obesity-related disease is concerned.

Assessing psychological versus physical concerns

As we say throughout this chapter, it's difficult, if not impossible, to separate the health issues caused by obesity and the psychological issues that drive binge eating, compulsive overeating, emotional eating, or any abnormal eating behavior along the eating disorder continuum. If you're thinking about making changes on your own or seeking treatment from professionals, chances are that it's for a combination of reasons discussed in Chapter 12 including, among others:

- ✔ Vanity or shame about how you look or how frequently you change clothing sizes
- ✔ Being fed up with the feeling of being out of control
- ✔ Being scared of present or future health consequences
- ✔ Fear of impacting others in your family, such as your children, who may learn such behaviors or maladaptive coping skills

Even though slowing and eventually stopping binge eating and compulsive overeating is a process that often includes psychotherapists, psychiatrists, dietitians and/or other specialists, if you're obese and suffering from life-threatening conditions such as heart disease, high blood pressure, or high cholesterol, you must see your doctor first and develop a plan to manage these health concerns. A carefully chosen professional team can evaluate and assess your medical conditions and not only determine if you're at risk for conditions you haven't developed yet exist but can also offer concrete, helpful steps toward change.

For many people, it's possible to manage high blood pressure, high cholesterol, heart disease, or any other medical issue brought on by obesity through an outpatient team, but there are some cases when a residential treatment program might be the best choice for you. For some, inpatient treatment may offer the contained, supportive structure that you need to move past old habits and take on new patterns for the long haul. In addition, sometimes medical monitoring is needed when making big changes in these ways. If this is something you're considering, please be sure your professional team helps you choose the right facility, taking into consideration populations served, logistics, cost, and reputation.

Balancing necessary nutrition needs with the delicate treatment of BED

Every binge eater is different and that means that each person's recovery plan is different. That's especially true if you're obese and trying to stop bingeing. If your health is at risk, your psychotherapist or dietitian may find some typically used techniques inappropriate in your case.

For example, intuitive eating is commonly promoted as a practice in the treatment of all eating disorders, binge eating in particular. *Intuitive eating* is an approach to eating that teaches you how to create a healthy relationship between your food, mind, and body by showing you how to recognize physical hunger and satiety cues, not just ravenousness and busting fullness. This recognition is a critical step in finding out how to regulate your food intake and not feel deprived in the process. With intuitive eating, food is not labeled good or bad, and no foods are forbidden. For many people struggling with BED, the idea of being able to eat something considered forbidden, like desserts or sweets, can be very empowering and a welcome relief to the all-or-nothing mentality that led to endless cycles of the swinging pendulum of overeating versus dieting.

But if you're obese and coping with serious medical conditions, you may need to prioritize dietary restrictions related to your health and well-being over psychotherapeutic techniques. Working with a therapist who's familiar with both obesity and disordered eating can be a critical part of moving forward toward less bingeing. Even if you're just getting started and working through some of the ideas in this book on your own, remember that your health is your first priority.

For example, if you're a binge eater who's obese and has insulin-dependent type 2 diabetes, having cookies or other sweets may be hazardous to your health. Even if you eat sweets in moderation, they'll affect your blood sugar, and you'll need to adjust your insulin. In this case, teaching intuitive eating won't necessarily work because your health depends on not eating sweets at all.

If you have the chance to work with a clinical team, try to find those who have worked with obese patients suffering from binge eating. Experience matters in these cases because knowledgeable professionals can offer a targeted and personality-specific variety of treatment choices that can help create a long-term health treatment plan at a pace that is manageable and, most importantly, sustainable for the long haul.

Part V

Providing Help: Advice for Family and Friends

Five Things Not to Do If You Want to Help Someone with BED

- ✔ **Don't focus on weight loss.** Asking "How much weight have you lost?" or "How much do you want to lose?" is a natural question, but weight loss isn't the point of treatment and may prevent your loved one from coming to you if she thinks that's the only measure of her progress.

- ✔ **Don't work harder at recovery than the binge eater.** The binge eater in your life needs to be doing most of the work and driving the process of recovery. It's not that you shouldn't help, but if you find yourself doing all the grocery shopping, keeping a calendar of treatment appointments, or having to cajole him to go to the appointments, it's time to re-evaluate. You probably have great intentions, but true recovery from binge eating requires that the binge eater himself find a reason to move forward and make progress.

- ✔ **Don't sabotage a binge eater by bribing her to stop.** Think twice about offering to trade less bingeing for some sort of reward. It may sound like a cliché, but the reasons for recovery have to come from the binge eater herself, not from outside sources. You may think you're helping by offering incentives, but in the long run, you may really sabotage your friend's or loved one's efforts.

- ✔ **Don't make paying for treatment dependent on results.** Getting treatment for binge eating can be somewhat costly and may not be covered by insurance. It's an act of kindness and generosity to pay for part or all of your friend's or loved one's therapy, but if you decide to contribute, making demands or expecting results just because of your financial commitment can be counterproductive.

- ✔ **Don't be the food police.** That your friend needs to stop binge eating may sound obvious, but telling someone to simply stop eating or doling out advice about what a binge eater should or should not eat always works against the binger's efforts, no matter how well-intentioned. It simply feels like judgment and criticism. Also, you're probably not offering any information your loved one doesn't already know. The core of the matter is that there is a disconnect between what she knows and what she does. That is the therapeutic work she must do for herself.

Go to www.dummies.com/extras/overcomingbingeeating for tips on how to help a recovering binge eater.

In this part . . .

✔ Finding ways to help a loved one with binge eating disorder (BED) is at hand. Information here tells you how to be most effective in aiding your loved one's recovery.

✔ Exploring ways family members can affect both the onset of BED and recovery from it can bring new insights. Family relationships are multilayered and sometimes multigenerational — a problem that afflicted your grandparent may have relevance for your child.

✔ Changing your routines around food to accommodate the needs of a binge eater can provide a healthier diet for everyone.

✔ Making sure that your own emotional needs are taken care of gives you the ability to offer meaningful support to a friend or loved one with BED.

Chapter 21

Helping Someone with Binge Eating Disorder

. . . .

In This Chapter

▶ Taking the first steps together

▶ Supporting a friend or family member who needs you

▶ Approaching someone keeping a secret about bingeing

▶ Protecting and caring for yourself when your offer to help is refused

. . . .

*F*or someone who binge eats, opening up to friends and family about eating issues may be one of the most difficult and important steps she can take toward recovery. And if you're the loved one or a close friend of someone looking for support and encouragement on her journey away from bingeing, emotional eating, or compulsive overeating, you may be wondering what you can do to help.

For a binge eater, having a support system can make all the difference in overcoming the disorder. Changing longstanding eating habits and examining the reasons she's been using eating as a coping mechanism can be a challenging process that no one should have to face alone. That doesn't mean that as a friend or family member, you need to or should do all the work. But more than likely, you can make small, but significant, changes in your relationship that will contribute in a constructive, long-term way. Most of all, just being there and staying positive and nonjudgmental is important.

If you know someone who's open about her binge eating and needs help, it's generally best to wait to be asked for your support. Even the most well-intended comments and efforts can easily be misinterpreted as judgmental. By the same token, binge eaters often feel that they're not entitled to ask for assistance or may simply be too afraid. You'll need to rely on your own assessment of your relationship with the binge eater to know if and when to start asking.

In this chapter, we discuss both general and specific ways you can help someone in your life who's a binge eater, touching on specific strategies as well as the dos and don'ts.

Telling the Truth and Making Progress Together

Eating disorders can be baffling and heartbreaking for the people suffering from them as well as for loved ones witnessing the struggles. If you live with or are friends with someone who binge eats, you may cycle through a complicated set of your own emotions toward the person and toward the eating behaviors you (and perhaps your friend or loved one) would like to see change. Sometimes you may feel sympathetic, sometimes angry, sometimes frustrated, or sometimes desperate — it's difficult to watch someone you love suffer.

But if the time has come to swing into action on behalf of your friend or loved one, it may also be the moment to set aside your own emotions and difficulties for a while. That's not to say that your feelings aren't valid or real, but helping someone recover from binge eating requires a single-minded focus, and you may need to seek out support for yourself as part of a therapy group or with an individual psychotherapist. There will come a time when you have a chance to voice your feelings, but at the beginning of this process a binge eater may be so overwhelmed by her own feelings of shame and guilt that she may not be able to take on relationship issues at the same time.

Being aware of a binge eater's world

Many people with binge eating disorder (BED) are embarrassed, ashamed, and secretive about their bingeing and their inability to stop on their own. Some believe that they've successfully kept the truth from friends and loved ones, and the idea of sharing their struggle can be terrifying. In particular, it's difficult for someone with BED to open up to someone who doesn't know what it's like to have an eating disorder of any kind — especially when it's not one of the better-known eating disorders such as anorexia or bulimia. Let's face it — so often this particular eating disorder is thought to be simply a lack of discipline, laziness, or the like.

Following are just some of the questions your loved one may be asking her-self as she contemplates sharing the fact of her eating disorder with you:

- How will he react?
- What will she say?
- Will he understand?
- Will she think I'm crazy?
- Will he be mad at me?
- Will she stop wanting to be around me?
- Will he leave me?

If you're afraid of asking about your loved one's binge eating, imagine how she must be feeling. Before confiding in even the most supportive and loving friends and family, someone who binge eats can spend days, weeks, even months trying to figure out what to say, how to say it, and how the other person is going to react to her confession. She probably has a very real fear of being rejected, judged, or misunderstood.

Keeping the basics of helping in mind

Helping someone with BED is complicated, and even if you have the best intentions, it may be more difficult than you imagined. You may be faced with the dual role of spouse, parent, sibling, best friend, or boss, and now also that of a primary support person in your loved one's recovery. Knowing your abilities and boundaries is crucial for helping someone else as well as keeping yourself healthy in the process.

The following list details techniques to help a friend or loved one who has an eating disorder:

- **Encourage him to get professional help.** The longer BED remains undi-agnosed and untreated, the more difficult it is to overcome, so urge your loved one to see a health professional right away.

- **Be a supportive listener.** Try to listen without judgment and make sure she knows you care. If your loved one slips up and binges on the road to recovery, remind her that it doesn't mean she can't get better. (Chapter 15 speaks about recovering from relapses.)

- **Offer support, not judgment.** Aim for positive comments only. Binge eaters feel bad enough about themselves already; using negative language only works against recovery efforts. Be optimistic by stating how much you care and ask how you can help in a constructive way.

✔ **Avoid insults, lectures, and guilt trips.** Lecturing, getting frustrated, or issuing ultimatums to a binge eater only increases stress and makes the situation worse. Instead, make it clear that you care about his health and happiness and that you'll continue to be there throughout the recovery process.

✔ **Lead by example.** By eating healthily, exercising, and managing stress without food, you indirectly help your loved one. Binge eaters (just like all people with eating disorders) need healthy examples. By being a healthy person in both mind and body, you're supporting her recovery.

✔ **Don't be the food police.** One thing is almost *never* helpful: monitoring what someone eats. Being told what to eat, how much to eat, being watched while eating, or hiding, limiting, or commenting on food choices can create a problem with food for just about anybody. Imagine how your behavior affects someone who is literally thinking about food all the time. Resist the pull to monitor, comment, or offer advice about eating. Even if you're asked to hide or limit food, or asked to say something if you see her eating too much, restrain yourself. You can't make someone eat or not eating something forever, so best not to start now.

✔ **Take care of yourself.** Know when to seek advice for yourself from a counselor or health professional. Helping someone deal with their BED can be stressful, and it will help you help them if you have your own support system in place.

Leaving all blame at the door

The most important thing to remember when you're trying to help someone who binge eats or who shows any signs of dangerous eating behaviors is to avoid placing blame — don't blame yourself and don't blame the person who binges. Instead, your collective focus and treatment itself should be on making the changes your loved one needs to get better.

Try to concentrate on what's keeping the unhealthy behaviors in place and what purpose binge eating serves in your loved one's life, as opposed to fixating on the origin of the problem. Discovering the origin and causes will slowly unfold over time and are a part of, but not the only aspect, of recovery or change. Ask yourself what function the eating disorder serves and pay attention to your own intuition and the feelings of your loved one. This means you need to focus on actively listening to each other and not get caught up in the blame game.

Helping Someone Who Asks for Help

If someone you love comes to you about binge eating or other kinds of compulsive overeating, she may or may not have an idea of what she needs from you. The request you hear may be as general as "I need help, and I'm not sure what to do" or as specific as "I've been struggling with this, and here's what I need from you."

Whether you're caught totally off-guard by the news that your loved one binges or whether you've been waiting for this moment for a long time, a direct request for help is an opportunity to make a big difference in someone's life and recovery. You may not be sure where to start, what to say, or even how to say it, but by approaching the situation with compassion and openness, the two of you can figure it out together.

Some examples of what to say are:

- ✔ I'm here for you, and I want whatever you want for yourself.
- ✔ I've been worried about you, and I'm glad you're talking to me about this.
- ✔ You're not alone, and it's not your fault. We're in this together if you think I can help.

The right kind of help is different for everyone. An open and honest conversation can lead to constructive, effective ways to support your loved one's journey to recovery. A few practical things you can do include:

- ✔ **Remove trigger foods from the home.** We cannot emphasize strongly enough that this must be a wholly collaborative process, one in which both you and your loved one decide together what to remove, when to remove it, and how to go about it. This must include a discussion of how you can eat the foods you want while allowing the person with an eating disorder to be in a healthier and more supportive living and eating environment.

One suggestion is to get single servings of the foods your loved one finds triggering and to purchase the food only when you know you're going to eat it. For example, if you're craving ice cream, grab a cone from your local ice cream parlor instead of buying a half-gallon from the supermarket and keeping it in the freezer. Buying single servings may not be as economical or convenient, but you'll truly be helping your loved one recover by avoiding unnecessary food triggers at home.

✔ **Help with providing distractions.** One technique many binge eaters use to prevent a binge is to make a list of activities they can use as a distraction when the urge to binge comes on. Let your loved one know that, if you're available, she can always call or spend time with you until the urge to binge passes. Talking about other things or doing something unrelated to food or eating is an excellent strategy to throw off the original temptation to binge.

✔ **Don't talk about dieting — anyone's dieting.** Diets most often set people up to binge. During the initial phase of recovery, a binge eater's goal is simply to decrease the frequency and amount of food consumed in a binge, and to eventually become binge-free. Even after recovery, it's important to keep the focus mainly on not bingeing rather than on losing weight.

✔ **Don't make comments about weight, shape, or looks.** Try not to point out how thin someone else looks in a magazine or on the street. The expectations that society puts on people in the media, and on women in particular, greatly contribute to the emotional and psychological reasons your loved one has an eating disorder in the first place. It's important to be part of changing, even to a small degree, your own and your loved one's perception of society's focus on image and being thin at any cost.

✔ **Arrange non-food related activities.** Many social gatherings revolve around food, but tons of fun activities exist that don't have much or anything to do with eating. Positive social experiences without a focus on food reinforce that there are many, many ways to spend time with a friend or family member without the risk of bingeing. Try taking a walk, attending a concert, relaxing at a spa, going bowling, or simply window shopping. You can include anything that's fun, relaxing, and doesn't involve food on the list of options.

Making the First Move

Talking to a loved one about suspected binge eating, emotional eating, compulsive overeating, or other eating disorders is important and courageous. But it's wise to keep in mind that even if someone needs help, she may not be able to ask for it for a variety of reasons. By beginning the conversation, you're letting your loved one know that you're paying attention, that you value your relationship with her, and that you care about her well-being. Even though some people can ask for help, others may never open up about binge eating without safe encouragement.

Using "I" statements in difficult conversations

Whether you're talking about binge eating or any other difficult topic, you can usually make more headway with a friend or loved one by using "I" statements rather than "you" statements.

An "I" statement focuses the conversation on the speaker and strips away the blame that comes through when you begin a sentence with "you." For example:

✔ **"You" statement:** You really shouldn't binge on leftovers in the middle of the night. You're going to kill yourself if you keep doing that.

   "I" statement: I'm worried about you. When you binge, I feel worried and sad.

✔ **"You" statement:** You promised me you'd go to the movies. When you get like this, you always let me down.

   "I" statement: I'd love to go to the movies tonight and I'd rather go with you than without you. When you retreat from doing things together, I feel sad not to be with you.

✔ **"You" Statement:** You always overreact to everything and make yourself binge.

✔ **"I" statement:** I can only imagine what you must be feeling. I'm sad and concerned when you hurt yourself by bingeing.

By using "I" statements, you're forced to articulate your own feelings in a way that can make both the speaker and the listener feel better. Oftentimes, if someone is in the midst of dealing with a particularly serious problem like binge eating, it may be more difficult for her to realize that her behavior is negatively affecting others. An "I" statement reminds her that what she does matters, and that other people love and cherish the relationship they have with her.

On the flip side, just because you're ready doesn't mean that you should dive head first into a heart-to-heart conversation. Having the right strategy and support team in place for you and the one you love is crucial. Asking about binge eating behaviors and talking about your concerns needs to happen in a thoughtful and considered way because your approach, however well-intended, could quickly backfire if your loved one is not ready to get help or if you begin the conversation in a way that's perceived as threatening.

Depending on how well you know someone, it may feel right to approach him individually to express your love and concern for his health and emotional and physical well being. Opening up about binge eating can be a painful and embarrassing topic, but if the two of you are close, allowing him a private opportunity to be truthful and to express the complicated set of emotions he has about bingeing can be a great gift.

Even if your initial talk doesn't produce immediate action, you may still have planted the possibility of change in someone's mind. Besides, keeping secrets takes time and energy, so having one person who knows the truth can be a great relief to a binge eater.

Before you can help someone else, remind yourself why you're doing this and prepare yourself for the conversation. Ask yourself these questions

✔ **Why now?** The earlier someone is able to address the underlying reasons and behaviors associated with binge eating or any kind of eating disorder, the easier it is to treat. In addition, someone who suffers from an eating disorder or who overeats as a way to self-soothe is probably in a lot of emotional and physical pain. An open conversation may be the first step in getting her on the road to recovery.

If you feel comfortable starting the conversation the first chance you get, by all means, go ahead. But if you don't, one of the easiest ways to begin is to look for an opening or some sort of change that might naturally lead to a discussion of binge eating. Some ideas are

- **Medical concerns:** Has there been a development in her medical history? If your friend has recently been diagnosed with high blood pressure, high cholesterol, heart disease, diabetes, or any of the many conditions associated with bingeing and/or overweight and obesity, it may feel more natural to segue from a conversation about the condition to one about the underlying causes. Be aware that although you may be concerned, there's no guarantee that you're loved one will be equally alarmed.

If you're thinking of raising your concerns about health problems as an opening for a discussion of binge eating, don't wait for the situation to deteriorate to the point of being life threatening.

- **A change in social functioning:** Many, but certainly not all, binge eaters have active social lives in spite of their eating behaviors. They're in romantic relationships, have friends, raise children, and go to work and school. If someone you love suddenly refuses to go to work or to school, it may be time to have an honest conversation about what's really going on. Furthermore, if you notice your loved one isolating for any reason, you may want to try a gentle attempt to get to the heart of the matter.

- **A disruption in the activities of daily life:** If you're close to someone, a dramatic change in what's known as *activities of daily life,* or *ADLs,* may be an important clue that her binge eating and psychological state has gone downhill. Perhaps you notice someone has stopped showering or that his house has gotten so messy you can't walk through the living room. Maybe his pets haven't been fed or his car has so much trash in it that it's impossible to drive. Any one of these and many other types of disturbances in ADLs may indicate a new, more serious issue.

✔ **Is this just troublesome to me or is this truly a problem?** We all have personal preferences and ways we choose to live our lives. We pursue a variety of careers, marry or don't, start families or decide not to have children. Our outlooks on life can be extremely different. For some people, occasional binge eating, while a concern for you, may not be a concern for them. If this is the case, you may need to simply acknowledge the binge eating and nothing more.

✔ **Why should I say something at all?** Because you care. If you're reading this, then there's someone in your life whose health and well-being concerns you. You don't have to be a parent, spouse, or relative to intervene; friends often play an important role in recovery. Don't underestimate the power of your love and commitment.

An open conversation is important because it breaks down the walls of denial and secrecy surrounding the eating disorder and begins to allow the person to accept help. Eating disorders are not about food. They are about underlying, unresolved issues about which food is being used to self-soothe.

✔ **What if the person gets angry with me?** It's common for someone who binge eats to get angry or deny that there's a problem when it first comes up. You should prepare yourself for this reaction, but don't let it deter you. That person's health is at stake, and her health is ultimately more important than her feeling upset with you. Even though the person may not be able to express it at first, underneath it all she may be relieved to have the truth out in the open.

✔ **What if it doesn't work?** No open, honest, loving conversation is a failure. At the very least, you've expressed your love and concern, which is a very powerful thing. And now the sufferer knows that someone else is aware of her problem and that help is available. Recovery ultimately depends on whether or not the sufferer is ready to begin the healing journey.

✔ **What if it does work?** If your loved one tells you she's ready to do something about her binge eating, it's important to have the right resources available. Even though you may not know where to start yourself, you can ask your physician if he knows someone. You may also want to go online before you talk and seek out resources not only for the best ways to have this conversation but also for referrals for therapists, therapy groups, dietitians, Overeaters Anonymous meetings, or any other help that you may think is appropriate and/or available in your area. More information about online resources is available at www.dummies.com/ extras/overcomingbingeeating.

If you're reading this book and don't suffer from an eating disorder yourself, you probably have a pretty strong suspicion that someone you love is in trouble. If you choose to begin a conversation with that person in an effort to help her, make sure to keep the focus on the specific concerns you have about the binge-like behaviors. Bringing up other behaviors that you think should be changed will seem critical and judgmental and will put your loved one in a defensive position.

Get help and support for yourself. Even if you really want to help, remind yourself that there's only so much you can do. Set appropriate limits and boundaries for yourself and seek help if you feel overwhelmed, depressed, angry, or sad by this process or by any of the situations it creates.

Coping with Someone who Doesn't Want Help

If your friend or loved one who struggles with binge eating isn't ready, there may be very little you can do. Of course, it's frustrating and sad to see someone you love deteriorating, but long-term success depends on internal motivation on the part of the sufferer. Bribes or other forms of external motivation may work for a while, ultimately those strategies backfire and do little to address the real reasons a binge eater uses eating as a coping mechanism.

Approaching a binge eater who's keeping a secret

Maybe you've noticed the trashcan filled to the brim with empty pastry containers and candy wrappers or perhaps you've woken up in the middle of the night alone and heard rustling in the kitchen. Even if someone you love acts like nothing is going on, if you live with a binge eater, you may already have a sense that something is amiss or you may even know the whole truth.

Unfortunately, if someone is a secret binge eater and not ready to openly discuss her struggle, there's little you can do to help. It's no surprise that binge eating, especially when kept secret, affects relationships. Over time, keeping any kind of secret alienates friends and family from each other. If you live with and love a binge eater, you may have experienced your loved one

- ✔ Choosing to stay home and binge rather than go out with you.
- ✔ Letting you go to bed alone, so she can binge late at night.
- ✔ Hiding food around the house, so he can eat it later without your knowledge.

Someone in the throes of an eating disorder often says he prefers spending time alone rather than with the people he loves or cares for. In addition, binge eating can also cause substantial financial pressures in a relationship if the disorder begins to keep someone from going to work or significantly inflates the household food budget.

In this situation, letting your loved one know you are there for her whenever she's ready maybe all you can do. In the meantime, until your loved one is ready, you may want to discover more about binge eating and other forms of compulsive eating, seek treatment for yourself, or attend a support group.

Taking a step back

At the end of the day, no matter how much support family and friends offer, the most successful recoveries depend on a binge eater's internally driven desire to stop bingeing. If you've talked with your loved one in a gentle, loving way, listened to what he has to say with compassion and understanding, and offered possibilities for change, that may be all you can do. If your loved one isn't willing to accept help from you, you may want to consider backing off for the time being.

Although you may be terribly disappointed, remember that in the long run, any treatment and recovery driven by friends and family may be short-lived. The binge eater herself has to be motivated to get better and to make permanent changes to his ways of thinking, habits, and lifestyle.

You may also want to consider that your loved one does want help, just not from you. If this is the case, the way you can help is to not try to help. It may sound strange, but sometimes it works because it may be too difficult for your loved one to accept your assistance. She may not feel comfortable talking to you about the situation for some reason, and in this case, distancing yourself and not trying to help is its own form of support. Continue to remind her that you're available if she ever needs you, and that until then you're taking a neutral stance and won't interfere.

In the meantime, make sure to take care of yourself and seek your own support system. Even though it's painful, you may also need to spend less time with the person who doesn't want your help.

Chapter 22

Finding Help with Family

· ·

· ·

*W*hether you live alone, are a divorced parent with children, an adult living with a partner in a committed relationship, a teenager living at home with your parents and siblings, an aging adult living with an ailing spouse, or in any of many other possible living situations, at some point on your journey to addressing your overeating, you may choose to seek the support of your family or relatives in your recovery. You may also be reading this not as a binge eater but as the family member of a loved one who is a binge eater. In either case, the aim of this chapter is to identify the ways in which families of all types can help and be helped.

Depending on your situation, your stage in life, and your family's willingness and ability to help you, they can be involved in your recovery in a variety of ways. For children, adolescents, or young adults still living at home, your family can be integral in helping you move towards a life that doesn't include binge eating or compulsive overeating.

It's neither possible nor advisable to treat young people without considering the entire family system. That's because more often than not the binge behaviors and other maladaptive coping methods affect and are affected by families. Families don't *cause* binge eating. However, it's possible that some families may contribute to the problem without realizing it. The good news is that these patterns can be properly identified in the right setting.

On a more practical level, it's also vital to involve the family of a young person, because more often than not parental figures are involved in food preparation, which may require integrating some more healthful changes to benefit not only the binge eater but the whole family.

Sometimes, it may not be a good idea to include family members in the therapeutic or healing process for any of a variety of reasons. For example, some may be too physically or emotionally ill or challenged to be of support. You may perceive someone you live with to be too negative or too anxious to be a helpful resource. Perhaps there are geographical or logistical considerations.

If you choose not to actually meet with certain family members in a therapeutic setting, you can still address even the most challenging situations without them being present via role plays and other psychodrama or therapeutic techniques designed to develop new strategies to deal with family and environments that may have been difficult or painful in the past.

In this chapter, we discuss what makes a family and how families can work together to help someone slow and eventually stop binge eating. We also talk about various methods of family treatment including couples counseling and what it can do for your relationship.

Looking at Various Types of Family

Families come in so many variations. When integrating family into a plan to help someone with any type of eating disorder, family may include anyone who can directly impact the binge eater, whether related by blood, by marriage, or those who are not related at all but serve as a "chosen" family.

For the purposes of family therapy, family can be defined as

- **Family of origin:** This is the family in which you were raised, your mother, father, grandparents, brothers, sisters, aunts, and uncles — anyone you lived with as a child. Some nuclear families are also blended families, which may include step- or half-siblings or parents. Oftentimes, the beginnings of many emotional habits, psychological patterns, and coping mechanisms, both good and bad, can be traced to childhood and adolescence.

- **Extended family:** Extended family includes both near and distant relations such as aunts, uncles, and cousins.

- **Chosen family:** There's no legal bond between you, but you've established a family unit based on emotional interconnectedness. Chosen families can include long-term roommates or any group of adults and/or children living together for an extended period of time who have joined together by choice.

Experts agree that it's almost impossible to successfully treat binge eating or any form of disordered eating without addressing the role family plays, whether actual and/or perceived. However, as you see in this chapter, family therapy takes many forms, and if your family is unavailable to you, be it physically or emotionally, therapeutic alternatives exist to help you deal with these issues without needing to reengage in relationships that may not be good for you.

Understanding the Need for Family Therapy

If you're just beginning your journey to identify, treat, and hopefully end the binge or emotional eating that has come to dominate your life, you may or may not be ready yet to consider involving your family in the process. As we have mentioned, for children, adolescents, and young adults, the family is an integral component of recovery, but an adult binge eater, who may have lived on his own for quite a while, may not need or want to address the complex, ongoing issues he has with his family. For a young adult, it may be enough to begin focusing on his own treatment and address issues related to family over time.

For children, adolescents, or young adults living at home, family therapy may begin early in treatment. For children in particular, it's difficult, if not impossible, to offer therapeutic strategies and solutions outside the context of the child's family. Children and adolescents can't and don't make decisions for the rest of the family, and even young adults who may be more emotionally independent but who are still financially dependent, can't fully recover from binge eating without the support of their parents and siblings.

In either case, whether family therapy is an integral part of your plan to end binge eating from the start or whether it's something you phase in over time if appropriate, it can be quite helpful in moving to curb and eventually cease binge eating or any kind of compulsive overeating.

There are many compelling reasons to consider and include family therapy as part of your long-term therapeutic plan:

- ✔ Family therapy is a proven therapeutic component of successful, long-term recovery.

- ✔ With a supportive family, therapy that includes them can be one way to mitigate the sense of isolation that so often plays a part in the life of chronic binge eaters.

- ✔ Binge eating can often be traced to certain triggers, both real and imagined, that occur within the family environment. In family therapy, a patient and her family can identify and seek to address those triggers together.

- ✔ Family therapy can be very practical and solutions-based so that you can get help with shopping, cooking, scheduling, and other logistics that better support the recovery or healing of the binge eater.

- ✔ Family-based strategies can help take the pressure off food-related family time. It's important to learn active ways to redirect any perceived stressors that exist during family mealtime.

These are just a few of the general reasons that involving your family can be good for the binge eater's psychological and physical health and for the rest of the family's as well. Many family members participate in a loved one's counseling only to find themselves reaping the benefits in unexpected ways.

You may have specific, very personal reasons of your own that drive you to include your own family on your journey. Whatever they may be, your goal is to get there together.

Creating a genogram — Marla's story

Marla is a 25-year-old binge eater who recently began treatment with a psychologist and a nutritionist. For her entire adult life, she's struggled with disordered eating, sometimes bingeing up to twice a day and sometimes not bingeing at all for several months at a time. Although things have been going well and Marla has not been bingeing regularly, she recently was passed over for a promotion, which sent her into a week-long episode. She missed two days of work because she felt she couldn't get out of bed.

This most recent crisis propelled her to call the psychotherapist whose number she'd had in her nightstand drawer for two years. Now she's been seeing that therapist for six weeks, and they're working together on a genogram so that Marla can begin to understand some of what drives her to binge.

Marla's family profile:

✔ **Rachel, mom, age 53:** Obsessive-compulsive tendencies although never diagnosed with OCD. Always dieting and slim but never treated for an eating disorder. She is a corporate lawyer, works 60+ hours/week. Rachel has always encouraged rigorous dieting and exercise. She does not eat dessert, not even birthday cake on her kids' birthdays. Mom is always mad at Dad; Dad ignores mom.

✔ **Jim, dad, age 57:** Emotionally distant, Dad travels frequently for work. He drinks four or more alcoholic drinks a day, although has never admitted to or been treated for substance abuse. He was diagnosed and successfully treated for testicular cancer in his 20s. When at home, he's loving toward his children and frequently showers them with gifts although he's never spent much time with them.

✔ **Toni, age 27:** The oldest child is a perfectionist, goes on diets with mom, has anorexia nervosa (AN) and sees a therapist weekly. Graduated summa cum laude from college, now in law school at Yale and is engaged to Jeff, another Yale law student. Toni is Mom's perfect daughter.

✔ **Marla, age 25:** The middle child, Marla is severely obese and binges daily after work. Her mother first put her on a diet when she was six years old. Marla has a good job at a marketing firm where she's worked since she graduated from college. Even though she was an above average student and is doing well professionally, she has always felt inferior to her straight-A, perfect sister. Mom still pays for Marla to see a diet doctor and nutritionist weekly. Marla is not losing weight.

✔ **Jeremy, age 22:** Jeremy has just graduated from college. An average student and a superb athlete, he is the apple of his mother's eye. He doesn't yet have a job and is living at home again where his mother coddles him. He's rarely reprimanded for his poor work ethic. He calls Marla "fat" in front of the family and is never corrected. He takes medication for attention deficit hyperactivity disorder (ADHD).

- **Aunt Joanne, age 51:** Rachel's sister, Joanne is single and is also a binge eater. Joanne has always struggled with weight and has been hospitalized several times for depression and suicidal thoughts. She suffers from high blood pressure, high cholesterol, and type 2 diabetes. She and Rachel had another sister who died at the age of four in a car accident, but the family has never talked about the death. Joanne is starting to explore this in therapy.

- **Aunt Jane, deceased 1962:** The eldest of the siblings, Jane died in a car accident at age four when Rachel was two and their mother was pregnant with Joanne.

- **Uncle Steven, age 49:** Divorced, an alcohol and drug addict, no one in the family has

seen Steven for ten years. In his 20s he was arrested for selling cocaine, after a brief time in jail, he was released and disappeared. The family knows little about him other than that he's still alive as he sends Christmas cards every year with no return address.

- **Carol, maternal grandmother, age 75:** Highly critical of the entire family, she isn't loving toward her children or grandchildren. She places a lot of emphasis on appearance. Had tuberculosis as a child and breast cancer when she was 60. She is considered cancer-free at this time.

- **Matthew, maternal grandfather, deceased 1966:** He committed suicide three years after his four-year-old daughter died when his surviving children were 6, 4, and 2. He was an alcoholic and drank daily. He was a nice drunk and never hurt his kids physically. His widow Carol tells people he drank himself to death.

With the help of her therapist, Marla created a genogram of her family relationships:

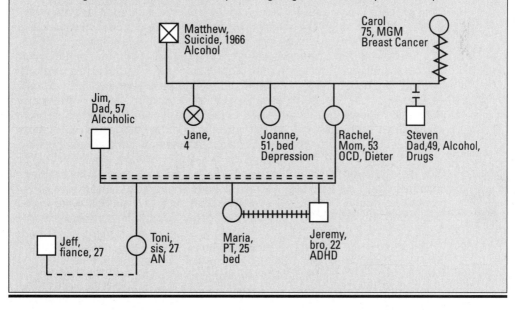

Breaking Down the Different Types of Family Therapy

Just as an individual therapist uses different methods, a good family therapist uses a variety of techniques and strategies depending on the overall objectives and what may be most effective. Many adapt approaches used in individual sessions such as talk therapy, cognitive behavior therapy, alternate coping skills for conflict resolution, and many other therapeutic tools. (We talk about therapeutic techniques in Chapter 10.)

Nevertheless, addressing the concerns and feelings of a group of individuals is a complex and layered process that takes patience, flexibility, and openness on the part of everyone involved. The results of working through emotional issues together and learning practical skills to help all of you move forward can be well worth the effort of family counseling.

Getting started with genograms

For anyone just getting started in counseling, it's not always obvious where to begin when you're talking about your family.

That's where genograms come in. A *genogram* is a visual representation of a family system much like a family tree but with opportunities to visualize emotional relationships, medical conditions, and behavioral patterns that may be passed down from generation to generation. It employs unique symbols to identify each type of family relationship. A genogram also graphically depicts the binge eater's perception of the emotional status of various family relationships, be they close, distant, supportive, conflict-laden, or otherwise. Figure 22-1 shows the symbols used to represent various relationships. Here, all the lines are black, but in an actual genogram the lines are various colors. Typing genogram into any search engine yields many colorful examples.

Not all psychological conditions or medical problems have a corresponding symbol in the genogram keys we include here. If necessary, feel free to create your own symbols to designate something that comes up multiple times in your own family.

Like a family tree, a genogram includes names, birth dates, dates of death, and basic family relationships. But a genogram can do so much more in terms of representing family and emotional relationships, and for the binge eater, showing other family members who may have suffered from eating issues, depression, anxiety, or any other related medical or psychological issues. (For an idea of what an actual genogram looks like, check out the nearby sidebar, "Creating a genogram — Marla's story.")

Emotional Relationships Legend

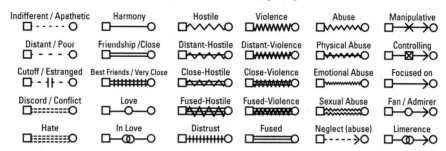

Family Relationships Legend

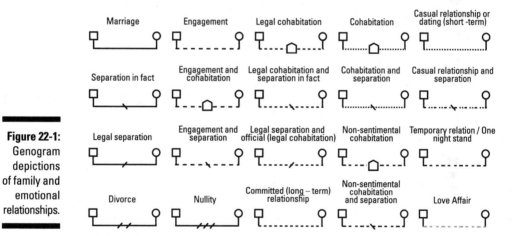

Figure 22-1: Genogram depictions of family and emotional relationships.

Some of the things you can include in your genogram are

✔ **Cultural information:** If a family member is a first generation immigrant, speaks a different language, or practices a different religion, make a note of that. Include any cultural information that may have played a part in family dynamics.

✔ **Deaths:** Make sure to include the age, date, and cause of death.

✔ **Eating disorders, addictions, or any other psychiatric diagnoses:** Even though you may be seeking treatment for binge eating, it's important to note whether or not your relatives have suffered from any kind of eating disorders, addictions, or other struggles. If possible, identify the substance(s) used, the duration of the addiction, and whether the family member ever recovered and/or relapsed.

✔ **Divorces and separations**

✔ **Education levels**

✔ **Occupations**

✔ **Parenting styles:** Indicate whether your parents were controlling or relaxed and if you know about the parenting style of your grandparents and/or siblings, include that information.

✔ **Quality of relationships:** Beyond the simple fact of being mother and daughter, sister and brother, and so on, to the best of your abilities, make note of both alliances and conflicted relationships. Were relationships distant, enmeshed, or healthy?

✔ **Trauma:** Trauma is a subjective experience, but record anything that seems relevant to you — big or small. A trauma could be the death of a loved one including a beloved pet, moving, job loss, divorce, bankruptcy, or many other painful experiences that create a disruption in the activities of daily life and prolonged feelings of denial, sadness, anger, and depression. It's important to remember that each person defines trauma differently; an event that has little impact on one person may be devastating to another.

Whatever you think you know about your own family, you may still have a lot to learn from seeing it diagrammed and represented in a genogram. Just drawing a genogram can provide a lot of food for thought.

Your therapist may have tips and suggestions for how to get started with making a genogram of your family, but you can do it on your own as well. Just follow these steps:

1. **Get a pencil and paper, or if you're more comfortable on the computer, you can use Word, Excel, or any of the programs available to build genograms such as GenoPro.** (www.genopro.com).

   You may end up doing several drafts, so don't worry too much about paper size at the beginning. You probably won't know at the start how extensive your genogram will be. You can transfer your genogram to poster board or butcher paper depending on how large it becomes.

2. **Familiarize yourself with the genogram keys in Figure 22-1.**

   You don't need to memorize the symbols but simply begin to become familiar with them. As you go, you can also reference a number of sites on the Internet for further information and guidelines on drawing your genogram and eliminating ambiguities, such as how to document multiple spouses. You can find standard genogram symbols many places on the web including http://en.wikipedia.org/wiki/Genogram or http://wellsk.faculty.mjc.edu/GenogramDetailed.pdf.

You can also find examples of genograms and a legend of genogram symbols many places on the Internet including www.Wikipedia.com and www.Pinterest.com.

3. **Start at the bottom of the page with yourself and add family members in order above your name.**

   • Your spouse, partner, or boyfriend/girlfriend

   • Your children, stepchildren, and/or the children of your partner if they're significant in your life.

   • Add any siblings you have and their partners and children.

   • Move to your parents and all your aunts and uncles. Include multiple spouses and stepsiblings if you have them.

4. **Add as many generations as you can.**

   In each generation, fill in as much information as you know about your grandparents, great-grandparents, and their siblings.

5. **Fill in as much psychological and medical information as you can about the family members in your genogram.**

   Refer to the standard symbol key in this chapter, but keep in mind that you can also make up your own symbols if you need to as long as you're consistent. If you prefer, you can also use words to describe a particular illness, relationship, or trauma if a symbol doesn't do the trick.

   Include information that you believe to be true, and don't worry if it can't be correlated or confirmed. After all, you're making a genogram and using it for your own psychotherapy, so your perceptions are an important part of understanding who you are and how you came to be that way. For example, even if your aunt was never diagnosed with anorexia, but she died of a heart attack in her late 30s and you remember her as far too thin, you may want to note that she was anorexic. Similarly, if your cousin is overweight or obese and she's been your eating partner at family reunions for as long as you can remember, you can make a note that she may binge or overeat even if you've never discussed it.

6. **Look for patterns.**

   You won't discover everything right away, but maybe you'll see certain similarities at first glance. Perhaps all first children were overachieving perfectionists, maybe all of the men in one branch of the family left their first wives after a second child was born, perhaps almost everyone in another branch works as a doctor or medical professional except for your uncle Harry, who's a musician.

   Give the patterns time to emerge from your genogram and consider revising and remaking your genogram on a regular basis depending on what you discover and how your thinking changes.

Seeing the family as a system

Even though many eating disorder professionals begin seeing patients on an individual basis, family counseling most often plays an important role in enhancing a binge eater or compulsive eater's recovery.

As are we all, binge eaters are both products of and active contributors to the family environments in which they are/were raised and live in. Family counseling seeks to untangle and understand both the good and the not-so-good aspects of those environments and helps binge eaters and those who love them recognize triggers and patterns that may be part of the drive to overeat as a way to deal with stress, anger, sadness, anxiety, and/or other negative emotions.

Although treatment for eating disorders may be the catalyst for family therapy, ultimately understanding and addressing any larger issues within the family system, irrespective of the eating disorder, can be a wonderful and unexpected benefit. For example, imagine a family in which a young woman seeks treatment for binge eating, and her long-divorced parents come together to support her recovery.

Perhaps their divorce was a bitter one, and both parents are now remarried, but the conflicts in their relationship were never resolved, and their current relationship is little more than civil. Over the course of several family counseling sessions with their daughter, the girl's father comes to realize how his drinking affected his daughter's childhood and how it may have contributed to her inability to cope with difficult situations. Upon reflection, he understands much more deeply than he did before the effect his behavior had on the end of the marriage, and for the first time, he apologizes to his ex-wife and to his daughter for drinking so much.

Although the apology may not initially seem as if it has anything to do with the young woman's binge eating or overeating, healing longstanding rifts has everything to do with the emotional health of an individual or family. Whether or not you know it explicitly, events that happened years before may directly and indirectly affect your behaviors today, and working through these issues with other willing family members can have unexpected, positive results for all of you.

Dedicating time to family nutrition

Some of the work you do on your journey is emotional and psychological, while some consists of picking up concrete, practical skills and techniques that can help you replace the impulses and habits that led you to binge in the first place.

No matter how far along you are in your personal plan to put a stop to binge eating in your life, it's often very helpful for you and your family to meet together with a dietitian for at least one family nutrition session.

These nutrition sessions are not family counseling per se, but they provide valuable communication time within the family that can be specifically about food. When a family takes the time to come together in a nutrition session, they can use this time for both logistical food and meal planning as well as strategic planning for supporting the binge eater at mealtimes.

Family nutrition sessions may include any or all of the following

- ✔ Meal planning for specific meals, holidays, restaurant outings, or any other special food-related occasions.
- ✔ Grocery shopping and how to prepare a grocery list for the entire family.
- ✔ Learning about relative portion sizes, which better facilitates putting together a healthy meal for each family member. For Dad the meal portion may be larger than for Mom, and Mom's portion is larger than a child's, and so on. This varies greatly depending on whether the binge eater is a child, teen, or adult.
- ✔ Extensive discussions about how not to be the food police, how to recognize if someone in the family is doing so without realizing it, and how to offer more constructive, non-judgmental support.
- ✔ Kitchen organizing. Sometimes the way a kitchen is organized can be impactful for a binge eater. Where certain foods are located in the cabinets, and having separate shelves for different family members may be valuable for some families. Locking cabinets or other food storage areas is never recommended, but there are ways to minimize trigger foods for the binge eater without depriving other family members of the foods they favor.
- ✔ Eating together with the dietitian observing and/or suggesting ways the family can organize meals so as not to trigger a binge eater.
- ✔ Setting food-specific ground rules such as no food-talk while at the table, who sets the table, who cleans up, and discouraging family-style dining so that all food is portioned at the stove or counter, leaving no extra food on the table.

Reconnecting as a couple

A subset of family counseling, couples therapy is a way to reestablish intimacy, respect, and/or trust in a committed relationship if it has suffered as a result of one or both partners eating in a disordered way. Over time, binge eating can take an emotional, physical, and/or psychological toll on any relationship, and couples counseling can be one way to work through some of the troublesome behaviors, secrets, and/or conflicts that may have arisen during the months and years in which binge eating has played a role in the relationship.

It may be obvious to you that your relationship is in trouble if binge eating or its consequences has made either of you consider walking away. But even if you and your partner aren't in obvious crisis, couples counseling may be worth considering if you're on a journey toward ending your disordered eating and are trying to establish healthier ways of thinking about yourself, your habits, and the way you and the people around you relate to one another.

If you're wondering if couples counseling might benefit you, consider the following questions

- ✔ Does the binge eater's changing body affect the romantic attraction of her partner?
- ✔ Does the binge eater's perception of his body lead to less intimacy?
- ✔ Does binge eating affect the couple's ability to socialize with other people at restaurants, dinners, events, or parties?
- ✔ Does binge eating affect the couple's ability to make simple decisions about food shopping, meal prep, and/or dining?
- ✔ Does binge eating affect the couple in that one partner is disappointed that the other can't or won't stop binge eating?
- ✔ Has binge eating taken a toll on the couple's finances? Have your health insurance premiums gone up? Does the price of groceries and/or treatment put a strain on your budget? Is one of you unable to work because of binge eating?
- ✔ If you have children, has binge eating made caring for your children difficult? Has your binge eating begun to affect their eating behaviors?

Whether you want to address practical concerns or more deep-seated emotional issues, counseling may help you and your partner.

Finding the right clinician is important, and you can find referrals though your individual therapist, a support group, the Internet, or through training institutes specifically devoted to couples therapy.

Family therapy at all stages of life — Juliana's story

Depending on your stage of life, family therapy can mean many different things. For a child, an adolescent, a young adult, a new parent, or someone in their 40s, 50s, or 60s, effective family therapy may be conducted in diverse ways.

Take Juliana, an obese ten-year-old girl who's binge eating. Concerned about her health and the fact that other kids are teasing her at school, her mom brings her to the pediatrician, who recognizes that she's gaining more weight than she should for her age. He refers her to a dietitian, who gives her and her mother meal plans and solutions to some of the daily struggles they both have with eating properly.

When several months go by and Juliana's nutrition and eating habits have not improved, the dietitian's impressions that the family is reluctant to change are confirmed. Juliana seems sad and quiet in their sessions, and the dietitian suspects that something else is at work since Juliana's parents are seemingly reluctant to adhere to the meal-planning strategies set forth, and Juliana is continuing to gain weight. The dietitian recommends that Juliana see a child psychologist, who discovers that Juliana is overeating to cope with the stress in the household and because she may be being experiencing emotional and verbal abuse.

If Juliana is lucky, the cycle ends there. She and her family get the counseling they all need, and Juliana is able to limit and eventually stop bingeing. She grows into a teenager and a young adult who has adequate coping skills and who hopefully no longer turns to food for emotional sustenance.

If, however, her parents are reluctant to accept any of the recommendations of the dietitian or therapist and/or they never really address the problem in any meaningful way, Juliana may make her way through middle and high school, getting further into the dieting-bingeing-gaining weight cycle and perhaps having social and emotional trouble due to her fluctuating weight and the developmental changes that occur during adolescence.

Perhaps she goes to college, but she has trouble making friends, getting her school work finished, and adjusting. To cope with the stress of her new environment, she's bingeing two-to-three times per week. In order to preserve her financial aid, the administration suggests she take a medical leave and seek counseling due to her eating, and she's forced to withdraw during the first semester.

The counseling, both individual and family-oriented, that occurs when Juliana is 18 would be somewhat different than what might have happened when she was a child. Although she's nearing adulthood, she's still financially dependent on her parents, and she's living with them, which would mean that they might be involved from the beginning. Again, if Juliana and her family stick with therapy, Juliana may return to college the following fall with better coping skills and less of an impulse to binge when life gets difficult. If not, perhaps Juliana makes her way through college, develops reasonable social skills that help her cope with her weight and appearance, and she graduates with honors along with her classmates.

All through college, she's made friends but never dated, and now that college is over, she moves to another city with her roommate from college and gets an entry-level job. Without the structure of her class and study schedule along with the regular social events she used to attend, she's bored and lonely in the evening, and her bingeing gets worse. In this moment,

(continued)

(continued)

she seeks therapy because she's sick and tired of feeling this way, and what she's putting her body through has become too much.

Now that Juliana no longer lives with her family, her therapeutic journey may be very different. She may seek out individual therapy and/or a support group, and perhaps she'll see a dietitian as well. If she does participate in family therapy, it may be less about emotions and more about practical ideas she and her roommate can implement to slow and eventually stop her binge eating.

If she doesn't seek therapy at this point or if the therapy doesn't work for her, she may continue on and stabilize to some degree. Perhaps she advances in her job and begins dating. Unfortunately, all through her twenties, she gains weight every single year. It becomes an issue because she's shopping for a wedding dress, and she's obsessed now more than ever with how she's going to look in the dress. She knows her fiancé loves her, but he's intimate with her less often. When her mother arrives for the final dress fitting, she makes a remark about Juliana's weight, and Juliana begins bingeing in the weeks leading up to her wedding and refuses to leave the house.

At that point, her fiancé must be part of the family therapy picture with Juliana's parents not so involved other than Juliana figuring out what she will say to her mother in the future if she belittles her. If instead of seeking counseling, Juliana goes on without it and gets married, she may later on find herself unable to get pregnant due to weight-related issues. As hard as she tries, she can't lose weight, and so she enters treatment because she wants to have a baby. In this moment, her parents are out of the picture, and she and her husband must work together on her binge eating behaviors without directly involving her parents.

At each stage of Juliana's life, seeking help and ending the binges could be critical, but the support she needs to succeed from family and friends is very different. One thing we know for sure is that the earlier binge and other disordered eating behaviors are addressed, the better the long-term outcome. It makes sense that self-destructive habits and patterns are more and more likely to become entrenched over time. That's not to say it's *ever* too late to seek help. In fact, quite the contrary. But the variations in Juliana's scenarios illustrate the idea that earlier is certainly more beneficial.

Chapter 23

Changing Family Habits and Routines

• •

In This Chapter

▶ Surrendering control in order to take it back

▶ Creating new ground rules for family and others in your life

▶ Thinking about the future together

• •

Much of this book focuses on what binge eaters themselves can do to slow and eventually stop using overeating as a coping mechanism, but family and friends also have an important role to play in recovery. If you're committed to helping your loved one make permanent changes to his eating behaviors and other ingrained habits and ways of thinking, it may not always be enough to let him do it alone without at least some awareness or attention to your own daily food habits and how they may either affect or be affected by your loved one's disordered eating.

Even though it can sometimes be difficult, working together as a family to help support recovery is crucial. After all, the journey to wellness is not just about the individual, it's also about the family unit, couple, or other family system in which the binge eater exists. This is particularly true because getting better can dramatically change one's behaviors, which inevitably affects how the family interacts and functions as a whole.

In this chapter, we provide some practical advice to help you and your loved ones decide on and implement changes to the whole family system. We'll discuss what works and what could backfire. Finally, we turn toward the future and what a life without binge eating might look like.

Recovering Step by Step

Binge eating, compulsive overeating, emotional eating or any type of disordered eating has the potential to tear a family apart. Although recovery is about the journey to better and sustained health, it's also about repairing the family system and making it stronger.

As we point out throughout this book, recovery is a step-by-step process. For every two steps forward, there's the possibility of one step back, not only for the binge eater but for the entire family. As in any relationship, the overall responsibility of recovery effort is most effective when shared by all.

The keys to success for the whole family are

✔ Collaborating, not trying to dominate.

✔ Supporting each other, not criticizing.

✔ Communicating honestly and responsibly.

✔ Not trying to catch each other doing something wrong, and realizing that it's better to pick your battles and not sweat the small stuff.

✔ Catching each other doing something right and acknowledging it.

Long-term success in ending binge eating depends not only on the binge eater's internal motivation, but also on the continuing support of friends, family, and a professional treatment team.

Controlling the Need to Control

We all know someone who likes to be in control. Maybe that person insists on picking the restaurant when your family goes out to dinner. Maybe he always wants to drive on family outings or she only sits on the aisle at movies or in the airplane. You may have come to tolerate some of these behaviors because you've decided that in all relationships, there's compromise and that in the scheme of things, you can live with these idiosyncrasies. However, a binge eater may perceive what seem to be innocuous behaviors as overly controlling, and those perceptions may then serve as a trigger for a binge.

Problems arise when those controlling behaviors begin to negatively impact others. For a binge eater, something that seems insignificant to others has the potential to set off a chain reaction that leads to a binge. Even if it seems unimportant at first, living with someone who thinks and acts as if she knows what's best for everyone can be difficult when it comes to starting the journey away from binge eating and toward a different life with more sustainable habits.

As a parent, spouse, partner, child, sibling, or anyone else who lives with and/or cares about someone who binges, you may think you're doing that person a favor by stepping in and creating rules and regulations designed to end the binges. But what seems like a logical, helpful act to you is not. Part of the process of recovery is for the person with an eating disorder to find her own way to handle her food issues in a healthy manner. Imposing your rules is counterproductive. Over time, your behavior may end up making the bingeing worse or creating distance in the relationship when what your loved one really needs is a neutral, non-judgmental person for support.

Although you can sometimes trick yourself into thinking otherwise, it's important to remember that the only person you can attempt to control is yourself. If someone you love suffers from binge eating and seems out of control, even if you have the best intentions, attempts to control the binge eater's behaviors will always backfire.

Defining controlling behavior

It may feel unnatural, and it may not even make sense to you at first, but for your friend or loved one to move forward toward a life without binge eating, you have to do your part and let go of your need to control him or any situation that may affect his binge eating.

Chronic binge eating leaves sufferers feeling out of control, but it leaves the people who love them feeling powerless, too. It's natural in these kinds of situations to try to control something in your life because you sense you can't make the bingeing stop, but control of any sort can undermine a binge eater's already weakened sense of self and integrity.

If you find yourself trying to organize and manipulate situations in any way so that your loved one doesn't binge, you must figure out ways to back off and let things take their course without your intervention. Yes, you may feel frustrated or frightened enough to think it's a good idea to lock up food or take control of decision making in other ways, but as the loved one of a binge eater, ultimately you can't keep someone from their own powerful psychological, emotional, and physical impulses to binge, and your efforts to do so will likely make matters worse.

By now, you may be thinking to yourself, "Are they crazy? Do nothing? Just sit around and let her eat everything in sight, gain weight by the minute, and put her health and our budget in danger?" In many ways, that's exactly what we're saying, but there are other steps you can take that can actually help.

The most important thing to keep in mind is that disordered eating behaviors are almost always metaphors or symbolic expressions of other emotions, behaviors, and thoughts, whether consciously or subconsciously. You may want to ask yourself the following questions as a way of finding some hidden triggers (not causes) that you can work on changing in order to have a more positive impact on the ones you love:

✓ **Do you consider yourself a perfectionist?** Expecting perfection from others and trying to enforce unattainable standards of behavior is always controlling even if you think that you just want everything to be as good as it can be. For perfectionists, constantly striving toward an ideal seems like an honorable pursuit, but it can be a way of controlling others and turn the perfectionist into a long-suffering martyr or a nag whose expectations are never met. Since perfection simply does not exist, it makes more sense to strive for excellence, allowing, of course, for human frailty.

✓ **Do you expect others to read your mind and anticipate your needs?** Everyone loves surprises, but good relationships work because the people in them are able to communicate their needs to one another. If you fail to ask for what you want but also feel and act unhappy that your loved one can't figure it out without your having to spell it out, you put an unfair burden on him to guess what you have in mind. You'll both just be disappointed.

✓ **Do you ask questions even when you already know the answers?** Asking too many questions, especially ones related to behavior about which someone might be ashamed, can put the person being asked on the defensive. This is especially true if you think you already know the answer. For example, if you ask your daughter if she ate the whole chocolate cake when it's only the two of you in the house, it may be that your question isn't quite as innocent as it seems.

✓ **Do you find problems to solve even when things are pretty good overall?** Everyone has pet peeves, and sometimes something is really so annoying that you can't let it go. However, if you discover yourself finding fault with small problems even when the big picture may be good, you can effectively block any discussion of other, deeper issues that may need to be addressed, and you divert attention from yourself and your own flaws or missteps. It's harder, but much more satisfying in the end, to catch someone (and yourself) doing something right rather than doing something wrong.

✓ **Do you talk a lot?** By talking a lot, we don't mean being bubbly, loquacious, or friendly. That's your energy and effervescence. What we mean is whether you tend to keep the focus on yourself in conversation, interrupt other speakers, continue a story even when you know others have lost interest, or otherwise monopolize most discussions. This is an uncomfortable one, but you may need to consider whether you're inadvertently controlling people by telling them too much about yourself and your own concerns.

✔ **Do you pretend not to hear or understand someone even when you do?**
You don't want anyone to think you're being rude, but you also don't
want to acknowledge something uncomfortable that someone's just said.
If you fall back on, "I'm sorry, I don't understand what you mean" really
often, you may be subtly controlling the relationship by denying someone
the opportunity to be heard. It takes courage to talk about feelings, and if
you pretend you haven't heard something that was difficult for someone
to say, the person talking to you may not get up the nerve to say those
words again.

✔ **Do you ever give anyone the silent treatment?** Whether all is going well
in a relationship or not, people depend on verbal cues and communication
to give them an idea of where they stand. If you use the silent treatment
when you're angry, frustrated, or sad, you keep the people around you in
suspense and unable to go about their days, whether you mean to or not.

Most relationships have a natural ebb and flow that hopefully, over time, set-
tles into a comfortable and happy situation full of compromise. Even in the
best relationships, it's normal to do some of these things at times, but if you
answered yes to some of these questions, you may want to consider whether
you need to relinquish some of the control you feel you need to have.

Of course, trying to control a binge eater can take far more obvious forms as
well. Consider the following examples

✔ **Bribery:** If you work but your wife doesn't, you may try to control her
binge eating by promising some sort of financial reward or gift. For
example, controlling behavior can be asking her to quit bingeing in
exchange for a fancy car, a trip, jewelry, or some other kind of present.
Bribery of any sort is a form of controlling behavior.

✔ **Placing restrictions:** If you're the parent of a binge-eating teen who can't
drive, you may try to control your child's life by restricting access to
friends, work, or school for reasons that may or may not have anything
to do with binge eating.

✔ **Hiding food:** If you've ever hidden food from a binge eater, you may be
trying to prevent a binge even when it's not your place. Unfortunately,
if someone is determined to binge, there's not much you can do about
it. They will, in fact, always find a way, and having to sneak around also
exacerbates their level of shame.

It's tempting to hide food in certain situations. For example, you may know
that a specific food is a trigger for your loved one. This may be a binge
food for her, and you know that having this food in the house could be
a set up for her to have urges and binge. However, this particular food
is one of your favorites and a quick and easy way for you to pack your
lunch or make a snack. Giving it up entirely may make you feel deprived

or angry. So you opt to buy that food and hide it so your loved one can't binge on it.

This well-meaning attempt to hide a trigger food from your loved one is an act of control. In this situation, you need to ask yourself

- Is it worth the chance that the binger will find it and possibly binge with it?

- What happens if she finds it?

- What would I say about hiding it?

Binge eating disorder or any type of disordered eating isn't really about food. It's about abusing food as a coping mechanism to deal with unresolved issues.

Although it may not be what you want to hear, you may have to shift your focus to finding compromises that meet most of everyone's needs and concentrate on moderation, not only where food is concerned but where control is a factor as well.

Identifying controlling behaviors specific to binge eating

When it comes to binge eating or any form of disordered eating (or many other situations, come to think of it) trying to control things on behalf of another person isn't helpful, even when it's meant to be. If you're the loved one of a binge eater, be on alert for controlling behaviors:

- **Hiding food:** Hiding anything, especially food, from someone who binges or overeats communicates distrust and lack of faith in his recovery.

- **Talking behind her back:** You may need to vent about how difficult life can be with a binge eater, and you probably have a lot on your mind that rightfully deserves discussion, but doing it behind someone's back is destructive — even when you don't mean it to be. This eventually leads to more hidden behaviors, not only for you but also for your loved one, because she doesn't feel comfortable confiding in you.

Venting can be a profoundly helpful coping mechanism if done in a healthy way. Try writing down everything on your mind in an unfiltered way, as if simply transcribing every one of your unedited thoughts and feelings from your head to the page. This can be quite cathartic if you let it all out until you're truly finished for that moment. Then either shred or rip the paper into many pieces. You can also make an appointment with a therapist to discuss the journaling and what's on your mind in general (we discuss individual therapy for family and friends in Chapter 24).

✔ **Reacting from emotions, not thoughtfulness:** If you have automatic responses to some situations and don't take time to evaluate what and why you're saying something, then you're acting from emotions and not thoughtfulness.

✔ **Blaming your loved one for not being able to stop binge eating:** No matter how well-intended, the last thing you want to do is accuse, judge, or manipulate the person you're trying to help end his binge eating. If it's all frustrating, frightening, and aggravating for you, imagine how your loved one must feel. Whether or not he ever seeks treatment, it's important to come to terms with the way things are rather than the way you would like them to be.

If you've engaged in any of these behaviors, it's important to begin to understand why you may have done so and what you can do in the future to make changes both in the way you act and feel. Just as the binge eater in your life may be making slow but meaningful progress toward ceasing the binge behaviors, this is the time for you to also set realistic expectations for yourself.

Living Life as a Family

Whether you've been living with binge eating for a short time or for as long as you can remember, something as complicated as disordered eating has probably come to dominate your life as a family or couple, or the essence of any relationship you have with a binge eater. Recovery, however incremental, is a chance to rethink what's possible for your relationship in the future, but with that opportunity comes a new reality that may have its own new challenges as well as triumphs.

There are as many stories as there are binge eaters themselves, but we're sticking to just two: one that illustrates the complexity of a family with children negotiating a child's recovery from binge eating and the other showing what it might be like to be in a couple when one person is a binge eater.

✔ **Young adult binger:** Stacy's been a binge eater since adolescence, and although she went away to college in the fall, after a semester, her bingeing got so bad that she decided to take a semester off to seek treatment. Stacy's little brother, Brian, just made the varsity basketball team this fall, and during the six months she was out of the house, he got used to being able to eat as much as he needed at mealtime and to keep sweets in the house for dessert. Now that Stacy's back and serious about treatment, their mom's cooking much healthier meals and refuses to buy sweets. Brian loves his sister and wants her to get better, but it's frustrating to be hungry in the afternoons before practice, and he's sometimes annoyed that he can't have dessert after dinner because it's a trigger for Stacy when it's in the the house.

✔ **Adult binger:** Alfonso started bingeing off and on in his 20s, but by the time he was 40, he was bingeing three to four times per week and often so depressed that he had trouble going to work. When he was 43, he had a massive heart attack, and his doctor told him that if he didn't lose weight and change his eating and exercise habits, the next one would surely kill him. Alfonso knew that the weight was a symptom of the depression and anxiety that had plagued him since childhood. When he left the hospital, he began to see a nutritionist and a psychotherapist. Although he didn't lose weight at first, over time his healthier habits resulted in his losing 50 pounds. He and his wife Maria also went to couples counseling, and their relationship is better than it's been in years.

Now the two of them are planning to start going out to dinner with friends again, and Maria's not sure what to do. She supported him through a long recovery, and even though it's been hard, their relationship is still strong. Maria fears the idea of any missteps at dinner, but she doesn't want to embarrass Alfonso in front of their friends.

Even though both Stacy and Alfonso are getting better, recovery changes how a person behaves and therefore changes the dynamics of day-to-day living in most families. The challenge is being able to adapt to these changes even if it's not always comfortable. You may have gotten so used to bingeing and the rituals and routine around it that when your loved one stops, there's almost a vacuum and often a sense of uncertainty about what to do next, like waiting for the other shoe to drop, so to speak.

What's right for your family or any other type of relationship is specific to you and your relationships, but as you figure out what your changing family life requires, remember to

✔ **Try to take everyone's needs into account.** At the start of someone's recovery, her needs may be first priority, but as you remake some parts of your family life, focus on balance and equilibrium for everyone.

✔ **Recognize that the situation is always evolving.** Recovery isn't a fixed process but one that develops and changes over time, what makes less bingeing possible at the start of someone's journey toward a healthier life may not be what works in the long run for the binge eater or for the people who love him.

✔ **Keep the focus on the binge eater and her drive to be healthier.** Slowing and eventually ending binge eating isn't easy. The best way to support the binge eater in your life is to be a gentle, loving, non-judgmental presence. Taking on the role of the food police or offering advice, however well-intentioned and knowledgeable, will only set your relationship back.

Finding Ground Rules that Work

If you've had the chance to work with a psychotherapist or family counselor on developing strategies to support the binge eater in your family, you may already have an idea of how to move forward. But even if you haven't, flexibility, realistic expectations, and an ongoing conversation about what works and what doesn't can help you and your loved ones figure out family ground rules that help put binge eating behind all of you. (We talk about the ins and outs of family and couples therapy in Chapter 22.)

Honoring and respecting each other's needs and requests ultimately furthers the healing process and sets precedents in how you live your lives from here on out. Although establishing some ground rules is simple and straightforward, others may take some time to develop.

Use these general dos and don'ts to help get you on track with ground rules that make the most sense for your family:

- ✔ Schedule a weekly family conversation to discuss this week's progress, struggles, and/or other topics that are difficult to talk about. The focus here is not on the amount of weight lost or gained or how many times one has binged or not binged. Progress is measured by such things as the safety of the family environment to not judge or be judged, the degree to which open and honest communication is fostered, and the ability to not take relapses or slips personally.

- ✔ Develop and refine a list of family food dos and don'ts. For example, do buy single serving containers of snacks for the kids' lunches, and don't buy the large, economy pack of that item.

- ✔ Come up with alternate behaviors to bingeing that each family member can engage in. For instance, if your brother's trying to avoid a binge, ask if you can help distract him by going for a walk with him or playing a board game together.

- ✔ Stay calm and speak from your own experience rather than judging or giving advice about what someone else should do. Use "I" statements that share your perspective, and focus on solutions to underlying issues rather than behaviors. See Chapter 21 for examples of "I" statements.

- ✔ Get rid of the bathroom scale, and don't ask about weight or weight loss.

Looking toward the Future

In the moment of insight and motivation when your friend or loved one who's a binge eater decides that enough is enough and it's time to embark on her journey towards better physical and psychological health, the recovery process begins. Some motivations can be as specific as the desire to go to a mall and buy an outfit that's not a plus size, while others may be something as compelling as wanting to avoid a heart attack or the onset of a variety of diseases, or simply feeling the gravity of being a healthy role model for other loved ones. Over time, it's going to take all of these reasons and new ones developed along the way to keep a binge eater's resolve to address and end bingeing strong.

Changing longstanding eating habits and confronting the underlying reasons for them isn't for the faint of heart. It often takes months and years to make permanent changes and find healthier, sustainable, and more peaceful ways of life.

Even if the binge eater you know and love is getting better, it's important to keep your expectations in check. Overcoming binge eating is a lifetime struggle, and even if, over time, your friend or loved one improves so that bingeing isn't a regular part of his life, when life becomes stressful, bingeing may still be an issue.

Don't expect recovery to be a perfectly linear, perfectly orderly path towards permanent improvement and no bingeing again ever. Instead, recovery is more like an EKG in which the spikes get shorter and the distance between them gets longer over the months and years. In other words, in the best-case scenario, someone who's a binge eater will have to deal with a recurrence less and less often and for a shorter period each time. Even though your friend or loved one can eventually arrive at a point when binge eating isn't a constant factor in his or her daily life, unfortunately it may never really go away permanently, and a sufferer will always have to be vigilant when it comes to the causes and triggers of bingeing.

Chapter 24

Taking Care of Yourself

· ·

In This Chapter

▶ Looking out for your own mental health

▶ Treating the family as a system

▶ Remembering the basics of self-care

· ·

*B*eing the friend or loved one of anyone with a serious psychological or medical condition can be exhausting both mentally and physically. Even though you may not be using overeating as a coping mechanism yourself, watching someone you love struggle takes a toll on you if you don't take care of yourself.

Families function as a system, and if one member of the family is unwell, the repercussions undeniably impact everyone. Although longstanding family patterns of communication and behavior, both positive and negative, may influence most of your interactions, that doesn't mean that you can't step back and start making changes to protect yourself and to improve your own life. It may be difficult to break the habit of familiar behaviors and ways of thinking at first, but keep in mind that if your loved one is in recovery or even just thinking about it, he will also need to change entrenched binge eating behaviors and discover different ways to manage the feelings that trigger them.

Your role may not only be to support your loved one in whatever way seems best for her, but also to find peace with the situation yourself even if the binge eater you love never seeks help or treatment. Although you may encounter periods when your loved needs more attention and encouragement than usual, in the long run, it's a worthwhile goal to find balance between your own needs — both physical and emotional — and the demands that come with knowing and loving a person who binge eats. Although this is easier said than done, by keeping yourself healthy and strong, you're indirectly benefiting your whole family and sustaining yourself in a way that makes your life better overall.

In this chapter, we discuss the benefits of various forms of emotional support for those affected by the disordered eating of another. We also cover the basics of self-care such as proper nutrition, exercise, getting enough sleep, and maintaining strong friendships that could sometimes fall by the wayside when life gets complicated.

Going for Individual Therapy

You're not the one with an eating disorder, but that doesn't mean that you're not suffering as well. A family is an interconnected system, and the way one person behaves or thinks produces actions and reactions on the part of other family members, whether they realize it or not.

It's normal to feel stressed, angry, sad, hopeless, and disappointed if someone you love struggles with binge eating or disordered eating of any kind. Regardless of whether your loved one has sought treatment, you may benefit from participating in your own counseling if you find yourself unsure of how to move forward with your loved one or in your own life.

Therapy is a way to increase consciousness, which in turn can help you understand your thoughts and feelings in relation to a problem or situation. This increased awareness allows you to find out about different options or choices for coping with life's stressors and develop new ways to help your loved one by keeping yourself healthy. No doubt this will help your loved one's long-term recovery and improve your relationship while keeping you grounded in the process.

Family therapy in the real world

Safrina has been suffering from various forms of disordered eating, including bingeing and emotional eating, since age 12. Now at age 20, she's finding it hard to finish college because she's become quite overweight. Day in and day out, she feels socially isolated and too unattractive to date. And to make matters worse, when she can't concentrate to study or write papers, she binges instead. In order to enter into any social situation, she now finds it necessary to binge drink at parties.

Her situation eventually led her to take a temporary leave from school, so she can get treatment and address the escalation of all of her self-soothing behaviors.

As part of Safrina's treatment, her divorced parents have been forced to come together to help their daughter. At the suggestion of the eating disorder therapist treating Safrina, she and her parents enter family therapy together to try and figure out ways to help her. During these sessions, Safrina's father starts to recognize the role his own drinking may have played in contributing to the situation and begins to attend Alcoholics Anonymous support groups. He then apologizes to both Safrina and her mother, now his ex-wife, for behaviors that affected the whole family.

As a result of this long-awaited acknowledgement of what his drinking meant to the family over the years, the relationship between Safrina's parents, each of them now remarried to other people, becomes much more collaborative, civil, and less contentious than it has been for many years. It's clear that there's more work to be done here, but Safrina's health crisis was a great motivation for her parents to coalesce to support her. The impact of her parents' newly found civility also effects Safrina's siblings.

Understanding the benefits of therapy

Therapy is a commitment to improve your emotional and physical life. Research shows that therapy produces long-term benefits in mental and emotional health, which ultimately decrease the demand for other health services.

Even with all its benefits, many people still view psychotherapy as an invasion of privacy or worry about it being "only for crazy people." Nothing could be further from the truth.

Therapy happens in an environment where you can go without fear of being judged. An open, communicative therapeutic experience can help release emotional tension and stress, thereby decreasing anxiety and opening the channels of communication between you and your loved one with binge eating.

Psychotherapists observe the same kind of confidentiality rules that physicians do, and anything you say in session stays between you and your therapist (unless you're planning to hurt yourself or others).

Hopefully, over time you come to trust your therapist with some of the things you cannot or may not be willing to say to outside his office.

Seeking therapy for yourself

Seeking help is a sign of courage and insight, even if you're not the one who binge eats or uses overeating of any kind as a coping mechanism. There are many reasons to decide to begin some kind of supportive therapy. You can view it as a learning experience or as an opportunity to improve something about yourself that will ultimately help your loved one. And of course, you'll be learning about and improving something for yourself too.

Depending on where your loved one is in the process of seeking or not seeking her own treatment, you may have various motives for finding help yourself, which can also change over time.

Even if your loved one is not able or willing to deal with his binge eating, it's still worth exploring the possibility of taking care of yourself by talking with a professional. Some reasons to consider:

- You're not really sure you can stay in a relationship with the binge eater you know and love. Her behaviors have become so worrisome that they're interfering with how the two of you interact on a day-to-day basis. You don't want to make things worse, but you're not sure you can just sit by and do nothing. In fact, it may be that you don't have the stamina to continue the relationship, and you're trying to figure out what to do.

✔ You're worried, embarrassed, concerned, angry, or experiencing any combination of emotions and you feel like you have to figure out strategies to persuade your loved one to engage or re-engage in some form of treatment. Even though it seems as if you're going to seek counseling to help someone else, in the bigger picture, you're looking for ways to live with, love, and help a binge eater without losing yourself in the process.

✔ You're doing everything right — not pressuring your loved one to get help, being a supportive, non-judgmental, loving presence, and resisting your urge to be the food police — but it's taking a toll. You're stressed, worried, and anxious, and you've noticed that you don't feel like yourself. You have to find support to figure out how to handle everything you're trying to manage and to keep yourself healthy.

✔ You're secretly worrying that you've had a hand in your loved one's binge eating. You want to go to therapy to understand more about your family history and to put any sense of responsibility to rest.

✔ You're worried about your own well-being. You know that addictive tendencies run in families, and as your loved one's binge eating has come to light, you've realized that you may have a problem yourself. Whether it's alcohol, drugs, shopping, gambling, or any other behavior or substance, including binge eating or another form of disordered eating, that could be dangerous or destructive, you have a feeling that you may be slightly out of control yourself.

If your loved one has already started treatment of some sort, it's likely that you'll be asked to participate in the process at some point as part of a cohesive, integrated strategy to address any longstanding issues that may have led to the bingeing and to give all of you techniques and ideas you can use to move forward day in and day out.

If professional treatment isn't available due to finances or geography, keep in mind that there are other ways to work on ending bingeing behaviors. Steady progress can be made with a combination of programs and groups such as Overeaters Anonymous and/or online and in-person support groups. Even if you don't go to a psychotherapist yourself, you may find relief and resources by attending Al-Anon meetings, which are designed to address the concerns of those who live with or are affected by those with addictions of all kinds.

Treating the Family

Every family is a complicated system with its own norms and patterns that sometimes need to be explored and often reworked for the benefit of all. As you may well know, family relationships can be a source of great stability and warmth, but they can also sometimes cause stress and bring challenges.

In the case of binge eating or other disordered eating, the eating behaviors themselves may have developed as a reaction to other situations or behaviors in the family but may also produce an equal or greater amount of tension as a result. The objective of family therapy is to identify and affect the patterns of psychological stress, binge eating, and other coping behaviors. (We discuss the benefits of family therapy in detail in Chapter 22.)

Some of the most important reasons to seek treatment as a family include

- ✔ Finding practical solutions to resolve longstanding behavior patterns that may be contributing to disordered eating.
- ✔ Putting to rest any questions of blame and allowing all members of the family to move forward with a sense of healing and peace.
- ✔ Establishing a collective goal for the entire family to move away from binge eating toward a focus on health and wellness.

Using Support Groups

Just as support groups can be an invaluable tool for binge eaters and those who suffer from other forms of disordered eating, they can also be extremely helpful for family members and friends looking for psychological and emotional support in a group setting.

If you feel you need additional help beyond individual counseling, if you haven't found a therapist with whom you feel comfortable, or if you're simply not interested in one-on-one counseling, you may want to consider a support group. They can offer

- ✔ **A chance to connect with other people facing similar issues:** Just as a binge eater can become very isolated and secretive, family members may also feel that they can't tell anyone about what's going on with their loved one because of shame, fear, frustration, and/or a concern about violating that person's privacy. A support group can cut through the sense of being alone and give you a community apart from your day-to-day life.

- ✔ **A source of new ideas and strategies for dealing with a binge eater:** If you're open to suggestions, the people in a support group can give you different and effective solutions for helping and supporting the binge eater in your life. Hopefully, you'll also hear ideas for keeping yourself healthy and sane as you deal with the stress.

> ✔ **A place to find companionship:** Support groups can provide a shoulder to cry on or a place to laugh about how difficult things can be sometimes. Whether the members of your group are going through exactly the same challenges as you are is irrelevant; everyone's looking for a supportive, non-judgmental environment where they can be themselves.

If your loved one is in treatment and you participate in counseling sessions as part of that treatment, you may be able to get a referral from the psychotherapist for targeted support groups in your area. If not, keep an eye out for signs advertising support groups at your community center, the grocery store, or anywhere you go throughout your day. Of course, you can also look online at sites such as

> ✔ Binge Eating Disorders Association (www.bedaonline.org)
>
> ✔ EDReferral (www.edreferral.com)
>
> ✔ Body Positive (www.bodypositive.com)
>
> ✔ Overeaters Anonymous (www.oa.org)
>
> ✔ Something Fishy (www.something-fishy.org)

Although these sites have general information and resources for binge eaters, many also include sections specifically dedicated to supporting friends and family of those with all kinds of eating disorders. In addition to in-person support groups, you can find more information about online support groups and chat rooms where you can discuss what you're going through.

Caring for Yourself in Other Ways

Directly addressing any psychological or emotional issues you have is one way to sustain and nurture yourself, but you can use other methods to keep yourself grounded and in good health. Developing and nurturing friendships and prioritizing your physical health are key components to a life that allows you to be your best and to support and, if need be, care for others.

Maintaining relationships

An urgent problem can easily take over your life. That's true of many different issues you face as you navigate work, family, friends, children, and getting older. Binge eating is certainly overwhelming for the binge eater, and it can easily dominate that person's relationships, especially if the consequences of chronic overeating threaten someone's health and safety.

The natural ebb and flow of any relationship means that sometimes your life and your issues will be more prominent and sometimes the other person's will. However, dealing with binge eating can be a full-time job, and if someone you love is facing the challenges of day-to-day life as a binge eater, it may feel as if that's the focus of your whole relationship.

First, keep in mind that this is hopefully just one phase of your relationship. In time, perhaps things will improve and become more balanced. In the meantime, don't forget to cultivate relationships with other people or to spend time with friends and family who can support you just as you're supporting your loved one who binge eats.

Affecting relationships in the real world

Johanna is a single mother of two, 12-year old-Josefina and 9-year-old Jack. She works full-time as a nurse, often picking up night work to cover the bills. During the past year Johanna noticed that Josefina has gained a significant amount of weight. At first she thought that Josefina was going through a growth spurt, but a few months ago she began to notice food missing from the pantry and empty candy wrappers in the trash. She and Josefina used to cook dinner together and watch a movie one night a week after Jack went to bed, but between her work schedule and Josefina's changing moods, that's stopped.

Johanna didn't do anything initially because she thought the way Josefina was acting was just normal adolescent behavior, but lately it's gotten worse. Josefina won't talk with her at all anymore, and she's spending more and more time in her room alone. Josefina's annual visit to the doctor revealed that she's pre-diabetic, and her pediatrician recommended that Josefina lose weight and stop eating sugar. During a recent conversation, Josefina admitted to Johanna that "eating a lot of food makes me feel better," but when Johanna tried to figure out exactly what she meant by asking a few more questions, Josefina burst into tears and ran into her room.

Johanna's first inclination is to not buy junk food, but after doing some research, she knows that it's probably not going to solve the problem. Obesity, diabetes, and heart disease runs in the family, and Johanna is scared that her daughter will suffer the same fate. Whenever Johanna tries to talk to Josefina about her eating she gets upset and angry. Johanna isn't sure what to do and tries to split her time between the two children equally but knows that Josefina probably needs more attention and affection than she's capable of giving given her responsibilities and their circumstances.

After a particularly rocky month when Josefina refused to speak to her most of the time, Johanna realized that her daughter needed professional help. She first spoke to the counselor at Josefina's school who recommended several child psychologists who offer sliding-scale fees. The counselor also referred her to several after-school programs for kids who need additional support for various reasons. The counselor felt that a program that offered a yoga class for kids would be a particularly good fit for Josefina. In addition, despite the cost, Johanna decided to enroll Jack in an art camp once a week so she can spend some more one-on-one time with Josefina. After considering her options, Johanna feels that spending time with her daughter is the most important step in rebuilding their relationship.

Making nutrition a priority

Maintaining a healthy diet is one of the most important things you can do for yourself. Eating healthfully

✔ Promotes a sense of well-being.

✔ Reduces the impact of stress.

✔ Improves your immune system.

✔ Decreases the risk of disease or even reverses some diagnosed diseases.

✔ Is a positive influence on your loved one who uses overeating as a coping mechanism.

Whether or not you're currently affected by any medical conditions, eating healthfully most certainly helps you feel better, which is important to maintaining your emotional and physical stamina and strength during the process of recovery from binge eating.

If someone you love is a binge eater, it may have forced you to reevaluate your own eating habits and to consider making healthier choices. Making changes to your own eating habits, and enlisting support from others can be a huge help to the person you love who binges or overeats in any way. Not only do you set a good example, but the more support you have in keeping yourself strong and healthy, the more support you can give. If you work together with other people who care about the binge eater in your life, it's easier to make changes that improve the health and well being of your entire family. Let the people you love know what you're doing, and ask them to learn about and to practice healthy eating with you.

Even though direct conversation about specific foods is often discouraged while in the presence of binge eaters for fear of triggering behaviors, it can be helpful and therapeutic when done in the right environment and under the right circumstances. For example, discussing the health benefits of high-fiber cereal may be part of a grocery shopping trip you take together. In this case, talking about nutrition for the purpose of purchasing the best product for you and your family, including the person who suffers from binge eating, is a way to integrate healthy food talk back into the family system and into overall recovery.

The benefits of healthy eating mostly revolve around three main topics

✔ Feeling better

✔ Living longer

✔ Looking better

When discussing nutrition, emphasize feeling better and living longer, *not* weight loss or other body-focused nutritional goals — even if you do want to lose a few pounds.

If you're just learning yourself how to talk about nutrition without talking about weight, remember that you may not get it right on the first few tries. If you can, stick with these concepts and practice, practice, practice:

- ✔ **Better sleep:** Balanced eating promotes deeper, more restful sleep, which helps you deal with stress and improves your energy levels.

- ✔ **Disease protection:** Optimal concentrations of nutrients in your body lower your risk of developing many diseases such as diabetes, heart disease, cancers, arthritis, and neurological diseases.

- ✔ **Improved energy levels:** If you always feel tired, part of the reason could be your diet. Energy production in the body is dependent on the food you eat, with healthy foods providing the components you need to keep you feeling vital and energetic.

- ✔ **Improved mood:** Foods greatly influence the brain's behavior. A poor diet, especially one consisting of excessive junk food contributes to depression and anxiety. The foods you eat control the levels of *neurotransmitters* your brain produces; these are the chemicals that regulate behavior and are closely linked to mood.

Sleeping well night after night

How you feel when you're awake hinges greatly on how well you sleep. Similarly, the remedy for sleep problems can generally be found in your daily routine. Your sleep schedule, bedtime habits, and day-to-day lifestyle choices have an enormous impact on the quality of your nightly rest. If you're supporting someone who binge eats or overeats for any reason, even though you may need sleep now more than ever, chances are you're not getting enough.

It's essential to create an environment that promotes deep, restorative sleep that you can count on night after night. Although it may not seem necessary, part of sleeping well is actually planning when, how, and where you're going to sleep. Discovering what works for you and also how to avoid any sleep preventers is critical.

Experiment with a variety of sleep-promoting techniques so that you can figure out your personal sleep hygiene prescription for a good night's rest.

You may be wondering how much sleep is enough. Sleep requirements vary from person to person, but most healthy adults need at least seven to eight hours of sleep each night to function at their best. But keep in mind that consistency is the most important quality of a good night's sleep. By keeping a regular sleep schedule, going to bed and getting up at the same time every day, you'll feel better than if you sleep the same number of hours at different times.

Use these tips for proper sleep hygiene to get a good night's rest:

- **Go to bed at the same time every night.** Plan to go to bed at the same time every night. Aim for a time when you usually feel tired so that you can fall asleep fairly quickly. Try not to break this routine on weekends, even when it may be tempting to stay up late because you can sleep in.

- **Get up at the same time every day.** If you go to bed at the same time every night and if you're getting enough sleep, you should naturally wake up around the same time every morning without an alarm. As with your bedtime, try to maintain a regular morning routine even on weekends.

- **Take a nap to make up for less sleep.** If you need to make up for a few lost hours, choose a nap rather than sleeping later. This way you can make up for lost sleep without disturbing your daily routine, which can quickly backfire and throw you off for days.

- **Fight drowsiness during the early evening.** If you get drowsy in the evening, particularly after dinner and well before your bedtime, do something stimulating to avoid falling asleep — call a friend, answer e-mail, or get ready for the next day. If you give in and take a nap this late in the day, you may wake up later in the night and have trouble getting back to sleep.

- **Turn off all technology including your television, computer, cell phone, and/or tablet.** Using television to relax or fall asleep at the end of the day is a mistake. Research shows that backlight devices suppress melatonin production, and these technologies stimulate the mind rather than relax it. Try listening to music or audio books instead or practicing breathing and relaxation exercises. If your favorite television show is on late at night, you're better off recording it to watch later.

- **Don't read from a backlit device in bed.** If you're a portable electronic device junkie, switch to an e-reader that's not backlit or, better yet, a regular book. Using something that requires an additional light source such as a bedside lamp does not stimulate your mind as much as a backlit device.

- **Make sure your bedroom is dark.** The darker your room, the better you'll sleep. Cover electrical displays, use heavy curtains or shades to block light from windows, and/or try a sleep mask to cover your eyes.

- **Don't drink too many liquids for about two hours before bed.** Drinking lots of water, juice, tea, or other fluids may result in frequent bathroom trips throughout the night. And caffeinated drinks, which are diuretics, only make bathroom trips more frequent.

Exercising as a regular habit

Don't underestimate the benefits of regular exercise. The American Heart Association recommends 30 minutes of moderate activity daily, but three 10-minute periods of activity are almost as beneficial to your overall fitness as one 30-minute session. This is achievable even for busy folks who are trying to support a family member who's struggling with disordered eating of any kind.

Regular activity, be it exercise or daily activity, relieves anxiety, depression, and anger. If you've ever exercised regularly, you may have noticed a feel-good sensation just after exercise. Most people also notice an improvement in general well-being and outlook on life as physical activity becomes a part of their routine. This is because exercise increases the flow of oxygen, which directly affects the brain. Your mental acuity, memory, and ability to deal with life stressors all improve with physical activity.

In addition to all its psychological benefits, regular exercise improves your physical health too by

- **Improving your immune system:** Regular exercise enhances your immune system and decreases the risk of developing diseases such as cancer and heart disease.

- **Reducing long-term disease risk factors:** Being active can lower blood pressure up to the same amount as medications. If you're under stress of any kind, including the concern and anxiety that may come about when supporting someone who binge eats, your blood pressure can easily rise. Exercise is an excellent natural way to curb that. Physical activity can also boost your levels of good cholesterol, which reduces the risk of heart disease.

Regular physical activity maintains muscle strength, stamina, and circulation among other benefits. In addition, for each hour of regular exercise you do, you'll gain about two hours of additional life expectancy, even if you don't start until later in life. Moderate forms of exercise, such as brisk walking, for 30 minutes or three 10-minute intervals per day has the proven health benefits in the preceding list as well as:

- Improving blood circulation, which reduces the risk of heart disease
- Keeping weight under control
- Improving blood cholesterol levels
- Preventing and managing high blood pressure
- Preventing bone loss

- ✔ Boosting energy levels
- ✔ Helping manage stress
- ✔ Releasing tension
- ✔ Reducing the risk of some cancers
- ✔ Promoting a positive outlook on life
- ✔ Reducing anxiety and depression
- ✔ Improving sleep
- ✔ Increasing and maintaining muscle strength
- ✔ Delaying or preventing chronic illnesses and diseases associated with aging and maintaining quality of life and independence longer for seniors

Physical activity is a great way to support your loved one who binge eats. Moderate activity is an ideal distraction for many people who may otherwise use food as a coping mechanism, and exercising together is also a great way to connect emotionally and to indirectly promote a healthier lifestyle. Engaging in family activities, including exercise, is one way to spend time together, improve communication, and support someone who binge eats.

Exercise should not be used as a way to lose weight or to compensate for binge eating. Even though it seems counterintuitive, activity, while a good distraction form binge eating, better serves improving mood and realizing health benefits than it does burning calories.

Part VI
The Part of Tens

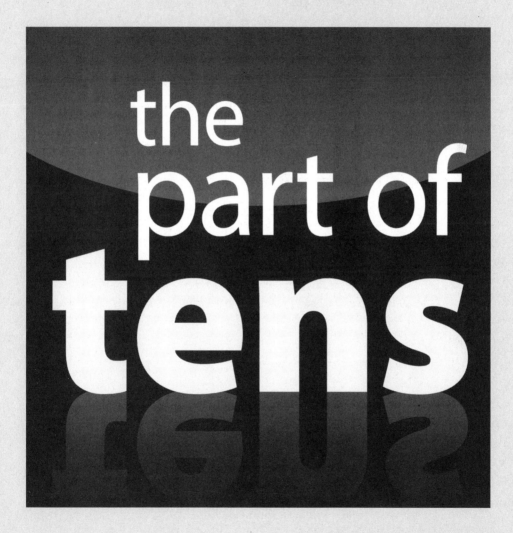

Visit www.dummies.com/extras/overcomingbingeeating for a list of helpful resources for binge eaters and those who love them.

In this part . . .

✔ Find helpful tips to use if you have binge eating disorder (BED). Get advice on seeking treatment, what to eat, and coping day to day.

✔ Dispel myths about binge eating and binge eating disorder. No, it's not all about willpower and dieting.

✔ Offer help and support to someone in your life with BED. Discover tips that work (patient listening) and tricks that hinder (becoming the food police).

Chapter 25

Ten Do's for Binge Eaters

*O*vercoming binge eating can be a long process, but if you're reading this book and recognize yourself in some of the descriptions of binge eaters and others with disordered eating, you may be ready to think about treatment and/or to make changes that can greatly improve your life and the lives of those around you. If you don't know where to begin, this chapter gives an overview of the most effective steps you can take to slow and eventually stop bingeing or other types of eating that may be harming your physical and psychological health.

Do Consult with a Medical Doctor

Seeing your doctor can be a first step toward recovery. Your primary care physician may realize something's going on before you even grasp that you have a problem yourself. If you know and trust your doctor, you may feel free to seek help from her if you suspect you need support in slowing and eventually stopping your binge eating, compulsive overeating, emotional eating, or any other eating behaviors driven by something other than physical hunger. Your doctor can begin to treat the physical health issues that may have arisen from your eating disorder and can refer you to other specialists to further the psychological and behavioral aspects of treatment.

Do Seek Treatment

Although it would be wonderful if every binge eater could simply decide to stop bingeing successfully on his own, the truth is that the journey to better health takes time, patience, a lot of support, and guidance from a team of experts. Binge eating comes about for many reasons, and although you may have some limited success on your own, for sustainable results and to truly move on with your life, you may well need therapy with a trained psychotherapist, along with nutritional guidance from a dietitian, medical monitoring by a physician, and, in some cases, the additional support of medication that's carefully selected and managed by a psychiatrist.

Do Keep a Food-and-Emotions Journal

Knowledge is power. By tracking your intake of specific foods and your thoughts or feelings before, during, and after eating, you can begin to understand some of the root causes behind what triggers you to binge. Although it may be difficult and uncomfortable at times, without getting to the bottom of the circumstances and personal history that led to your disordered eating, it can be hard if not impossible to make the necessary long-term changes. Ideally, by keeping a food-and-emotions journal, you can identify and implement concrete strategies to deal with the eating behaviors you want to change at the same time that you're exploring what drives it all.

Do Allow Yourself to Eat

The inevitable pendulum swing between starving yourself and bingeing is a dangerous cycle that jeopardizes both your emotional and physical health in the long run. That's why eating an individually tailored and well-balanced diet every single day is key to making meaningful changes that will improve your overall well-being.

Restricting your food intake may even be just part of what got you started down the path of overeating in the first place. One of the keys to recovery is to begin establishing healthier, more sustainable, more moderate eating habits that can last a lifetime — the gray in the world of black-and-white thinking and eating. Labeling foods as good and bad, and starving yourself all day only results in the kind of all-or-nothing thinking that fuels your binges.

Do Focus on Your Inner Qualities

Focusing on how you feel rather than on how you look is crucial to recovery. There's more to you than how and what you eat, and if you can set aside any negative feelings you may have about bingeing and how it may have affected your weight up until this moment, you'll have time and motivation to remember who you are and all that you have going for you. Even though it may seem like a cliché, if you can recognize your positive attributes psychologically, spiritually, intellectually, socially, and otherwise, your physical appearance reflects this energy that radiates from within.

Do Be Patient with Yourself

Recovery is a step-by-step process that takes time — just as it takes time to gain weight and to discover and admit that you have a problem. But the passage of time can feel less onerous when you create specific benchmarks for progress. Even though you may crave a quick fix, it's critical to develop and practice problem-solving techniques and coping skills to help you manage the urge to binge. Remember to focus on each and every individual success along the way. That includes being able to avoid even a single binge after a stressful day, or stopping a binge after eating only half of what you routinely binge on. Long-term change starts with day-to-day adjustments that you can celebrate. (We talk about coping techniques in Chapter 10.)

Do Expect Your Recovery to Have Ups and Downs

. . . and we don't just mean on the scale. You can expect emotional ups and downs while on this journey. It's a normal part of the process when attempting to unseat long-standing behaviors and their root causes. Just keep in mind that even when treatment feels a bit challenging, you're still making progress as you learn to integrate healthier coping skills and seemingly new reflexes. Also, remember that a relapse may be just what you need to move forward in your recovery. (Chapter 15 offers advice on how to handle a relapse binge.)

Do Find People who Support Your Recovery

Having a support system in place is a crucial part of the process. Even just one or two people who know you're making changes or who you can tell about your struggles can make a huge difference in your outlook and your progress. Over time, you'll quickly be able to tell the difference between the people in your life who are in fact supportive and those who are less supportive, whether intentionally or not. You'll become eager to surround yourself with friends and family who cheer you on rather than bring you down. Ending destructive relationships and developing positive ones is just one of the keys to continued success during your recovery. (Chapter 14 talks about finding a support team.)

Do Distance Yourself from Relationships that Bring You Down

Saying no to a relationship, a person, or an activity that triggers your binge eating is a positive step toward taking care of yourself. That's not to say that you need to be alone and isolated all the time. In fact, the opposite is true. It merely means being more discerning about the people, places, and ideas that serve you best. As you begin to make changes in your life, some friends or loved ones will either continue to criticize your eating or weight or may even seem to become angry, defensive, or threatened by your attempts to get healthier. No matter how much you love and care for someone, you must keep the focus on your own needs and work on making positive changes during your recovery. Even though it may not be easy or comfortable, distancing yourself from unhealthy, unsupportive relationships may be one of the most important things you do for yourself.

Do Remind Yourself that You Are Not Alone

Although you may feel you're alone at first, in truth, you're really not. Many people struggle with binge eating, emotional eating, compulsive overeating, and other forms of disordered eating. If there's someone within your circle of friends, family, and acquaintances who's recovering from binge eating, you may want to reach out to that person for support and companionship on your journey. But even if you don't know anyone personally who struggles with the same issues, with a little research you can find so many others, either online or in local support groups. Online communities are a great place to find inspiration, encouragement, and friendship.

Chapter 26

Top Ten Myths about Binge Eating Disorder

In This Chapter

▶ Looking at the full spectrum of binge eating

▶ Defining what binge eating is and isn't

▶ Understanding there's no quick fix for binge eating

*M*any myths persist about the circumstances and factors that contribute to binge eating and what it means to be a binge or emotional eater. Only time, continued research, and greater acceptance from the general population and the medical community will help dispel some of the myths identified in this chapter.

All Binge Eaters Are Obese

This is perhaps the greatest myth about binge eaters. Weight is not a measure of binge eating disorder (BED). Binge eating, emotional eating, and compulsive overeating don't always result in obesity. Whether or not someone struggling with certain aspects of binge eating is obese, he may still fight other symptoms of the disorder including depression, guilt, and other negative emotions.

People with BED Have No Willpower

Willpower has nothing to do with overcoming BED. If only it were that easy! If you're on a dieting-bingeing-weight fluctuation cycle, it's very difficult to break this pattern on your own. You have likely come to depend on overeating as a way to self-soothe and to get you through the day (or night), and although this may have worked for a long while, you now find that it causes more problems than it solves. In order to make changes to improve your physical and psychological health, you need tools, techniques, and support to break old habits and establish newer, healthier ones.

Binge Eating Is not a Real Eating Disorder

Until recently, many people weren't sure how binge eating disorder fit into the spectrum of eating disorders and professionals were forced to define binge eating and other types of overeating as an *eating disorder not otherwise specified,* or EDNOS. However, in May 2013, the fifth edition of the *Diagnostic and Statistical Manual of Mental Disorders (DSM-V)* identified binge eating disorder as its own diagnosis for the very first time. This classification is so very important not only because it may start to destigmatize people who suffer from binge eating, but also because it may promote more equitable reimbursement by managed care for related services. (The EDNOS classification no longer exists, and a new classification, *other specified feeding or eating disorder,* or OSFED, has taken its place.)

Binge Eaters Just Need to Exercise Some Will Power and Go on a Diet

The last thing a binge eater should do is go on a diet. The dieting-bingeing-gaining-weight cycle is one of the hallmarks of binge eating disorder and a symptom of the all-or-nothing thinking that gets binge eaters in trouble. While seeing a dietitian and following a healthful, structured eating plan can be helpful for some binge eaters, going on a diet specifically designed for weight loss is generally not recommended.

Weight Loss Surgery Can Cure Binge Eating Disorder

Even if you lose weight after bariatric surgery, weight-loss surgery doesn't address the reasons why you binge. Often times, whatever reasons drove you to binge in the first place remain unaddressed and often creep back up once your body adjusts to the procedure.

In fact, according to the American Society for Bariatric Surgery, the average person who has bariatric surgery loses 40 to 70 percent of excess weight after one to four years but does not reach her ideal body weight. What may be more disappointing is that up to 70 percent of those who have the surgery, especially laparoscopic banding and similar procedures, often regain some or all of the lost weight in just a few years following surgery. These statistics suggest that you should carefully balance the medical indications for surgery against the risks, costs, and discomforts of the procedure and recovery.

Only Women Binge

Unlike other eating disorders that affect mostly (but not only) women, binge eating disorder affects almost as many men as it does women. About 40 percent of binge eaters and compulsive overeaters are men, and the numbers may be on the rise. Though men typically begin bingeing later in life than women, there are more similarities than differences between men and women who binge. If you're a man who binges, effective, specialized treatment is available to you as well to help you understand and control the urge to binge or overeat.

Binge Eaters Are always Hungry

Bingeing and overeating have nothing to do with physical hunger. You may want to read that sentence again. In fact, all forms of disordered eating have little to do with eating or food; food is just the weapon of choice, so to speak. For a chronic binge eater, eating beyond physical hunger or satiety has become a way to self-soothe in moments of stress, sadness, depression, loneliness, anger, and other negative emotions. Effective treatment for binge eating aims to get to the bottom of why you binge eat, promote alternate coping skills, and help you learn how to tell the difference between physical and emotional hunger. They are quite different.

Only Adults Are Binge Eaters

Even though children are not often diagnosed with binge eating disorder, rising childhood obesity rates across the United States and the industrialized world suggest that young people are at risk for developing binge eating disorder or other types of disordered eating as they get older. Children become overweight and obese for a complex set of reasons and circumstances that we discuss in Chapter 17. However, one of the most important things to note about children and disordered eating is that it's not possible to treat children without treating the entire family.

Medical Doctors Are the Go-To Experts for Binge Eating

Although your medical doctor is likely an excellent resource for medical problems that arise as the result of binge eating and may well be your first stop clinically, your doctor is unlikely to have the time or expertise to coordinate the many aspects of your treatment for binge eating. To get better and healthier, it's just as important to consult with a psychotherapist or psychiatrist and a dietitian who also specialize in treating disordered eating. Working with professionals who have expertise and insight into BED helps ease behaviors and symptoms and also ensures that you get accustomed to recognizing the feelings and emotions that drive the compulsion to overeat.

After You're Diagnosed with BED, You'll always Have BED

It's important to remember that BED is not a life sentence. As with any psychological condition, with the right treatment and support, you can find ways to manage and overcome this disorder. Sustained recovery may take a long while and likely require your time and attention to varying but hopefully lesser degrees for most of your life. The difference is that it need not be a lifelong burden but rather just a daily set of choices you make for yourself.

Chapter 27

Ten Best Ways to Help Someone who Binges

. . . .

In This Chapter
▶ Knowing all you need to know to help
▶ Maintaining a supportive but appropriate distance
▶ Remembering to be a friend first

. . . .

*I*f you're the friend or loved one of a binge eater, you may be wondering what you can do to help. The right kind of support can be critical as someone begins the journey to overcome binge eating and begins to make healthier, more sustainable choices about food.

Educate Yourself about Binge Eating

Becoming familiar with the basics of binge eating disorder (BED) is the best place to start if you want to help a loved one suffering from it. It's painful for people who use overeating as a coping mechanism to explain the ins and outs of their behaviors. If you take time to read and learn about the thoughts and feelings that go along with binge eating, you're better equipped to help.

Let Your Loved One Take the Lead

Those who binge or chronically overeat can't expect to get better without seeking out treatment and/or making changes themselves. You can be there for support, but it's up to the sufferer to tackle the problem in his own way and in his own time. If the binge eater seeks treatment for you or because he "should," his efforts to stop binge eating will be short-lived.

Listen without Judgment

At times, we all need someone to sit down and quietly listen to us without expectation or judgment. And someone who binge eats probably needs a sympathetic ear now more than ever. If your loved one suffers from disordered eating, she wants to be understood, to find ways to express what she thinks and feels, and to come up with ways to stop the madness. Eating disorders are personal, so lending an unconditional and understanding ear is critical to helping someone recover.

Know Your Limits

No matter how supportive you hope to be, don't feel that you must take on the role of therapist. Even if you've done your research, therapeutic advice should come only from a trained professional. People develop binge eating and other eating disorders for a complicated set of reasons and circumstances, and treating these disorders can be complex and sometimes precarious. Effective long-term treatment often depends on a collaborative approach from a team of eating-disorder professionals.

Practice Patience

As people come to terms with their disordered eating, it make take a while to open up to friends and loved ones. It's scary to admit to anyone that food and eating have taken over their lives, and some people may also be frightened by the thought of trying to change their behavior. If someone comes to you to talk about binge or emotional eating, let him know that you understand how serious the situation is and that when he's ready, you'll be there to help in whatever way you can and are available for the long haul. And have patience because the process will, in fact, take time.

Remember that Recovery is Day to Day

Every eating disorder is different, and each person who binge eats is unique. Although there are certainly some promising tried-and-true approaches, there isn't a standard treatment plan that applies to every person and every situation. Focusing on the here and now, literally one bite at a time, will ultimately help your loved one in the long run.

Do Not Suggest Your Loved One Go on a Diet!

Tempting as it may be to offer a solution to someone you care about, dieting is actually a frequent contributor to binge behaviors for many people because it creates a pendulum swing due to its restrictive nature. Instead, suggest that your loved one start by getting proper evaluations and creating structures for support and slow but steady insight and change. Understanding her triggers and examining the root causes of her disordered eating is the first set of primary tasks.

Help Tackle Some of the Day-to-Day Stressors for Your Loved One

One significant way to reduce triggers for many bingers is to keep life simple. By helping your loved one reduce his daily stress, you can ultimately make a huge impact. Work together to see what may be helpful in freeing up some time for him to start the process of healing and treatment. Often the little things make a big difference.

Don't Talk about How Other People Look

Those with BED are generally very self-conscious about their appearance. Even though many of us do it, by pointing out others' sizes, whether large or small, you may be unintentionally triggering a binge by contributing to your loved one's self-consciousness.

Allow Yourself to be a Distraction

Boredom is often cited as the number-one trigger for bingeing, so one great way to help your loved one is to try to keep her occupied when she may be at risk. Of course, there's a lot more to it than that, but at the outset, that's what it seems.

One common therapeutic technique is to create a list of activities that bingers can turn to when they feel urges. Let your loved one know that if you're available, you can be on call for her and that you can spend time on the phone or in person until the cravings pass. By all means, suggest but do not pressure her into pursuing a list of alternate activities. If you nag, you may start to be perceived as a trigger yourself. The idea is for someone to slowly become self-motivated and to know that no matter what, you can be counted on for nonjudgmental support.

Make Positive Comments Only

Pointing out the negative, even when your intentions are well-meaning, just make a difficult situation more difficult. Try to refrain from asking questions like, "Did you eat the whole chocolate cake last night?" or "I thought we had more peanut butter in the cabinet. Did you finish it?" Chances are this will only embarrass, shame, or anger your loved one even if you don't mean to be mean or hurtful. Binge eaters feel bad enough after the numbing effects of a huge binge quickly wear off; the last thing they need is someone else, particularly someone important to them, inadvertently contributing to their feelings of guilt, shame, and helplessness.

Plan Fun, Food-Free Activities

Many social gatherings revolve around food, but you can find tons of fun things to do that don't involve food including going for a walk, attending a concert, or making an appointment at a spa. Anything that's fun, relaxing, and does not involve food should be included on the list of options. Make sure to ask your loved one what he would like to do.

Don't Become Overly Involved

It's commendable to want to help someone recover and live a healthier life, but you can't make someone else change. Once your loved one has committed to working towards recovery, it's best to take a backseat and take your cues from her.

One exception to this rule is to know what to do in an emergency should one arise due to your loved one's disordered eating. Be aware of community resources and gather information about resources for treatment.

Index

• *E* •

• *Y* •

About the Authors

Jennie J. Kramer, MSW, LCSW, is the Founder and Executive Director of Metro Behavioral Health Associates Eating Disorders Centers located in New York City and Scarsdale, New York. The centers offer comprehensive outpatient treatment for all forms of eating disorders along the spectrum.

Ms. Kramer has been treating eating disorders for many years and served as the Director of the Renfrew Centers for Eating Disorders in both New York and New Jersey for five years. Prior to entering this field, she served as Chief Operating Officer for Dr. Robert Atkins and was a management consultant to the healthcare industry with a special interest in integrative medicine.

Ms. Kramer received her training from Adelphi and Fordham Universities. She serves on the Board of The Westchester Group Psychotherapy Society and enjoys membership and affiliation with organizations including The National Eating Disorders Association (NEDA), The Academy for Eating Disorders (AED), The Binge Eating Disorder Association (BEDA), the Eating Disorders Coalition (EDC), the International Network of Integrative Mental Health (INIMH), the Eastern Group Psychotherapy Society (EGPS), The American Group Psychotherapy Association (AGPA), The National Association of Social Work (NASW), New York Academy of Sciences (NYAS), The NY State Society for Clinical Social Work (NYSSCSW), and the International Association of Eating Disorders Professionals (IAEDP).

Marjorie Nolan Cohn is a Registered Dietitian Nutritionist, Certified Personal Trainer, speaker, and author of *The Belly Fat Fix: Taming Ghrelin, Your Hunger Hormone, for Quick, Healthy Weight Loss.* Her work as a national spokesperson for the Academy of Nutrition and Dietetics has reached millions. In addition to her network TV appearances, she has appeared in almost every major publication and medical website in America, including *Glamour, Shape, Fitness, Self, Marie Claire, Men's Fitness, The New York Times, U.S. News & World Report, The Boston Globe, The Wall Street Journal, USA Today, Better Homes & Gardens,* WebMD, AOL Health, iVillage, and more.

Marjorie has worked in many facets of the nutrition and fitness field with a primary focus on eating-disorder treatment, addictions, and medical nutrition therapy. She owns a consulting practice in New York City where she works with individuals, groups, and corporations teaching nutrition and fitness. She's also Director of Nutrition at Metro Behavioral Health Associates. She was part of the Renfrew Center for Eating Disorder NYC and Philadelphia teams for more than five years where she worked in the inpatient and outpatient programs treating patients with binge eating disorder, anorexia, and bulimia.

While writing this book, Marjorie was a newlywed. She enjoys spending time with her husband, Scott Cohn, and their two cats, Bunny and Ghrelin.

Dedication

To anyone who has ever struggled with binge eating, emotional eating, or compulsive overeating. Know there is a light at the end of the long, dark tunnel.

Authors' Acknowledgments

Jennie J. Kramer: This book would not have been possible without the guidance of our editors at Wiley, Kathleen Dobie and Anam Ahmed. Many thanks for the vision and perseverance of our literary agent, Claire Gerus. My heartfelt appreciation is due for the indefatigable expertise and collaboration of my coauthor, Marjorie Nolan Cohn, as well as the unwavering assistance of Julie Mosow. For technical review, much gratitude is due for the expertise and guidance of Dr. Jeffrey DeSarbo. Most importantly, I am inspired by the extraordinary courage, insight, and inspiration provided by all of our patients, families, and blog readers who have provided us with their stories and their honesty as they seek to find answers and alternatives to binge eating and all forms of eating disorders. And to all of my family and friends, thank you for your cheerleading and moral support, and yes, I am now back in circulation (as is the book!).

Marjorie Nolan Cohn: I'd like to thank Jennie J. Kramer, Founder and Executive Director of Metro Behavioral Health Associates Eating Disorder Centers, for making this project happen and doing an amazing job. I'm proud to be her Nutrition Director, colleague, and friend. I'd like to acknowledge Julie Mosow for her collaboration and for helping shape this book into something of which I'm immensely proud. Thanks to Dr. Jeffrey DeSarbo, our technical reviewer, for painstakingly evaluating the facts and opinions in this book. I am humbled by your knowledge and professional accomplishments. A huge thanks to Kathleen Dobie, our project editor. Your guidance, patience, and commitment were evident, especially on those Sunday mornings when you answered our questions despite having your own life. Thanks, Anam Ahmed, for months of discussing my initial concept of *Overcoming Binge Eating For Dummies.* This book is available to those struggling with binge eating because you were open to hearing, perusing, and pitching the initial concept to your colleagues at Wiley. To my husband for being the most important person in my life. There are no words that can thank you enough.

Publisher's Acknowledgments

Acquisitions Editor: Anam Ahmed

Development and Copy Editor: Kathleen Dobie

Technical Editor: Dr. Jeffrey DeSarbo

Sr. Project Coordinator: Kristie Rees

Project Manager: Lindsay Humphreys

Cover Photo: ©iStockphoto.com/Tsuji

EDUCATION, HISTORY & REFERENCE

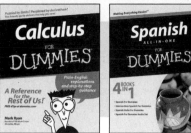 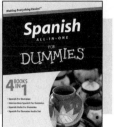

978-0-7645-2498-1   978-0-470-46244-7

Also available:
- Algebra For Dummies 978-0-7645-5325-7
- Art History For Dummies 978-0-470-09910-0
- Chemistry For Dummies 978-0-7645-5430-8
- English Grammar For Dummies 978-0-470-54664-2
- French All-in-One For Dummies 978-1-118-22815-9
- Statistics For Dummies 978-0-7645-5423-0
- World History For Dummies 978-0-470-44654-6

FOOD, HOME, & MUSIC

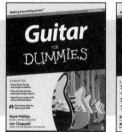 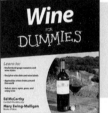

978-1-118-11554-1   978-1-118-28872-6

Also available:
- 30-Minute Meals For Dummies 978-0-7645-2589-6
- Bartending For Dummies 978-0-470-63312-0
- Brain Games For Dummies 978-0-470-37378-1
- Cheese For Dummies 978-1-118-09939-1
- Cooking Basics For Dummies 978-0-470-91388-8
- Gluten-Free Cooking For Dummies 978-1-118-39644-5
- Home Improvement All-in-One Desk Reference For Dummies 978-0-7645-5680-7
- Home Winemaking For Dummies 978-0-470-67895-4
- Ukulele For Dummies 978-0-470-97799-6

GARDENING

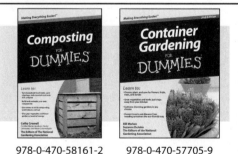

978-0-470-58161-2   978-0-470-57705-9

Also available:
- Gardening Basics For Dummies 978-0-470-03749-2
- Organic Gardening For Dummies 978-0-470-43067-5
- Sustainable Landscaping For Dummies 978-0-470-41149-0
- Vegetable Gardening For Dummies 978-0-470-49870-5

Available wherever books are sold. For more information or to order direct: U.S. customers visit www.dummies.com or call 1-877-762-2974.
U.K. customers visit www.wileyeurope.com or call 0800 243407. Canadian customers visit www.wiley.ca or call 1-800-567-4797.

WILEY

GREEN/SUSTAINABLE

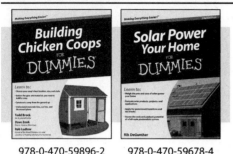

978-0-470-59896-2   978-0-470-59678-4

Also available:

- Alternative Energy For Dummies 978-0-470-43062-0
- Energy Efficient Homes For Dummies 978-0-470-37602-7
- Global Warming For Dummies 978-0-470-84098-6
- Green Building & Remodelling For Dummies 978-0-470-17559-0
- Green Cleaning For Dummies 978-0-470-39106-8
- Green Your Home All-in-One For Dummies 978-0-470-59678-4
- Wind Power Your Home For Dummies 978-0-470-49637-4

HEALTH & SELF-HELP

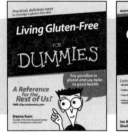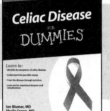

978-0-471-77383-2   978-0-470-16036-7

Also available:

- Body Language For Dummies 978-0-470-51291-3
- Borderline Personality Disorder For Dummies 978-0-470-46653-7
- Breast Cancer For Dummies 978-0-7645-2482-0
- Cognitive Behavioural Therapy For Dummies 978-0-470-66541-1
- Emotional Intelligence For Dummies 978-0-470-15732-9
- Healthy Aging For Dummies 978-0-470-14975-1
- Neuro-linguistic Programming For Dummies 978-0-470-66543-5
- Understanding Autism For Dummies 978-0-7645-2547-6

HOBBIES & CRAFTS

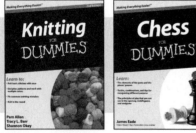

978-0-470-28747-7   978-1-118-01695-4

Also available:

- Bridge For Dummies 978-1-118-20574-7
- Crochet Patterns For Dummies 97-0-470-04555-8
- Digital Photography For Dummies 978-1-118-09203-3
- Jewelry Making & Beading Designs For Dummies 978-0-470-29112-2
- Knitting Patterns For Dummies 978-0-470-04556-5
- Oil Painting For Dummies 978-0-470-18230-7
- Quilting For Dummies 978-0-7645-9799-2
- Sewing For Dummies 978-0-7645-6847-3
- Word Searches For Dummies 978-0-470-45366-7

HOME & BUSINESS COMPUTER BASICS

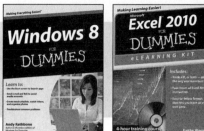

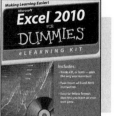

978-1-118-13461-0   978-1-118-11079-9

Also available:
- ✔ Office 2010 All-in-One Desk Reference For Dummies 978-0-470-49748-7
- ✔ Pay Per Click Search Engine Marketing For Dummies 978-0-471-75494-7
- ✔ Search Engine Marketing For Dummies 978-0-471-97998-2
- ✔ Web Analytics For Dummies 978-0-470-09824-0
- ✔ Word 2010 For Dummies 978-0-470-48772-3

INTERNET & DIGITAL MEDIA

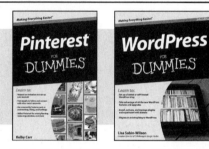

978-1-118-32800-2   978-1-118-38318-6

Also available:
- ✔ Blogging For Dummies 978-1-118-15194-5
- ✔ Digital Photography For Seniors For Dummies 978-0-470-44417-7
- ✔ Facebook For Dummies 978-1-118-09562-1
- ✔ LinkedIn For Dummies 978-0-470-94854-5
- ✔ Mom Blogging For Dummies 978-1-118-03843-7
- ✔ The Internet For Dummies 978-0-470-12174-0
- ✔ Twitter For Dummies 978-0-470-76879-2
- ✔ YouTube For Dummies 978-0-470-14925-6

MACINTOSH

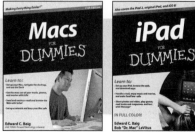

978-0-470-87868-2   978-1118-49823-1

Also available:
- ✔ iMac For Dummies 978-0-470-20271-5
- ✔ iPod Touch For Dummies 978-1-118-12960-9
- ✔ iPod & iTunes For Dummies 978-1-118-50864-0
- ✔ MacBook For Dummies 978-1-11820920-2
- ✔ Macs For Seniors For Dummies 978-1-11819684-7
- ✔ Mac OS X Lion All-in-One For Dummies 978-1-118-02206-1

PETS

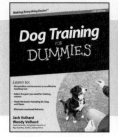

978-0-470-60029-0

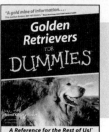

978-0-7645-5267-0

Also available:
- Cats For Dummies 978-0-7645-5275-5
- Ferrets For Dummies 978-0-470-13943-1
- Horses For Dummies 978-0-7645-9797-8
- Kittens For Dummies 978-0-7645-4150-6
- Puppies For Dummies 978-1-118-11755-2

SPORTS & FITNESS

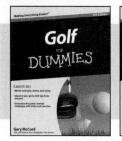

978-0-470-88279-5

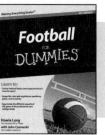

978-1-118-01261-1

Also available:
- Exercise Balls For Dummies 978-0-7645-5623-4
- Coaching Volleyball For Dummies 978-0-470-46469-4
- Curling For Dummies 978-0-470-83828-0
- Fitness For Dummies 978-0-7645-7851-9
- Lacrosse For Dummies 978-0-470-73855-9
- Mixed Martial Arts For Dummies 978-0-470-39071-9
- Sports Psychology For Dummies 978-0-470-67659-2
- Ten Minute Tone-Ups For Dummies 978-0-7645-7207-4
- Wilderness Survival For Dummies 978-0-470-45306-3
- Wrestling For Dummies 978-1-118-11797-2
- Yoga with Weights For Dummies 978-0-471-74937-0

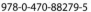